P9-DEL-665

PRAISE FOR

American Indian Healing Arts

"Conservation and appreciation of plants and animals are essential to the practice of American Indian healing arts. However, to carry Good Medicine requires an understanding of the more complex spirit-creatures of the ancient Indian world. Barrie Kavasch knows these creatures well and she carries with her their Good Medicine."

—*Melissa Fawcett, Tribal Historian, The Mohegan Tribe*

"Barrie Kavasch has given voice, meaning, and practical wisdom to Native American thought, beliefs, and ceremonial systems. Not only does the work provide depth of understanding of the potential applications of Native healing, but Barrie never forgets to present such compelling knowledge in a most entertaining and deliciously personal manner."

—*Alberto C. Meloni, Executive Director,*
The Institute for American Indian Studies

"A great many of us are hungry for information that can help us reconnect to the soil as well as to the rhythms of our own lives, and I am extremely grateful to E. Barrie Kavasch and Karen Baar for giving us this fascinating, accessible, and suggestive survey of American Indian wisdom and ritual."

—*Jean Hegland, author of* Into the Forest

"Written in a highly reverent tone, this book goes beyond most popular herbals by helping the reader experience the richness of the rituals connecting the people, the herbs, and their uses into one complex, interwoven fabric."

—*Mark Blumenthal, founder and*
Executive Director, American Botanical Council

American Indian Healing Arts

Herbs, Rituals, and Remedies
for Every Season of Life

E. Barrie Kavasch
and Karen Baar

BANTAM BOOKS

New York Toronto London Sydney Auckland

AMERICAN INDIAN HEALING ARTS
A Bantam Book / April 1999

Portions of the royalties for this book will go to support the
American Indian College Fund of thirty American Indian colleges,
and numerous American Indian museums and health organizations
and community groups in the United States and Canada.

Library of Congress Cataloging-in-Publication Data
Kavasch, E. Barrie.
*American Indian healing arts: herbs, rituals, and remedies for
every season of life / E. Barrie Kavasch and Karen Baar.*
p.   cm.
Includes bibliographical references and index.
ISBN 0-553-37881-3
*1. Herbs—Therapeutic use. 2. Indians of North America—Medicine.
3. Traditional medicine—North America. I. Baar, Karen.
II. Title.*
RM666.H33K39   1999
615.8′8′08997073—dc21   *98–43985*
CIP

Published simultaneously in the United States and Canada

*Bantam Books are published by Bantam Books, a division of Random House, Inc.
Its trademark, consisting of the words "Bantam Books" and the portrayal of a
rooster, is Registered in U.S. Patent and Trademark Office and in other countries.
Marca Registrada. Bantam Books, 1540 Broadway, New York, New York 10036.*

PRINTED IN THE UNITED STATES OF AMERICA

To American Indian and Native American People,
your amazing history, contemporary lives,
and bright futures, and for
the many generations yet to come.

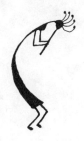

Contents

INTRODUCTION:
HEALING THE TRADITIONAL WAY

It may be that some little root of the Sacred Tree still lives. Nourish it then, that it may leaf and bloom and fill with singing birds. Hear me, not for myself, but for my people; I am old. Hear me that they may once more go back into the sacred hoop and find the Good Red Road, the shielding tree.

—BLACK ELK, OGLALA SIOUX HOLY MAN AND MEDICINE MAN

This book explores the healing arts of American Indians. Our native tribes had and still perform a dazzling array of healing rituals; they also know and use hundreds of herbs, fungi, lichens, and other natural materials. Although many of these practices are ancient, they remain vital. Today healers from all over the world—Europe, Australia, India, and China—come to the United States to learn how to use our native medicinal plants. But ironically, many Americans have not yet tapped into this distinctively American tradition, instead choosing European herbal medicine, homeopathy, or acupuncture in their quest for alternatives to conventional medical treatment.

But American Indian healing goes well beyond treating disease. As we approach the end of the twentieth century it offers a rich resource for people who want to connect, both collectively and individually, with their spiritual selves. Throughout their sweeping history, American Indians have held the spiritual side of life to be primary and sacred. Their belief system provides them with a deep and nurturing connection to the earth and the spiritual realm.

The Good Red Road

American Indians understand life as a special path, the Pollen Path for the Navajo and many other tribes, the Good Red Road for others. This road is part of a sacred circle with no beginning or end, a continuing cycle of survival that goes beyond the individual and the group. It is deeply interwoven with nature and the world of the spirits; everything in creation is interrelated. Entering this world, with its deep sense of connection to the universe, brings richness and meaning to every aspect of daily life. And it can help all of us touch the sacred and divine within ourselves, pointing the way to deep personal healing.

American Indians, like many other traditional people, have a holistic view of health that is gaining credibility as we realize the limitations of conventional or Western medicine. Conventional practitioners have long considered infection by bacteria or a virus, or sometimes genetic disorders and disabilities, to be the causes of disease. American Indian beliefs take these factors into account, but also see illness as a disharmony or imbalance that may be directly related to spiritual causes.

Throughout Indian America, healing strategies are closely tied to spiritual beliefs. In the imaginative and highly evolved worldviews of native peoples, everything is linked. Life, death, and all things connected to them are part of the Great Mystery. In fact, most native languages possessed no traditional word as such for medicine; rather, it was called "the mystery."

The intricately interconnected concepts of body/mind and nature/spirit govern tribal views of wellness and illness. American Indian healers look beyond symptoms to discover the roots of an illness, which may lie in the spiritual world. The power of American Indian healing cannot be isolated from its spiritual and magical content and close integration with the natural world.

Harmony and Balance

Harmony is the overall theme governing health and wellness and their absence. Life is perceived as a balance, and illness is an upset of that balance. A person's equilibrium can be lost as a result of grief, sadness, or personal wrongdoing; the purpose of healing is to assess what has to be rectified to bring that person back into balance, to the Good Red Road.

Most American Indians believed that illness or disease had three possible origins: natural, human, or supernatural. The sources of disease were complex, and within one tribe individuals might disagree on the exact cause of a particular problem. For example, different tribes understood supernatural causes to entail soul loss, spirit intrusion, taboo violation, or unfulfilled dreams. Sorcery and witchcraft were prevalent in many areas and continue to be reason for concern among many people.

But many traditional people also believe that the only time a person is vulnerable to a bad use of power—such as that employed by a Hopi nightwalker, for instance—or other causes of illness is when her personal and spiritual energy is so low that the bad power can affect her. The best defense against this and all illness is prevention: keeping one's mind, body, and spirit strong and pure.

When someone does fall ill, restoring balance in several dimensions—both within the patient and without, in the family, group, and place—is central to American Indian healing. Native healing practices are diverse, colorful, and fascinating, frequently involving the use of ritual and ceremony. Treatment is often a family-based process; sometimes it includes the entire tribe. This is because each person is part of the whole; if one spoke is frail, the whole wheel is weak.

Healing Rites

Although treating an illness or disorder is a primary purpose of every healing ritual, it is not the whole focus. Sweat lodge rites of purification, spirit feasts, prayers, and much more are all part of the healing spectrum. Herbs and medicines are used, but only as a small part of the entire process, which frequently succeeds without the use of any medicines whatsoever. Often, in fact, native herbalists are reluctant to prescribe herbs and healing regimens unless the patient is willing to make some lifestyle changes as well.

Rituals feed the body, mind, and spirit and draw people back into personal balance. And Mother Earth is at the heart of many healing ceremonies. Some rituals, such as Navajo sand paintings, literally take place on the earth. Others are linked to the summer or winter solstice or to harvest time. A large number of ceremonies end with a roast or a feast, a meal geared to feed the family, relatives, friends, and healers who have come together. Often the earth serves as the oven. People make long trenches and barbecue in them; this is also the origin of the clambake.

Besides treating the patient, healing rites strengthen everyone attending by linking them to their origins and reaffirming their commitment to tradition. Contemporary scientific research has validated this idea, demonstrating again and again that feeling connected to a support network of family, friends, and community prevents illness and speeds recovery.

In earlier times, there was no real separation between life and religion, temple and spirit, or food and medicine for most native people. The rhythms of human worship were present everywhere. Everything on the earth and in the universe possessed its own special spirit, and this was acknowledged with respect at every turn.

The Life Cycle

The cycle of human life was and is a part of this larger, universal circle. Rites and rituals, songs and prayers, and spirit foods and celebrations evolved to recognize and honor individuals during important life passages. Many of these ancient ceremonies are still performed today. These rites of passage are the markers that delineate the vital links between a person's life and that of the family, clan, band, and tribe. And in performing these rituals, the tribe also calls in nature and the spirits to ensure that a person enjoys a long, healthy life.

The human life cycle is the backbone of this book. In Chapters 1 through 9, we look at each major stage of an individual's life—both what it symbolizes and how it is celebrated—from different tribal perspectives. We focus on the healing rituals—prayer, incantation, song, and dance— as well as herbs, fungi, and other materials that help people through important rites of passage and prevent and heal illnesses. We've woven in a mixture of historical and contemporary descriptions of the most interesting and relevant native healing rituals performed from birth through old age and death. And we've included hands-on techniques and remedies:

Scattered throughout the book are more than sixty easy-to-prepare American Indian–inspired recipes and a host of variations to treat health problems that are of particular concern during each period of life.

In addition, in every chapter we provide fascinating tidbits of native knowledge in histories, legends, personal quotes, interviews with and reflections from patients, American Indian herbalists, singers *(hataalii)*, shamans, and medicine people. Because special foods and ceremonial preparations invariably accompany many rites, we've included some healing foods and beverages in addition to botanical remedies.

"Hollow Bones"

Although healers are at the heart of many ceremonies, the best healers lead patients to their own healing. Sharing their knowledge has been difficult for some individuals, but many give it generously. Some of the greatest holy men have thought of themselves as conduits, or "hollow bones," through which the Great Mysteries flowed to the people. "The power and ways are given to us to be passed on to others. To think or do anything else is pure selfishness. We only keep them and get more by giving them away, and if we do not give them away, we lose them," said Frank Fools Crow, ceremonial chief of the Teton Sioux, nephew of Oglala Sioux healer and holy man Black Elk.

No one healer has the whole repertoire. Individual healers often have precise and idiosyncratic knowledge; when a medicine person dies, it is as if a whole library were lost. Many herbalists know as many as three hundred substances, but as you move around an area in the same region or even the same village, two herbalists may be familiar with different sets of herbs and mushrooms. They may also specialize; in some cases, one healer may refer a patient to another who has specific expertise in a particular area. It is not unusual for a patient living on the Akwesasne Reserve in upstate New York to drive six hours to see a healer at Six Nations in Canada.

We hope that as you read the first nine chapters, you will allow your imagination to take hold, creatively adapting the rituals and making them your own. In Chapter 10, "An American Indian Medicine Chest," we provide more hands-on applications. Here you'll find directions for making lotions, healing salves and ointments, tonics, tooth powders, and digestive remedies, as well as additional gifts from Mother Earth that embrace all stages of the life cycle.

The appendix features a lexicon of the herbs, fungi, and minerals most frequently used by American Indians. This section supplies key information about the ingredients used in the recipes and remedies throughout the rest of the book. We've also provided a list of sources for these ingredients.

Tribal North America is the heart of this book: American Indians and Native Americans (those indigenous groups who do not consider themselves to be Indians, such as the Aleuts, G'wichin, Inuit, Inupiat, Yupik, and others of our northern latitudes). We occasionally reflect upon some of the cultures in Mexico and Central America. Because North America is an enormous patchwork of more than 540 native nations in the United States and more than 600 indigenous groups in Canada, we have had to be selective in our choice of rituals and practices, discussing only those that are most relevant to today's needs.

"Ghost Prints"

The illustrations depict more than eighty different plant species that are significant in native healing. The pencil rubbings are spontaneous "ghost prints" of freshly harvested leaves. Leaf rubbings are a good way to learn more about a plant's spirit, characteristics, and personalities, and such details can help you identify plant species. But plants alone are only a small part of American Indian healing. The illustrations of pictographs and petroglyphs from various native prehistoric sites and other objects and symbols suggest its broader scope.

Healing Past and Present

Although American native healing arts are centuries old, much has come forward in time virtually unchanged, because the healing virtues are there. American Indians may seek symptomatic relief from modern medicine, but they often turn to their traditional healers not only to treat symptoms, but to find and remedy the true cause of an illness. These healers or medicine people may work alone, or they may coordinate with other doctors. But often, as with other alternative caregivers, they treat people for whom conventional medicine has nothing more to offer. For example, Sara, a Mohawk woman who had worked for many years off reservation in the Syracuse area, was diagnosed with cancer in her lung, bones, and several other parts of her body. Her doctors gave her no more than one to three years to live, and urged her to retire and enjoy her last few years. Taking their advice, she moved back to the reservation with her younger sister. She was treated by medicine men using traditional healing, and lived an additional twenty years, well into her late seventies. These were vital, active years during which she traveled, enjoyed her family, and accomplished a great deal.

American Indian healing today often functions in settings where it is grudgingly accepted, if not actively scorned, by conventional medicine. But encouraging signs of acceptance and cooperation between American Indian healers and conventional practitioners are emerging. Mainstream doctors call upon Indian medicine men and women to assist in treatment not just in reservation hospitals, but also in university hospitals and in cities where there are large Indian populations. In the Southwest, Apache and Hopi healers as well as Navajo herbalists, hand tremblers, and crystal gazers (seers who perform healing by divining the sources of illness) are being brought into medical centers; in and around Cornell University, the same is true for people from the Algonquian and Iroquois tribes. A complement to this is that spiritual leaders are also turning to American Indian people to share their prayers, rites, and ceremonies in order to expand the fabric of reverence for life.

Many conventional Western physicians have begun to realize that where the traditions are alive, even seriously ill patients survive better when native healing is incorporated into their care. This is because American Indians believe that illness is caused by more than "germs." While an orthodox doctor may be consulted for treatment, only a native healer can help discern the spiritual and tribal causes of an illness and suggest the appropriate remedies. These healers work with herbs, prayer, tinctures, and teas not only to treat disease but also to enhance the immunity of their patients, who include people from infancy to old age. And increasingly, non-Indian people are requesting native healers.

This cooperation benefits more than the patients. Native healers are proud to be invited in and happy to offer their services; through their work with conventional doctors and scientists, they deepen their own knowledge of the pathways of disease and disorder. At the same time, research in the biological sciences continues to explore the keys to native healing strategies. So promising are the results that they guarantee American Indian healing a place in the next century.

For example, recent research has validated the use of cranberry juice in the treatment of urinary tract infections; cranberry, like its sisters blueberry and bearberry, has long been employed by native peoples for kidney and bladder complaints. Similarly, scientists are synthesizing pharmaceuticals such as taxol—used to treat cancer—from yew, which was used by American Indians as an astringent and a tumor treatment. And chili peppers, used by the Maya and Aztecs for pain relief thousands of years ago, are being processed to extract capsaicin, which is used to treat patients with mouth and esophageal cancer at major medical centers. This same substance is an important remedy for the poor circulation of old age, as well as arthritis, rheumatism, and other joint discomforts. Some of the herbs most widely used in this country and around the world today—echinacea, ginseng, arnica, evening primrose, and saw palmetto—have been pillars of American Indian health and disease prevention for centuries.

The Circle Continues

America's history with the Indians has often been violent and troubled, a painful legacy of guilt, misunderstanding, and resentment. In bringing American Indian healing out of the shadows, we hope, through our shared human interest in healing, to help bridge the gap that still clouds our relationships. Regardless of our ancestry, the gifts that native healing traditions have to offer are one of our greatest living legacies.

We hope you will return to this book again and again, seeing yourself in all of the cycles and realizing that the circle continues.

ACKNOWLEDGMENTS

Our gratitude first to each of the countless American Indian people who have made this work possible. Their voices and good energies are embraced within these pages. Our families and friends endured our long hours of research, experiments, writing, and rewriting. They have our love and gratitude always.

Barrie sends loving praise to her mother, Vera, and her two grown children, Chris and Kim, her daughter-in-law, Fran, and four grandchildren, Derek, Sarah, Jeffrey, and Brooke, plus our extended families and relatives. You illuminate my work and enrich my life in more ways than you know.

Karen thanks her parents, Isabel and Eli Baar. To Emma and Kate Baar-Bittman, who brighten all of my days, hugs and kisses. And special love and thanks to my partner Mark Bittman, who provided more support and encouragement than anyone could possibly expect.

The great team at Bantam has won our affection and respect, especially Toni Burbank, Robin Michaelson, Marely Cheo-Bove, Matthew Martin, Chris Pike, Sue Warga, Maggie Hart, and our book designer Ellen Cipriano. Thank you for your vision, enthusiasm, and professionalism.

Grateful praise to Bill Milne, Jim Plumeri, and assistants for our stunning cover. Our enduring gratitude to Angela Miller and Betsy Amster for believing in us and this idea and enabling us to reach the goal. Working with all of you is a powerful gift.

Our work grows from the work of many talented, knowledgeable people, yet in the end we take full responsibility for any omissions or errors. Please treat this information with respect for the many different lifeways and practices glimpsed within these pages. Do not self-medicate. Seek the responsible opinion of your doctor and/or herbalist, nutritionist, naturopath, homeopath, and/or medicine wo/man. As we continue to learn from talented individuals, we can take charge, in a fuller sense, of our own good health and spiritual wellness.

In peace and love,
E. Barrie Kavasch and Karen Baar

And when we no longer walk the circle of life
Maybe other life will still feed on our skeleton remains
And know that in our struggle
Those tears that we dropped into the oceans
And those echoes we left on the mountains
And those footprints that fade on the paths
Someone has acknowledged our creation
And thanked us for still following our ways
The traditional ways the spiritual ways the earth ways
The ways our ancestors in humility and gratefulness
Sought to honor the sacredness of the earth mother
For it is she who gives birth
And it is her breasts which give us life
And we are taking care of her, because we care

—*From "The Earth Way,"*
by ssipsis, Penobscot elder

American Indian Healing Arts

CHAPTER ONE

Birth and Infancy

"THANK YOU FOR COMING TO OUR VILLAGE"

✦✦✦✦✦✦✦✦✦✦✦✦✦✦✦✦✦✦✦✦✦✦✦✦✦✦✦✦✦✦✦✦✦✦✦✦

When a new baby is born among the Six Nations of the Iroquois Confederacy, the Clan Mothers welcome the newborn by saying: "Thank you for coming to our village; we hope you will stay with us."

—KATSI COOK, MOHAWK MIDWIFE
FROM AKWESASNE AND A RESEARCH FELLOW IN
THE AMERICAN INDIAN PROGRAM AT
CORNELL UNIVERSITY IN ITHACA, NEW YORK

Black raspberry
Rubus occidentalis

✦✦✦✦✦✦✦✦✦✦✦✦✦✦✦✦✦✦✦✦✦✦✦✦✦✦✦✦✦✦✦✦✦✦✦✦

Dewberry
Rubus pubescens

The cry of a newborn child is music to which all people respond. American Indians place special emphasis on welcoming a child not only into the family but also into the tribe and the world. When a baby is born, he emerges from his mother's womb into the womb of Mother Earth.

Of course, childbirth was not always such a smooth transition. In early societies women frequently gave birth outside the village in less-than-ideal or even dangerous situations. Often they were alone and exposed to the elements. But most American Indian women were well equipped to manage within their environments. They were in vigorous good health and quite fit throughout their pregnancies, so that birthing was fairly spontaneous and without much trauma or pause from their normal work. Early records tell of women giving birth in challenging circumstances and then walking great distances with their newborns on their backs.

But not every birth was comfortable or successful. Infant deaths and abnormalities occurred, and mothers died in childbirth or of infections or complications immediately after giving birth.

Across the continent, as native people settled into village life they developed a broad array of ceremonies, rituals, prayers, and special herbs and medicines to protect and sanctify this important life passage. Each tribe used its own sequence of prayers and offerings of sacred substances to ease labor and delivery for the mother and help ensure the infant's survival.

Today, as long as there are no complications, many American Indian mothers choose to give birth at home or in specially prepared family settings. Birthing outside of the hospital allows women to continue to honor their traditional tribal rituals. But even hospital birth need not impede some of the smaller, more private ceremonies. And because some rites take place before labor begins as well as after the baby arrives at home, many people can avail themselves of these special blessings.

In some tribes, rituals for the birth mother begin just before or dur-

Red raspberry
Rubus idaeus

ing labor and delivery. Among the Diné or Navajo, for example, a woman can request that a Blessing Way, or "No Sleep," be done for her before she leaves for the hospital or as she prepares for the birth at home. The name "No Sleep" means a one-night sing; it is much like a vigil. The medicine man sings for her from late evening until "the dawn has a white stripe" in order to ensure that her labor and delivery will be normal and as easy as possible, and that her baby will be healthy and whole.

Birthing practices during and immediately after the birth frequently combine the sacred and the practical. Often part of the midwife's work during labor is to sing to and massage the laboring woman, bathe her in healing herbs, and ritually wash her abdomen, breasts, arms, and legs. In many cultures women do this for themselves, continuing a practice they began during the latter part of pregnancy. The midwife uses sacred herbs and important herbs of childbearing such as sweetgrass, hawthorn berries, or leaves of raspberry, strawberry, bearberry, or juniper submerged in either river or lake water. Not only do these herbs bless the process, they also relax the mother, ease the delivery, and nurture a pure, strong spirit in the baby. In some tribes midwives use other mild herbs, such as blue cohosh root, to gently speed the birth.

After the delivery, the focus is on the baby. A birth attendant ritually bathes the baby in a sacred herbal wash. Relatives may look the infant over for any unusual markings or other signs. For example, among the Delaware, knowledgeable elders read a birthmark as a special sign that means—depending on its size and configuration—good luck or a long life. Sometimes the mark may be attributed to the mother's or father's dream; in other cases it is an indication that either or both parents experienced difficulties with other people.

On occasion family members attending the birth may see an ancient wisdom in the infant's eyes or recognize the soul of an ancestor. In special instances it becomes clear at birth—or sometimes even before—that this particular baby has been blessed and summoned to a specific calling. In the past, a boy might have been dedicated to the path of a great warrior or directed to follow a favored uncle into a secret society. A girl infant might be consecrated to fertility, to skill in tanning, or to the mineral, animal, herbal, and fungal wisdom of the earth.

Families, especially those suffering from the previous loss of one or more children, feel a special urgency about strengthening a just-born member of the family in this way. Many Indian children rebel against this

Spiderwebs, the Earliest Dream Catchers

Today's popular dream catchers have their roots in ancient amulets called spiderwebs. Loving family members—parents, aunts, uncles, and siblings—created these graceful ephemeral designs of quill and beadwork on hide. The spiderweb, which can also be seen on early birch-bark scrolls, was a charm meant to hold good energy. And like a true spiderweb, this one could catch everything, especially harm coming from the spirit world or anywhere else, before it reached the baby.

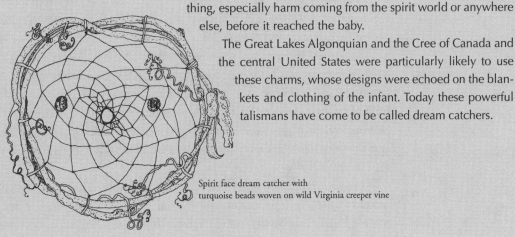

The Great Lakes Algonquian and the Cree of Canada and the central United States were particularly likely to use these charms, whose designs were echoed on the blankets and clothing of the infant. Today these powerful talismans have come to be called dream catchers.

Spirit face dream catcher with
turquoise beads woven on wild Virginia creeper vine

idea, refusing to follow the life path that the tribe has chosen for them. But there are amazing stories of individuals who eventually come around to occupy the roles envisioned for them at birth.

Welcoming a new child does not always involve elaborate ceremony. Paula Dove Jennings, of the Turtle Clan, is a Niantic-Narragansett oral historian. Among her people, traditions center on women. Growing up in Charlestown, Rhode Island, she recalls being told that when she was born, on July 3, 1940—the first daughter of Pretty Flower and Roaring Bull—her father walked out onto their street, raised his arms, and shouted, "Now I am a man!" to celebrate her birth. Her older brother, Red Earth, was a well-loved toddler, yet the importance of having a girl had to be publicly proclaimed.

Sometimes a rite is a small but significant act, such as the sprinkling of sacred cornmeal. Quiet prayers and other private practices, such as making a medicine bundle, dream catcher, or other special amulet, are sometimes all that are needed to work a bit of magic.

For example, Kwakiutl mothers, who live on the Northwest Coast of the United States, perform the Girl Child Prosperity Ceremony so that their baby girls grow to be healthy, industrious, and accomplished women. After preparing special birth amulets, which her infant daughter will wear or carry close until she is nine months old, the mother prays: "O, supernatural power of the Supernatural One of the Rocks, go on, look at what I am doing to you, for I pray you to take mercy on my child and, please, let her be successful in getting property and let nothing evil happen to her when she goes up the mountain picking all kinds of berries; and, please, protect her, Supernatural One."

American Indians weave prayers—large and small—into many aspects of their lives. This is especially true when it comes to the rituals, ceremonies, and other symbolic events that mark passages through an individual's life. Each tribe and culture group has its own unique way of praying. While a great deal has changed because of Christian influences and missionaries' work over the past five hundred years, the strongest traditions are still alive.

Prayers are usually long, melodic, and haunting. They are frequently offered to the sky, the Creator, and the universe. Many prayers use one or more of the most highly valued sacred substances—tobacco, cornmeal, pollen, bearberry, sweetgrass, sage, and cedar. Prayers unite the finest tribal traditions and beliefs with an individual's most personal feelings. The supplicant speaks, cries, or sings the prayer, shouting or loudly emphasizing certain parts. Many prayers are filled with earnest tears of sadness, love, beseeching, or even anger. And while birth-related prayers naturally are directed at the safety of the newborn, they also embrace all of the individuals present, whether a tiny family, a single individual, or an entire community.

The Long-life Ceremony of the Jicarilla Apache

Many of the ceremonies that native peoples perform at birth recognize, either explicitly or symbolically, that babies face many risks and that many children die during infancy. The Jicarilla Apache, who now live in north-central New Mexico but once roamed a much larger territory, note this in their cosmology, or religious beliefs. They believe that their people emerged from the underground, a peaceful, idyllic world where rituals were unnecessary because there were no diseases or other troubles. When that world began to die, they chose to move into the next world, which brought them here, onto the earth, with its attendant dangers. As they emerged, the gods gave them the Long-life Ceremony for protection. This ceremony, handed down over many years, is one of their most ancient traditions, imbued with special significance.

The native name for the Long-life Ceremony has been translated to mean "Water Has Been Put on Top of His Head." This practice blesses and strengthens the infant, much like an early Christian baptism. It takes place as soon as possible after birth, before anything untoward can happen. As practiced by Apache holy people, the paternal elders, or the parents themselves, it is meant to carry the child safely until the puberty ceremony. What actually occurs is highly personal and variable, depending on the families and circumstances, but it usually involves lightly touching sacred water and cornmeal to the baby's head while uttering special prayers.

The Omaha Ceremony of Turning the Child After the First Thunder

Other tribes recognize a birth more publicly and perform rituals connected to healing in the broadest sense. They call in all the help they can to bless the baby and strengthen his journey on the path of life. For example, on the eighth day of life the Omaha ceremonially announced a newborn's birth to the universal entities, uniting his life force with all of nature. Their petitions sought safe passage for each infant as he traveled the four hills, which for the Omaha symbolized life's major stages of infancy, childhood, adulthood, and old age.

Today many Omaha traditional families continue this ritual or perform similar ceremonies that have evolved from it.

As the infant grows, the Omaha perform another ritual that formally introduces her to the tribe and recognizes her as a member. This

Ho! Ye Sun, Moon, Stars,
all ye that move in the
 heavens,
I bid you hear me!
Into your midst has come
 a new life.
Consent ye, I implore!
Make its path smooth,
that it may reach the brow
 of the first hill!

—*Omaha prayer for infants*

rite, which is called Turning the Child, takes place in the spring after the first thunders have come. It includes all children who are nearly ready to walk alone. The barefoot child stands on a symbolic stone; as the family and other tribal members sing prayers and songs, they put new moccasins, blessed with sacred herbs, on her feet and help her take four steps. Symbolically she has been "sent into the midst of the winds," commemorating that she has made it through infancy and into childhood. Her baby name is thrown away, and a new name is announced to all of nature and to the crowd of people who have gathered for the occasion.

The new moccasins the child receives at the Turning the Child ritual have a small hole cut into one of the soles. According to the Omaha physician La Fleshe, this is a way of preventing the child's death: If a messenger from the spirit world comes to snatch the baby, the child can say, "I cannot go on a journey because my moccasins are worn out."

Traditionally, the Abenaki and certain other Eastern tribes also leave a tiny hole in the moccasins they fashion for each young child, but its purpose is different. If a messenger from the spirit world comes to invite the child back over, this symbolic hole allows the tiny spirit to slip out of the body if it so desires. Among these peoples, there has always been an implicit understanding that if a child's spirit does not wish to remain on earth, it should be blessed and allowed to depart.

The Navajo First Smile Ceremony

Not everything that happens at birth is invested with such gravity. Among the Navajo, the First Smile Ceremony, a short, private ritual that occurs shortly after a child is born, reveals a lighter, more humorous sensibility. The maternal grandmother usually does the honors, but another female relative attending the birth, the midwife, or the mother herself can carry it out. Holding the newborn child, she strokes its face with a finger or a little feather, teasing the baby to get it to smile and bring its soul to mirth. The Navajo seize on this fleeting moment, acknowledging the smile as a sign of blessing and a reassurance of a long, happy life.

A bit later the Navajo also honor the first laugh. Their understanding is that the person who first gets the infant to laugh wins the honor of preparing a big feast for the little one. Frequently this is a person who plays an important role in the child's life.

Birthing Customs: The Umbilical Cord and Afterbirth

Tribe members seize every opportunity to strengthen the newborn's connection to them and to life. Besides the special rites and rituals attending each new birth, the treatment of the umbilical cord and the afterbirth was and is extremely sensitive and sacred. In some cultures, tribal taboos dictated who could handle them as well as how they could be discarded.

Each tribe has always had its own particular customs regarding the umbilical cord. Among the Hopi, one of the midwives or the baby's father would take the umbilical cord out to the edge of the village and discard it in a specially designated spot. People from certain Northwest Coast tribes sometimes fashioned the cord into a bracelet for the infant to wear for the first few months of life. The bracelet brought good luck, strength, and long life. It also had the power to help set the child on her consecrated life path.

So precious is the umbilical cord among the Plains peoples and certain tribes of the Northeast that it often was and still is transformed into a piece of sacred art. Traditionally, the mother or grandmother, frequently before the child was born, fashioned a tiny, exquisite amulet case. The case was usually made out of leather, with beading, quill work, or moose hair embroidery. It might take the form of a lizard, turtle, or other animal totem; it could also be a sacred medicine figure. Each bead and every stitch held a special prayer, so even the tiniest amulet was filled with immense power.

After the birth, both the baby's navel and the severed umbilical cord were blessed and dabbed with pollen or the spores of *Lycopodium clavatum* (club moss) or mushrooms; these treatments also hastened healing. The umbilical cord was stitched up inside its unique case and attached to the cradleboard above the infant's head to provide a special blessing and train the child's gaze to beauty and strength.

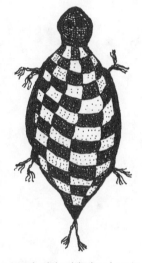

Sioux beaded umbilical-cord case in turtle effigy

If the child died, she was buried with the precious talisman. Otherwise, as she grew up she kept it, wearing it around her neck or placing it in her sacred bundle or medicine bag. Native people still make these sacred pieces, and many are copied as collectors' items or displayed in museums.

Although today most people usually discard the afterbirth, native people treated it with respect and even reverence. It was part of the life force, and to deal with it carelessly could cause injury to the mother or infant, or both. Where and how one buried or otherwise disposed of it was strategic. In some cases, a tribe member placed the placenta high up in a split tree to keep it from being scavenged. This act reflected the belief that the split in the tree might heal and close around the placenta, also symbolically preventing either infection and/or another immediate pregnancy. Some people continue this traditional practice today.

The link between birth control and disposal of the afterbirth was not unusual. Among the Cherokee and some other Plains tribes, the birth father or a chosen uncle carried the placenta a great distance from the village before reverently burying it. He made it a point to walk over several hills, because each hill he crossed would ensure that another year passed before the next baby was born. Among northern tribes, the grandmother took the placenta and filled it with porcupine quills as insurance against further pregnancies.

Once the birth and its aftermath are safely over and the tribe has welcomed the infant, it then becomes important to secure him in the tightly knit web of family and tribe. Having one's own clearly designated place is a key element of well-being and strength for American Indians. This task begins in the days and weeks following birth.

Pueblo Traditions

The Isleta Pueblo stretches across the fertile bottomlands of the Rio Grande River valley twelve miles south of Albuquerque. This pueblo, one of nineteen in the southwest United States, is named after a Spanish mission that was established in 1710. A child born in this pueblo goes through a number of rites to define his position in the tribe. This will en-

Corn

 Corn—as food, medicine, and an ingredient in ritual—is omnipresent in American Indian life. Many ceremonies incorporate perfect ears of corn because the cycle of corn, the life sustainer, symbolically reflects the cycle of the seasons and the fertility of the earth. American Indians from corn-growing tribes throughout the country, but especially those from the pueblos of Arizona and New Mexico, use the corn plant to make traditional art, musical instruments, and masks for healing rituals.

Sacred cornmeal in various colors is also part of many rites. The Hopi traditionally value the blue and the Zuni the black cornmeal. While both of these tribes raised corn in all the known colors, they carefully chose particular shades to use in specific ceremonies.

Besides its ritual and dietary uses, American Indians have always esteemed corn for its use in many spiritual and practical treatments. During childbirth, highly knowledgeable midwives used the ripe spores of corn smut fungus, *Ustilago maydis,* to activate uterine contractions and ease discomfort. Many tribes use corn smut fungus for ceremonial purification. Others apply it as a topical skin treatment and use it to clear and cure the rashes of infancy, birth marks, and other skin abnormalities. They also dust cornmeal, cornstarch, and corn pollen on the body, using these ingredients as talcum and for sacred ceremonies.

able him to fully participate in a lifelong series of rituals that are key to his survival.

At birth the child is linked to a moiety, a greater extended family. The first child is part of the father's moiety, the second belongs to the mother's, and so on in alternating fashion. When spring comes, each newborn receives his or her moiety name. This traditionally occurs during the spring ceremony when irrigation ditches are opened or during one of the first semiannual retreats and purification rituals. The critical link between the individual, agriculture, and the earth is the underpinning of Isleta Pueblo life. It recurs in rituals and ceremonies throughout the child's lifetime.

Each newborn also becomes a member of a Corn Group, a ritual unit that functions in the personal rites, such as baptisms, of the pueblo. This group also sanctifies the relationship of the new baby to corn, an attachment that is essential to a healthy life among the Isleta Pueblo and a host of other tribes.

The Sun Child Ceremony of the Zuni and the Hopi

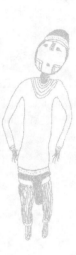

Just as important as the child's place in her family or tribe is her position in the universe. The poetic and beautiful Zuni Sun Child Ceremony invests birth with a broader meaning, recognizing the child's link not only to her earthbound community but also to the spirit world.

The Zuni Pueblo, located in northwest New Mexico, is one of the most ancient centers of habitation in the Southwest. The Zuni are distinguished by their diverse clan systems and complex system of sacred kachinas. Kachinas are a powerful race of supernaturals that touch all aspects of pueblo individuals' lives. The Zuni are governed by solar influences; their pueblos are controlled half the year by the winter people and the other half by the summer people. The Sun Child Ceremony is an age-old rite of welcome and passage.

On the eighth day of an infant's life, close ceremonial relatives, usually the aunts from his father's clan, wash the child's head, place sacred cornmeal in his hand, and, just before dawn, carry him outdoors. Facing the east at the moment of sunrise, they present him to the sun, which they consider the most powerful of the heavenly energies. They sprinkle more cornmeal on the infant's head as well as toward the sun, to honor it. The infant's paternal grandmother prays to the sun, the life sustainer, to bless the child.

The Hopi also have a tradition of presenting the infant to the sun. In their ceremony, which takes place twenty days after birth, the paternal and maternal grandmothers and aunts attend the baby. After ritually washing and purifying her in yucca suds and bestowing a family blessing, they carry her to face her first sunrise. After a further blessing with sacred ceremonial cornmeal, she becomes a full family member.

Naming Rituals

The naming ceremony is another thread that firmly attaches the newborn to the life-sustaining web of her ancestors and tribe. Some Inupiat peoples (Eskimos) in Alaska give the newborn the name of a respected elder who has recently died. Many American Indians believe that the spirit and wisdom of the elder for whom a child is named will return, carrying special privilege into the baby's life. Other people hold that children are ancient souls carrying the spirit of a treasured ancestor.

In some tribes, naming takes place at birth or soon thereafter. The child's name itself has great significance, and bestowing it is an honor. Often a grandparent or tribal elder has this privilege, although a parent, aunt, or uncle may assign the name. This early name is sacred and special, but not carved in stone. Among some native peoples, if a baby is unusually cranky in early infancy, the relatives come together again to give the child a new name. They believe that the child is irritable because he is unhappy with his name. A family gathering like this also provides support to parents struggling with a difficult baby. And in some tribes, a child receives new names at different stages in her life.

In some cases babies are not official members of their tribe until they have had their naming ceremony. Among the Mandan, for instance, the child is not considered part of the village before her naming. Instead, she remains linked to the Baby Hill from which she came. The Baby Hill is like an earth lodge, where an old man cares for the babies' spirits before they are born.

Naming rituals are joyous occasions, and they are often accompanied by feasts and other celebrations. Among the Cheyenne, when a baby girl receives her name a respected elder woman conducts the ritual. The baby's ears are pierced and adorned with round abalone-shell or bone earrings made by her father. Following the rite, the baby's family hosts a feast, where they distribute gifts. Relatives reciprocate with toys and dolls for the new baby to help her along the path to womanhood.

Much the same is done for boys. People make various effigies, often of animals, that they give to the baby as special blessings, to convey personal energy, and to bring about particular prowess. Many native peoples esteem dolls and toys for specific ceremonial uses, rather than as playthings.

Our child
It is your day.
This day,
The flesh of the white corn,
Prayer meal,
To our sun father
This prayer meal we offer.
May your road be fulfilled
Reaching to the road of
  your sun father.
When your road is fulfilled
In your thoughts (may we
  live)
May we be the ones
  whom your thoughts
  will embrace,
For this, on this day
To our sun father
We offer prayer meal
  to this end
May you help us all to
  finish our roads.

—*From the Zuni
Sun Child Ceremony*

The Cradleboard

Healing is not only connected to special events; it is imbedded in the everyday. Many practical objects have spiritual significance. Take, for example, the cradleboard, a nearly universal symbol of American Indian infancy.

According to some beliefs, a child has many nurturing influences. The first is the earth, who gives life to all beings; the second is the woman who gives birth to him; and the third is the father, who makes life possible. Finally, there is the cradleboard, which nurtures and protects him during his earliest days.

The cradleboard is key to a baby's well-being. The forerunner of today's baby carriers and backpacks, it is the first major object in an infant's life, a piece of furniture in a strikingly nonmaterial culture. Because male influence is critical for each child's healthy development, the birth father, or in some cases the adoptive or foster father, usually creates the infant's cradleboard. This also reflects the widespread belief that Father Sky oversees everything and everyone in a constant exchange with Mother Earth. Other family members sometimes contribute their special energy to the cradleboard. Older siblings or young clan relatives may add tiny amulets or other embellishments, perhaps a packet of sacred herbs tied onto it.

Cradleboard styles are as diverse as the artists who create them. Yet they are so distinctively connected to their tribe and region that you can almost "read" some cradleboards to see who made them and which tribe they came from. Nez Perce women, as well as many Ojibway and Great Lakes tribal artists, are famous for the fine, detailed beadwork on the tops of their cradleboards. The Navajo fashion their cradleboards from a solid piece of Ponderosa pine, with soft buckskin lacings. They often stain the cradleboard with red ochre. Jicarilla Apache basket weavers create some of the best woven cradleboards in the Southwest. And on Iroquois and Penobscot wooden cradleboards, carvers sculpt a symbolic tree of life and paint ornate pictures of key medicine plants across the backs. One of their primary medicinal plants—the jack-in-the-pulpit's beautiful hooded spathe and flowers—is a recurring theme.

Whether plain or fancy, carved of wood and decoratively painted or woven of willow, dogwood, tule, or cattail, cradleboards generally have a firm, wide, flat back, a small footrest, and a broad, rounded headpiece that bows out above the infant's head to provide shade. This piece also acts like a roll bar to protect the baby's face and head in case of an accident. A mother carries the cradleboard on her back or suspends it from

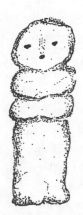

Clay figurine resembling a baby in a cradleboard wrapped and tied snugly

her forehead or shoulders using beautifully woven tumplines, or burden straps.

In early times, the cradleboard was vital to the Indian infant's first months of life, providing warmth, security, and portability, as well as a firm, protective frame for the baby's spine. Many tribes believed that the cradleboard prevented humpback, bowlegs, and bad posture. While the mother worked in the dwelling, village, or field, she could stand the cradleboard nearby or hang it from a sturdy tree. Some women nursed their babies while they were in their cradleboards. Frequently Indian women or other tribe members used them to safely carry babies on horseback during long journeys, making them a forerunner of car seats as well as backpacks.

Babies went into their cradleboards generously padded with fresh, dry sphagnum moss, cattail fluff, or shredded bark, which served as valuable disposable diapers. Some tribes, notably the Navajo, practiced an early form of recycling. These mothers cleaned and dried the padding, usually made of the shredded bark of juniper or cliffrose, in the sun and reused it. Not only were all of these materials naturally antiseptic, they also served to insulate and protect the baby's skin.

The baby was laced securely into the cradleboard with soft leather, her back and head well supported. Some Northwest Coast tribes also firmly bound their infants' heads with a soft, broad headband in order to gently shape a flatter, elongated forehead, which was considered a desirable feature among their ruling elite.

A soft piece of hide can be stretched or draped across the top of the cradleboard to act as a screen against the wind or sun. Suspended from the top, sacred amulets such as protective herbs, beaded umbilical-cord cases, and dream catchers or medicine wheels catch the baby's attention and train her eyes to focus.

Today cradleboards are treasured both as works of art and as useful baby carriers. They are passed down through many generations of American Indian families and continue to be significant objects of love and supportive protection. Older children enjoy carrying their infant siblings in their cradleboards, and Indian girls often want small ones for their dolls. Frequently cradleboards are security symbols. Many mothers recall their older toddlers running to hold or sit with their cradleboards during anxious times.

Pet Guardians for the Newborn Child

Newborns are vulnerable to many forces, including illness and everyday events as well as malevolent energies from the spirit world. Among the Delaware and some other Eastern tribes, a new baby is given a pet, usually a puppy or a kitten, to be its guardian spirit. The animal grows up and lives with the family, who treat it kindly and with respect. They speak to it frequently, encouraging the animal to stay close to the child, to sleep nearby, and to play with the baby as it grows.

Often the newborn's parents attach a small bag containing charcoal around the pet's neck. The Delaware and other tribes perceived charcoal to be purifying—an energized, protective substance. Interestingly, charcoal today is still used as a purifier or cleanser in many circumstances.

If the child is threatened by illness, the animal takes it on instead. As recalled by Mohegan elder Gladys Tantaquidgeon, the animal is thought to say: "I am only a dog. The child is more precious. Take me."

When the pet died, the family buried it with a ceremony that released it from the child. They also immediately gave their child another animal. If the child fell ill and died, they placed a string of wampum around the child's neck, thus freeing the animal.

Death and Grieving

The threat of infant death was always there. Legends and practices acknowledge the harsh reality of infant deaths, which, along with stillbirths, continue to occur, although not to the same extent as they did centuries ago. Historically, American Indian people lived close to nature and saw death frequently, in countless forms. Through many of their ceremonies, rituals, and talismans they attempted to allay their fears and provide protection for the newest member of the tribe.

Even in their mortuary practices, some tribes strove to provide shelter for the baby. The Oklahoma Seminole, Shawnee, and Kickapoo wrapped stillborn infants and placed them in hollow trees. By giving the small body to the soul of a tree, they placed the child out of harm's way and closer to the creator.

Ultimately, American Indians respected death as an inevitable state of transition and a metamorphosis leading to rebirth. As Chief Seattle said, "There is no death, only a change of worlds." People in many tribes felt that a young spirit unwilling to remain on earth should be allowed to slip peacefully away. Still, whenever a baby dies, it is a source of deep sorrow.

There are many ways to express grief when a newborn dies. Although it is expressed differently from tribe to tribe, grief is usually public and overt. Many tribal members, not just those who have actually suffered the loss, actively mourn; the shared grieving contributes to the healing that must take place. In some tribes, people give up a sacred personal object or cut their hair short for a period of mourning that can go on for as long as seven years. Death chants, "crys," ghost feasts, and spirit plates are traditional mourning rites; we will discuss them in Chapter 9.

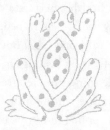

American Indians took advantage of their environments, using naturally plentiful substances to heal the ailments of infancy. Cornstarch, cornmeal, pollen, the fine talc dust from soapstone (steatite), and the dusty spores released from the distinctive ball-shaped white fungi known as puffballs were commonly used as topical skin treatments. (There is a dark puffball, *Sclaroderma* spp., that is poisonous.) They also had natural therapies for heat and diaper rashes, insect and spider bites, and various forms of dermatitis. Sphagnum and other leafy mosses, which possess antiseptic properties, made useful diapers and were also employed for padding and insulation. And along with the mosses, lichens and fungi have long been valued as wound dressings.

American Indian infant health care made extensive use of puffballs, which are abundant in many areas. Native people used small, underripe white puffballs as a styptic—torn open and bound securely in place over the newborn infant's navel—to assist healing. In fact, so common was this practice that Cherokee people sometimes referred to the small white puffballs as "baby's navel." Underripe white puffballs or the darkened spores from ripe puffballs were also applied to burns, birthmarks, or rashes. And suspended from the cradleboard or, as the child grew older, worn around the neck, puffballs served as an inhalant to treat respiratory distress and asthma.

Strawberry and raspberry leaves were and still are used in many ways, as a warm cleansing herbal wash for the infant or as a mild tea to treat digestive problems such as diarrhea, which can be dangerous in infants and young children. Nursing women also drank these teas as digestive aids for themselves and when their infants suffered from diarrhea, demonstrating an early understanding that mothers pass substances on to their babies through their milk.

The long creeping roots and rhizomes of the moisture-loving, aromatic perennial known as sweet flag, *Acorus calamus,* also known as sweetgrass, muskrat root, calamus root, beewort, and sweetroot, were one of the most valuable native root medicines. Indeed, this plant was by itself almost an entire medicine chest to some tribes, and it continues to be

Wild strawberry
Fragaria vesca

a highly respected health aid, an ingredient in many herbal bitters and other native formulas.

Useful at every stage of life, sweetgrass was especially important for infants and children. The Cheyenne called this *wi'ukh is e'evo* (bitter medicine), and traded with their Sioux neighbors to obtain the plants. They used it as a talisman or amulet, tying a small piece of the dried root onto their children's necklaces, clothing, blankets, or cradleboards to keep away the night spirits and bless their dreams. Along with the Cheyenne, many other tribes braided or wound the long, shiny green leaf blades into the infant's trappings for good luck and as an aromatic insecticide.

Gladys Tantaquidgeon, Mohegan medicine woman and respected elder, remembers that many eastern Algonquian peoples often carried or wore calamus root as a disease preventive. A worthwhile digestive aid when chewed or steeped in water, calamus root was the most reliable treatment for infant colic and stomachache. Indians also made teething necklaces from small sections of dried sweet flag roots; although they had to be used with caution, especially during the first year of life, they effectively numbed teething pains.

Honey and other bee by-products were also readily available and widely used. Long before European settlers brought the honeybee, *Apis mellifera,* to America in the seventeenth century, the early Maya and Aztec Indians kept bees and collected honey from wild bees, of which there are more than 3,500 species in North America. Honey is one of the purest sweets found in nature: it is twice as sweet as cane sugar. It is also 35 percent protein (it contains one half of all the amino acids essential for human life) and is considered a complete food. But besides its obvious nutritional value, honey is a beneficial wound dressing and medicine.

American Indians used honey or maple syrup to treat a variety of babies' needs. If an infant was cranky, they placed a small amount on her lips or tongue to calm and nourish her. Alternatively, they might give an irritable infant mildly sweetened water or particular herbal teas to pacify her and help her sleep. **Note: Raw honey should not be given internally to infants or babies in their first year out of concern for health problems such as allergic reactions or the possibility of infection.**

Perhaps the most beneficial treatment for infants was the use of honey as an antiseptic salve. This was made with honey alone or with propolis, the resinous substance that bees collect from various plants and

Common strawberry
Fragaria virginiana

Sugar maple
Acer saccharum

mix with beeswax to construct their hives. The salve can be used to soothe scratches, burns, and skin problems, as well as to kill bacteria.

What follows are recipes based on American Indian practices. In addition to treating a variety of ailments, you can use these light skin preparations and herbal tea washes while massaging your baby. Gently massage the infant's chest and abdomen as well as her back, buttocks, arms, and legs to promote good circulation and stimulate good muscle tone and development. At the end of each day bathe your infant with pure, clean water to remove any residue from these treatments. After drying, dust your child with a clean herbal powder.

EARTH MOTHER HERBAL POWDER

Like parents today, many Indian mothers used massage to naturally bond with their children and to exercise their babies after many hours spent in their cradleboards. They often used protective powders like this one as part of the process.

You can also use this mild powder both to keep creases and other moist areas of your baby's skin dry and to soothe the irritation from lingering rashes. It is especially useful when you put it on your baby's bottom, under his arms, or in other spots where heat rash flares up. Sage is a purifier and it also adds a light fragrance. Use the powder by lightly sprinkling it onto the baby's skin and gently rubbing it in.

Combine 2 cups of fine cornstarch and $1/4$ cup of fine ground sage. Blend well. Cover and store in a small, clean jar.

White sage
Artemisia ludoviciana

DRY-ROASTED CORNMEAL TALC

Here is an alternative to cornstarch powder that you can also use as a skin treatment and to absorb moisture. It's best to make this frequently—once or twice a week—so that it stays fresh. It's easy to do.

Roast 1 to 2 cups of fine cornmeal on top of the stove in a clean, dry skillet, shaking frequently to prevent burning. Or spread the cornmeal on a clean cookie sheet and roast at 325 degrees for 15 minutes or less. The cornmeal is done when it becomes light brown or honey-colored. Store it in an airtight container.

STRAWBERRY/RASPBERRY LEAF TEA

This herbal tea and its variations are mild and can be used, in moderation, for infants. Massage any of them onto your baby's gums to ease teething pains. If you're a nursing mother, you can use the tea as a digestive aid. And if your baby is colicky or has diarrhea, drink some yourself and give the baby some, lukewarm, a small spoonful at a time.

Strawberry/raspberry leaf tea also makes a pleasant, mild skin wash for infants. To treat scalp irritations such as cradle cap, use this tea, with a small amount of honey added, once or twice a day. Lightly sprinkle the tea on your infant's head and gently rub it in. Leave it on for ten minutes to half an hour, then rinse with plain water or unsweetened tea to lubricate the skin and wash away any stickiness.

In a clean pot, pour the boiling water over the herbs. Cover and steep for five minutes or more. Strain and use as needed, warm or chilled; add maple syrup to sweeten, if desired.

VARIATION: Use ⅛ cup to ¼ cup dried mint leaves for a cooling analgesic effect.

VARIATION: Use ⅛ cup fresh or 1 tablespoon dried slippery elm bark or willow bark. When made into a light tea, the smooth young inner bark of these trees is a good pain reliever; rubbed on the skin, it relieves heat or diaper rash.

TO MAKE ONE POT:

½ cup fresh raspberry and/or strawberry leaves, or ¼ cup dried
(Note: If you are picking your own, be sure to select clean, nonmildewed, healthy leaves that you know have not been sprayed or otherwise polluted. Never pick from plants growing by the roadside.)
16 ounces boiling water

Red raspberry
Rubus idaeus

HONEY-WATER LOTION

1 tablespoon natural honey

1 cup strawberry/raspberry
tea or plain hot water

1 teaspoon bee propolis
(optional)

¹/₂ teaspoon lemon juice
(optional—it adds a
cleansing benefit)

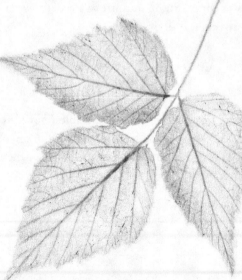

This is a soothing lotion that calms burns and rashes; it is also antibacterial. But it should not be used on highly sensitive skin or where there are open wounds. Apply the lotion on the skin as needed, one tablespoonful at a time, and gently massage it in. For diaper rash, use some with each diaper change; if your child has highly sensitive skin, use it only once a day.

You can also use this lotion to treat digestive problems by applying it to the baby's abdomen and softly massaging clockwise and then counter-clockwise.

MAKE THIS LOTION WHEN YOU NEED IT; IT DOESN'T STORE WELL.

Melt the honey in hot water along with the bee propolis and lemon juice. Stir until thoroughly blended and dissolved. Pour into a sterile 8 ounce bottle or jar.

VARIATION: For diaper rash, substitute black tea or green tea for the liquid. Their tannins will calm the inflammation.

Black raspberry
Rubus occidentalis

Caitlin

The story of baby Caitlin, whose survival was in doubt, demonstrates some of the mysteries of healing and urges us not to give up despite the sometimes hopeless prognoses we get from conventional medicine.

Celeste, a young woman of Choctaw, Mexican, and Irish heritage living in Florida, conceived a child despite having been told by doctors that it was highly unlikely. Unfortunately, she began to have early signs of miscarriage. After several examinations her doctor told her that her body was rejecting the pregnancy and that she should go home and allow nature to take its course. But she wanted to have the baby and knew it might be her only chance.

Her mother, grandmother, and other American Indian friends far away in the Northeast prayed for her and sent sacred herbs, such as red cedar, sage, tobacco, and sweetgrass, in tiny red packets (red, which represents the heart, blood, and heat, is a color frequently used in healing rites and sacred offerings) for the baby.

After a few months of confinement she delivered Caitlin, a very premature baby, who weighed only 1 1/2 pounds. Again the doctors held little hope. They were very cautious about the baby's survival, telling her family that if she lived, there was an 80 percent chance of blindness, loss of hearing, and very likely brain damage or some degree of cerebral palsy. Once more family and friends went to work with prayers, creating a special medicine bag, a dream catcher, and other accouterments for Caitlin.

In her tiny isolette in the hospital, Caitlin's heart was stopping many times a day. Doctors would say only, "Wait and see"; they thought it would be only a matter of time until she died. Her grandmother asked the nurses to put the medicine bag in with the baby. Trying to humor her, they put it in a Ziploc bag and taped it to the isolette. The baby's mother was very pleased but quite surprised

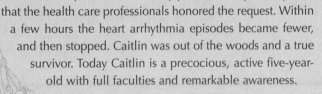

that the health care professionals honored the request. Within a few hours the heart arrhythmia episodes became fewer, and then stopped. Caitlin was out of the woods and a true survivor. Today Caitlin is a precocious, active five-year-old with full faculties and remarkable awareness.

CHAPTER TWO

Childhood

CONSECRATION OF
THE BOY TO THUNDER

⌇⌇⌇⌇⌇⌇⌇⌇⌇⌇⌇⌇⌇⌇⌇⌇⌇⌇⌇⌇⌇⌇⌇⌇⌇⌇⌇⌇⌇⌇⌇⌇⌇⌇⌇⌇

Sassafras
Sassafras albidum

The life of man is a circle from childhood to

childhood, and so it is in everything where

power moves. Our tipis were round like the nests of

birds, and these were always set in a circle, the

nation's hoop, a nest of many nests, where the

Great Spirit meant for us to hatch our children.

—BLACK ELK, OGLALA SIOUX HOLY MAN AND MEDICINE MAN

⌇⌇⌇⌇⌇⌇⌇⌇⌇⌇⌇⌇⌇⌇⌇⌇⌇⌇⌇⌇⌇⌇⌇⌇⌇⌇⌇⌇⌇⌇⌇⌇⌇⌇⌇⌇

Sassafras
Sassafras albidum

Like all parents, American Indians want their children to reach their maximum potential, and so they work to develop the child's mind, body, and spirit. Whenever possible, the extended family carefully guides the shaping of the child's earliest years. As she grows, they bolster her awareness of her personal strengths as well as her commitment to her family, her tribe, and the earth of their beginnings. Slowly and deliberately they introduce metaphysical lessons about life, illness, and death.

Naturally, childhood is a time of play, fun, relaxation, and enchantment. In the old days, and to some extent today, a great deal of teaching took place each evening around the fire, where many people, including some of the children themselves, told stories. The storyteller's role was to coax, illuminate, and galvanize young minds, revealing their roles and commitments in the life that lay ahead.

Sassafras
Sassafras albidum

Along with everyday learning and activity, the tribe pays careful attention to practices and observances that nurture young minds and enfold children into the broader community. Children are remarkably self-centered during their first few years of life. As they learn to walk and talk they are sometimes completely absorbed in their own developmental tasks. Often tribal ceremonies serve to draw children out of themselves, linking them closely with their relatives and natural surroundings.

Sometimes small moments are celebrated as great events. One charming example is the Cree Walking-out Ceremony, done to strengthen a child's feet on the pathway of life.

The Cree Walking-out Ceremony

The Cree Walking-out Ceremony and Feast is a unique ritual that touchingly commemorates a major event in a young child's life—her first experience walking outside the confines of her own home and intimate family circle. This ceremony also reinforces the strong traditional and personal commitment the family and tribe make to each individual.

The Cree, whose homelands stretch across southern Canada from James Bay to Saskatchewan, are the most broadly dispersed of the southern Canadian tribes. There are many tribes among the Cree, and within these tribes there is an extensive clan system. Like the Scottish clans, these are tightly knit groups of people who are related to each other, usually through lineage and marriage. Clans clearly delineate the extensive relationships an individual child has with his mother's and father's relatives. By custom, a child is born into his mother's clan. The maternal side is the guiding, shaping influence in a child's life as well as in the politics and hierarchy of the tribe. A child has his strongest physical, hereditary, and spiritual ties to his mother's clan, and no one can marry within his own clan.

The Walking-out Ceremony has long been traditional among all of the Cree. It is held around the time of a baby's first birthday, when she is about ready to walk or possibly already toddling. The Cree mark these first tiny footsteps as a major milestone, blessing the child and positioning her on a life path where she will be healthy, happy, and able to reach her goals. "You can compare the Walking-out Ceremony to Christian baptism," says Louise Saganash, of Waswanipi. "It's like a person's official entry into life, marked by respect for the environment and nature, of which the child is an integral part."

In going through the Walking-out Ceremony, the child symbolically enters the real world. Before it takes place, he is not allowed to walk outside of his home; he must be carried. At dawn on the chosen day, parents, family, and friends gather around the toddler (or toddlers, since it can be a joint ceremony for several children) in a big tent. They move from east to west around the interior, "from the sun's rising to its setting, from birth to death, greeted by the guests." Then, helped by his grandparents or parents, each child crosses the threshold to the outside. They follow a path strewn with fir branches to a tree (which symbolizes nature), circle the tree, and return to the tent. Back inside, the gathered guests joyously welcome, honor, and congratulate the toddler at a special feast given by the elders.

Underlying even those ceremonies that celebrate the smaller rites of passage is the consciousness of a connection to greater forces. All through life, American Indians see themselves as children of the Creator and of the creative energies in their natural universe. In this respect they are woven together in their beliefs, even though their cultures, languages, and rituals are strikingly different.

The Omaha Consecration of the Boy to Thunder

Childhood rituals often emphasize these spiritual and natural connections. Among the Omaha, the Consecration of the Boy to Thunder, which follows the infancy ritual of Turning the Child (see Chapter 1), marks the time when a lock of hair is cut from a boy child's head. But the significance of this ceremony lies far deeper than celebrating the first haircut. It dedicates the boy's life to thunder, the power that controls the life and death of a warrior.

Thunder and lightning have always been highly significant, especially among the many tribes of the plains and prairies. Because thunder, wind, and lightning are the voice, the breath, and the touch of the Creator, they are major forces to contend with.

As a messenger from the Creator and Father Sky, Thunder often warned that lightning was coming. Being struck by lightning and surviving meant you had been touched by the Creator or the Creator's energies, and often people who had this experience with thunder and lightning were "turned" by it, undergoing deep emotional changes.

People feared lightning and held it in awe, but they also greatly admired it. Although it could bring death and destruction, it frequently carried blessings. Wood struck by lightning was considered by many American Indians to be enhanced with special healing powers and medicinal virtues. Schaghticoke (Connecticut) councilwoman Erin Lamb believes that "lightning-struck wood has been kissed by the spirits." Artists often seek lightning-struck wood to make special amulets, and healers grind it into healing formulas to be used as wound dressings or taken internally. Some people wrap it in red flannel to keep in their medicine bundles. But some tribes, including the Navajo, feared lightning-struck objects and would not touch or use them.

The Consecration of the Boy to Thunder invokes the awesome energies of lightning and thunder. What further intensifies the ritual is its connection to hair. Especially among many of the Plains Indian cultures, hair

O our Mother the Earth,
O our Father the Sky,
Your children are we, and
　with tired backs
We bring you the gifts
　you love.
Then weave for us a
　garment of brightness;
May the warp be the white
　light of morning,
May the weft be the red
　light of evening,
May the fringes be the
　falling rain,
May the border be the
　standing rainbow.
Thus weave for us a
　garment of brightness
That we may walk fittingly
　where grass is green,
O our Mother the Earth,
O our Father the Sky!

—*Tewa Pueblo prayer*

has great beauty and power and must be treated especially carefully. In the past, young men grew their hair very long, sometimes even longer than the women of the tribe. They didn't cut it except when required by ceremonial tradition or for a mourning rite after the death of a loved one. During the Consecration of the Boy to Thunder, once the lock of hair is cut, it is tied and put into the child's medicine bundle or warrior's paraphernalia as a source of personal strength.

Because warriors had an exalted status, the Consecration of the Boy to Thunder is an old, highly esteemed ceremony. In the early days every man had to be a warrior to defend his tribe and family. Valiant and admired warriors, resplendently dressed, performed special feats of endurance, bravery, and cunning and became legends. Today, for the most part, these warrior skills are no longer demonstrated on the battlefield, except in the armed services. But this ritual, like the deeper meaning of the warrior spirit, lives on.

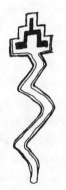

Zuni lightning symbol

Translated into modern-day life, the warrior spirit is a resolute commitment to your own particular path. Having the warrior spirit means being the best you can be, whatever your endeavor. Those with a desire to do something they believe in, who train for it and devote their lives to it, have the warrior spirit, that special determination to succeed.

Today children learn that both men and women can be warriors. A woman warrior is an achiever who works to overcome the odds against her. These days many American Indian tribes are headed by women chiefs. American Indian women are college professors and presidents, corporate officers and attorneys, and they successfully fill many other roles in society as well as in their homes, families, clans, and tribal realms. Their spirit, determination, and warrior's courage give them this strength.

The Consecration of the Boy to Thunder aims to instill endurance and perseverance in children of both sexes. Honoring the idea of the warrior spirit keeps the ceremony vital.

The Warrior Spirit

All through childhood, selected individuals were groomed to be warriors. To some extent this continues today. But the familiar pictures of belligerent, aggressive American Indian warriors painted by movies and television

Thunder Beings and Thunder Societies

*The Creator instructed the Grandfather Thunders to put
fresh water into the rivers, lakes, and springs to
quench the thirst of life. So with one mind we give our
greetings and thanks to our Grandfathers.*

—From the opening prayer of the Thanksgiving address
at the Akwesasne Freedom School, Mohawk Nation, Akwesasne

Throughout Native America the seasonal occurrences of thunder were associated with the strong, sometimes violent, forces of change and renewal. These awe-inspiring energies could affect everything in life, especially across the Great Plains and the desert Southwest. Thunder, Thunderers, Thunder Beings, and Thunderbird are some of the many names American Indians gave to this natural phenomenon.

Many children were afraid of thunder. It was an unearthly, sometimes fearful sound from the Sky World. It could portend many things, but it was always powerful. Adults tried to calm children's terror at thunder by explaining it in colorful ways. Sometimes it was embodied in otherworldly beings who were described by George Bush Otter, a Teton Sioux, like this: "Some of these ancient Thunder People still dwell in the clouds. They have large curved beaks resembling bison humps; their voices are loud; they do not open their eyes except when they make lightning."

Children also learned that they might be especially honored by the Thunder Beings. At their whim, these omnipotent powers might select and relate to chosen individuals, especially the young. This is not a rare occurrence: Many tribes had (and some still have) special thunder societies. The only people admitted were those who had dreamed of thunder or lightning and those who had been touched by lightning. Chosen members held special powers in league with the supernatural forces.

Thundercloud altar

fly in the face of true American Indian warrior traditions. Children learn that violence is not always part of the equation; a warrior can be gentle and calm. Parents and elders teach young people that a warrior possesses traits such as kindness, and that a macho attitude has to be balanced with a sensitivity for life and nature.

Historically, the best warriors were highly trained individuals who avoided most conflicts but because of their integrity and great skill won those that had to be fought. Codes of war, like the chivalric codes in medieval Europe, existed among the more than twenty Plains Indian tribes known as the "horse cultures"—the Sioux, Cheyenne, Pawnee, Omaha, and Crow, among others. For instance, the touching coup honored someone who touched his enemy but did not kill him. Warriors carried a coup stick, an elaborate, intricately designed, often feathered staff. The goal was to ride close enough to your enemy to touch him before he touched you. Childhood games of skill honed children's ability to pinpoint targets for fighting, hunting, and prowess in competition.

These warrior codes were not simply rules of war, either; they governed well-being and health. Violating them could bring devastating consequences. Respect for right living and following one's traditions was a part of staying balanced. A warrior who disobeyed or defied his rules of conduct disturbed this equilibrium and might sicken or even die.

Dreams and Visions

Thunder can interact with different levels of the world: Mother Earth, Father Sky, and the Spirit World. Dreams and visions give human beings similar mobility.

Dreams matter a great deal at all times, but childhood visions and dreams are said to be more powerful. Children, by virtue of their youthful innocence, are closer to the Creator, and dream spirits, Thunder Beings, and others from the metaphysical realm can reach children more readily.

Many tribes actively discuss and interpret childhood dreams, believing that the Creator sends valuable information to the people through their children. In earlier times dreams were spoken aloud and analyzed every day if possible, and they were considered sacred in many native societies. There are countless records of young American Indian girls and boys having dreams in which the spirits revealed new healing arts or foretold events that eventually came to pass.

American Indian children sometimes experience spontaneous visions. But people don't think visions are frightening; instead, they are considered normal and desirable among many tribes, especially those of the Great Plains. (Later in life the vision quest, puberty rituals, Sun Dance, and other special rites of passage provide structured ways to communicate with sacred beings.)

Perhaps the most famous examples come from the Oglala Sioux holy man Black Elk, who had his first vision during a thunderstorm in 1869 at the age of five, while out playing with his new bow and arrows. At the age of nine he received a great vision in which he foresaw changes for his people and their way of life. Black Elk had this vision after he had been seriously ill for several days. This is not unusual: Psychic, visionary, and shamanistic experiences often come at times of illness or grief.

Visions are linked to healing practices. Dreams, reaffirmed by visions, often set an individual on a healing path or reinforce a person's commitment to a particular career. Occasionally they provide information and special powers from sources that cannot be explained. According to Navajo legends like this one, some of their healing sand paintings began as knowledge mystically provided to a child:

> A Navajo boy was walking along the side of a lake when he was drawn into the water. He swam toward a floating log, which was joined by three other logs, making a sacred cross, which began spinning, creating a whirlpool that dragged him to the bottom of the lake. Without being harmed, he was given intricate sand painting designs and the right songs and ritual prayers to treat arthritis and rheumatism. When he had completely learned these holy rites and rituals, he was brought back to the surface of the lake and allowed to go back to his people.

Today among the Navajo, sand paintings like the one in this story are still an important tool for treating disabling conditions. Contemporary Navajo sand painters study most of their lives to hone their talents. A sand painting, which can take many hours to complete, can only be composed

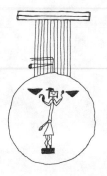

Pollen Boy on the Sun

on the earthen floor of the hogan, the eight-sided dwelling of the Navajo. Once it is done, the patient is blessed with sacred cornmeal and seated on the painting. As the Navajo medicine person and the patient's family sing the accompanying songs, prayers, and chants, the patient's illness is drawn down into the colored sand, after which the entire painting is destroyed, scooped up into a blanket or a piece of skin, carried east, and released into the desert where it cannot harm anyone. Often the patient retains a pinch of it in his own personal medicine bundle. While some people combine this traditional healing with mainstream medical practices, for others this is their only treatment.

Sand paintings, replicated on fiberboard with epoxy, have also made their way into the contemporary art world, where they are cherished collectibles. But a sand painting made as a piece of art must never copy one of the ritual healing paintings, which are invested with tremendous and mysterious power. Otherwise it will bring harm to the person who created it.

The dreams and visions of children are the wellsprings of important healing practices among other tribes, too. For example, people in the Iowa tribe tell how a little boy called Lone Walker ran away to follow his father and the other men riding off to hunt buffalo. Distraught at being left behind, he saw them kill a buffalo bull and ride on, planning to get it when they returned. As the little boy, sobbing and crying, ran up near the carcass, the bull spoke to him. "Ah, so it is you, Lone Walker? I'm glad you came, for I've recovered and am just about to get up again. Now I am going to tell you what to do from this time on." Afterward the buffalo taught him which roots and healing herbs his people could use to cure illness.

And the Medicine Bow Society, a secret society of the Sioux, began after a young Sioux boy experienced a profound and spontaneous vision while hiding among sheltering trees during a frightening thunderstorm. In his vision, he was given a white horse with special thunder powers and the medicine bow and its rites.

Many of the Medicine Bow Society's rites are not performed in public. Like the society's medicine bundles, they are private. Throughout Native America there are many secret healing societies. The veil of secrecy strengthens the mystical and actual healing power of their medicines and rites, which can occasionally come close to the miraculous. Members do not hide these practices to withhold knowledge, but to guard it and elevate it to a higher level, much like some of the deepest religious practices of the Judeo-Christian and Islamic traditions.

Sound and Music

Right from the beginning, sound and music are a vital presence in every young American Indian's life. Singing, chanting, or the methodical beat of a drum or sound of the rattle can relax and reassure an upset child, helping her to sleep. And sound and music frequently accompany healing.

Young children often make small wind instruments called bull roarers that they twirl over their heads or in front of them to feel the dynamics of wind and sound. In many American Indian cultures this innocent form of play has sacred overtones. The earliest bull roarers were ceremonial instruments whose mystical connection to wind, or the breath of the Creator, could effect healing. Bull roarers are still vital instruments of healing. They are used, especially by Pueblo peoples, to call in the winds for healing rites and other ceremonies.

Although it is a part of everyday life, sound in all its forms is also a vital link to nature, the Creator, and the Spirit World. The human voice, alone or collectively, through prayers, chanting, and singing, is a mainstay of major ceremonies such as the potlatch, the powwow, and kachina rites. People can achieve altered states of consciousness and heightened awareness through the repetition of particular sounds. And the human breath, directed over hallowed objects, patients, or sacred herbs or blown into holy whistling pots or musical instruments, is central to healing and restoring balance.

Childhood training in sound and music begins early. Some say that babies begin to learn about drumming and other musical instruments while they are still in the womb. Often, before they even learn spoken language, children are taught ceremonial chants and vocables, the nonword sounds that are ubiquitous in American Indian music.

Northwest Coast Practices

Dense populations of dynamic tribal groups lived in the lush environments along the rugged coast of the Pacific Northwest, stretching from

Drums and Rattles

American Indians use drums, rattles, whistles, flutes, and zithers. Many of these wind and percussion instruments are designed to echo aspects of nature. Their primary function is sacred, for use in ceremony, prayer, and healing rites.

The drum simulates the Earth Mother's heartbeat, or it can imitate thunder and pounding rain. Played very softly, it can sound like breath, wind, running water, or game animals. Much depends on whether one strokes or rubs it with the palm or fingers of the hand or uses a drumstick. There are many different types of drums—the small, sacred single-faced water drum of the Delaware and Iroquois in the Northeast; the large double-sided cottonwood drums of the Plains; the various hand-held, single-faced shaman's drums found in many regions—but all convey the vitality of the drum in native life.

Rattles, like drums, are complex, and their type, construction, and ornamentation speak volumes about which tribe made them and for what purpose. In the East, people pierced deer toes (the dark horn tips) and strung them close together with rawhide or sinew; tribes in northern sub-Arctic regions did the same with bony puffin beaks. These clusters of musical rattles were carried or worn by dancers or shamans. People also use rattles made of gourds, folded bark, horn, or bone as well as rainsticks to call in the rain spirits and other environmental energies needed for prayers, celebrations, and curing ceremonies.

northern Oregon all the way to southern Alaska. They have become known as the "totem pole" and "potlatch" cultures. Some of the most distinctive art, healing practices, and ceremonial rites in all of Native America radiate from their amazing tribal traditions.

While many childhood ceremonies connect the child to nature and the Creator, others secure and demonstrate her place in society. Fitting closely into the web of family and tribe ensures her a healthier life. And perpetuating the tribe's customs and traditions secures the health and well-being of the entire community.

Unlike most other tribes, the Haida people of the Northwest Coast had a social hierarchy and unique symbols to distinguish its ranks. They traditionally honored female children, who signified the continuation of the matrilineal line. Although it's no longer much in evidence, the Haida used the lip labret, an ornament placed through a small incision in the child's lip, as a marker of a girl's rank and status. The labret increased in size according to the rank and the fecundity of the woman wearing it.

The Haida also commonly practiced ear piercing and tattooing. These important symbols of beauty revealed key aspects about the child's family and who the child was in the family. Both male and female infants had their ears pierced, and if they were of high rank they were tattooed on their arms, hands, and legs, and sometimes chests and backs.

Wealthy parents gave potlatches to celebrate these ceremonies. A traditional Northwest Coast potlatch is a grand, well-planned feast and ritual of sharing and giving, held when a child is named and at other key moments in the life of a family. Nothing else in Native America matched the wildly imaginative Northwest Coast potlatch. It was an elaborate display of wealth staged to impress—and, it was hoped, overwhelm—friends and relatives as well as enemies. Only an affluent chief with a great many valued objects to give away could afford one. Some chiefs and their families would save for years, collecting and buying blankets, creating artwork, and gathering the goods for the potlatch.

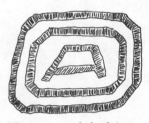

Tlingit spruce root basket design element

The potlatch originally had religious overtones. It included sacred rites and stories, and often began with emotionally charged oratories and special prayers owned by the family that could be spoken only at these events.

A potlatch was awesome and highly theatrical. It took place inside a huge firelit plank house. People wore elaborate masks and dance regalia. Ornately carved and strikingly painted wooden puppets and marionettes—multijointed octopi, frogs, and crabs—skittered across the floor, startling children as they sat, awestruck, in the flickering light.

Missionaries feared and misunderstood potlatches. They successfully convinced lawmakers to outlaw them in the United States, and in Canada potlatches were illegal for almost a hundred years before the ban was removed. Today many Northwest Coast tribes are returning to their traditional potlatching and other practices.

In addition to being an extravagant giveaway, the ancient potlatch was also a sacred time during which healing events could take place. Today, across the face of Native America, giveaways have become the simple counterparts to the old potlatching custom. Giveaways occur at certain prescribed times during the year and throughout an individual's life cycle.

Giveaways recognize the societal importance of giving back. Sometimes they take place during powwows or other Indian social events. Often they are explicitly connected to healing. For example, when a local child needed surgery, the dancers at a Connecticut powwow performed a special Blanket Dance. Dancing to a welcoming song, they held a blanket and circled the gathering, taking contributions from the audience.

Some tribes use giveaways to honor and pay medicine people. Or people might organize a giveaway when someone is recovering from a serious illness or after a woman endures a difficult but successful birth. Practices we see today, like a community drive to garner donations of blood for a child's bone marrow transplant, hark back to traditional American Indian giveaways.

Schooling, or Setting the Feet on the Pathway

Throughout an individual's life, maintaining balance is the key to staying well. One of the best ways to do this is to live in harmony with tribal traditions—to walk the Pollen Path. Among American Indians, teaching their children this lesson is of the utmost importance. Not only does having a strong connection to tribal beliefs, customs, and practices help people maintain equilibrium, it also provides critical support when a natural disaster, illness, or other unexplainable upheaval occurs. Childhood teachings of many kinds—not just those explicitly about healing—are thus seen as essential to properly setting young feet on the path and assuring good health.

Centuries ago, before the advent of formalized schools and education, many American Indian tribes developed methods to educate their children. Called childhood teachings, this nearly universal system of American Indian traditional education includes prayers, lectures, and storytelling. It carries children through childhood and into adolescence. Childhood teachings ensure not only the children's proper development but also the continuing survival of tribal customs.

The Winnebago, one of the Algonquian cultures of the Great Lakes, use their childhood teachings to give their children a strong sense of self and a solid grounding in tradition. They call this "setting the feet on the pathway." Because the tribe's well-being, especially in the past, depended upon leading their lives in as open and harmonious a vein as possible, the teachings admonish children never to harm anyone or do contrary things, so they can establish a clean life path. Stories teach and reinforce right thinking, honoring traditions and respecting taboos. Many of the Winnebago's neighbors—the Cree to the north and the Ojibway/Chippewa, the Menominee, the Sauk, the Fox, the Potawatomis, and the Shawnee around the Great Lakes—use similar childhood teachings.

American Indian stories are profound teaching tools. They frame the child's experience and work to explain the otherwise unexplainable. They are often told in a carefully delineated sequence to add to their impact. Some stories can be repeated only at certain times of year. For example, one can tell Coyote stories only in the dead of winter between the last and first thunders, when the nights are longer and when, in the past, the family huddled around the interior fires. Because Coyote is a trickster, if you tell Coyote stories outside of this time period, you might endanger yourself or your listeners.

While Coyote is an almost universal symbol, other tricksters exist in many cultures. Among the peoples of the Plains and some other Great Lakes tribes is found Iktomi, the mischievous spider. He sometimes performs valuable deeds and healing, but more frequently is a clown or changeling who behaves grossly.

The stories of many Northwest Coast peoples include the wily rascal known as Raven. Many say that Raven is still working on the order of things, and this is one reason why he is treated with respect.

These stories do not draw a line between religion and education. Like American Indian songs and ceremonies, they provide a key to everyday behavior, but they also reveal aspects of a tribe's worldview and religious philosophy. Stories spin this web of traditional beliefs around the children. They are often carefully designed to show correct behavior, such as the importance of being respectful to elders. But they are woven together with such charm and performed with such entertaining theatrics that children ask to hear them again and again. And, of course, the reiteration helps the storyteller solidify the message.

Often storytellers use props. Many create story baskets and bags in which they keep their props and special amulets they use to tease or trick the story out. The Iroquois no-face dolls, made of corn husks or leather, serve to reinforce certain moral values. By leaving the face blank, the doll can take on a number of different personas.

The Seneca explain their doll with no face by telling the story of a long-ago corn husk doll whose face was so beautiful that she became very vain and could think of nothing but her personal beauty. Distressed by

During my childhood it was traditional to be sent to live for a time with the elders of each clan we are related to. These elders eagerly looked within us to see if we carried their seeds and, if so, began to water us with teachings.

—Nosapocket
(Ramona Peters),
Wampanoag artist, dancer,
and traditionalist

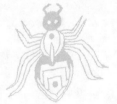

Raven Steals the Sun

This story is based on a Tsimshian Legend from the turn of the century. In the earliest earth time, people on the Northwest Coast existed without light. It was difficult for them to find their food, take care of their families, and see one another. People kept bumping into each other. Because of this, the people appealed to Raven to help them. Raven has always been a clever and mystical being, capable of changing himself into a giant or a glossy black bird or a little child.

Raven flew down from the Sky World, and as he flew over the ocean he dropped a little stone from his feathers into the sea. This turned into a large rock, which became land. He flew out over this and scattered salmon roe and the roe of other fish, so that every creek, river, and ocean would have all kinds of fish. He opened a seal bladder filled with the first fruits and sprinkled them generously over the land so that his people would have plenty of valuable foods to eat and herbs to heal themselves. But the world was still covered in darkness, and the people could not see how to gather these riches.

So Raven flew back up to the Sky World and landed near the smoke hole of the Sky Chief's lodge, where he and his wife kept many of the treasures of the Sky World. In order to learn more about what they had, Raven transformed himself into a little child, appearing on a soft mat in the center of their dwelling. The chief and his wife were very pleased with this little boy. They enjoyed watching him crawl around and play. Soon, though, he began to cry and ask for things from the chief's sacred box.

The chief got down the box in which he kept the Sun, and the little boy opened it. For days he enjoyed playing with the Sun, rolling it around inside the magnificent heavenly home of the great chief. The Sky Chief and his wife were amused, and they soon grew comfortable seeing the little boy play with the great ball of light.

When the boy felt he had a chance, he ran out the door with the light, changed back into Raven, and flew away with the giants of the Sky World chasing him. Because Raven is fast and cunning, he quickly flew through the hole in the Sky World to the earth below. As he flew he threw the sun high in the sky with such force that it continues today to circle the world below. The people from the Sky World realized they could no longer contain the Sun or Raven, so they retreated to their homes, leaving the Sun to the earth people.

this, the Great Spirit took her facial features away. The doll had to make a long and frightening journey through the woods to find the Great Spirit to restore her facial features. Assisted by her spirit helpers, she learned many things as she traveled, principally the virtues of humility and courage and the value of contentment. This story, one of the favorites of the Seneca, has clear parallels in Greek and Roman myths, especially the story of Narcissus.

Aleut Teachings and Practices

Along the great Aleutian Islands archipelago, a series of about a hundred rocky islands strung like dark pearls from the tip of the Alaskan Peninsula westward across almost 1,200 miles of the Bering Sea to Siberia, live the Aleutian people. The Aleuts, who also have a vibrant storytelling tradition, have inhabited the northern Arctic regions for seven thousand years, and their economies have always been based on the sea. Today, many Aleuts also live in native villages on the mainland. They call themselves the Alutiiq people and Unangan people to distinguish themselves from their Aleut ancestors, but they continue to regard their ancient traditions as the vital threads that weave their lives together.

Aleut childhood practices and teachings embrace centuries of customs that continue today, though they may vary from village to village and from one family to another. Children grow up with legends about natural forces, creation and origination stories, and amusing trickster tales. Along with these stories, a growing child learns songs and dances that affirm his sense of self, place, and duty within his village and family group. Dancing is especially important in Aleut social and religious life and is often employed in healing rites.

The Aleuts used dolls carved of driftwood, bone, or ivory as teaching devices for both boys and girls. Boys played with small dolls, which they placed in a toy umiak, kayak, or baidarka. These were models of the hide or oiled-skin boats that adults used to glide rapidly across the water as they pursued various marine animals. Similarly, Aleut and Inupiat (Eskimo) girls learned many tasks of everyday life by playing with their dolls, often beautifully fashioned

Dolls

Early American Indians made many different types of dolls, but scholars believe that the earliest native dolls were probably not play toys. Simple dolls fashioned of roots, stone, coral, or clay were probably first used in medicine, fertility, or birthing rites.

It's likely that tiny symbolic dolls served as companions to sick or dying children and accompanied them into the afterlife. People also created small symbolic dolls from roots, wood, or bone to serve as love dolls. Along with love medicines, these dolls, carefully wrapped and securely tied together, were supposed to ensure successful unions between two people. On a more sinister level, some dolls were no doubt created for the purposes of witchcraft or harm. In every tribal group there were powerful personal safeguards against the dark side, or black medicine.

Loving parents and relatives also made various fetishes and dolls for their children to amuse and comfort them. And they created miniature kayaks, tipis, cradleboards, and travois. By playing with these precise and detailed toys, Indian children learned how to make and use the full-sized models as they grew up.

Some American Indian dolls were classic works of art, dressed in soft buckskins or cloth with delicate quill work or beaded details. These special childhood dolls, including Hopi kachinas, Eskimo dolls, and Iroquois and Cherokee corn husk dolls, have long been coveted by collectors. When American Indians saw that their play toys could be sold to appreciative white tourists, it added another dimension to their doll making. They began to create dolls to suit the fancies of adults and children from other cultures.

Certain Indian dolls grew out of particular periods of our nation's history, like the skookum dolls of the late 1800s. Often sold from railway platforms along train routes and through early catalogs, these were contrived to entice early travelers to venture across the American West. Fine buckskin dolls, lovingly adorned with beaded attire, accompanied by tipis, toy horses, and travois, moved from the hands of the Plains Indian child into those of museum ethnographers and wealthy private collectors. Today the development of modern tourism has done much to sustain the craftsmen who make native dolls, from the bright palmetto of the Florida Seminoles to the clay storyteller dolls of the Pueblo Southwest.

Pueblo storyteller doll

for them by their mothers, aunts, or grandmothers. Little girls eagerly learned to trap ground squirrels and voles so they could skin them to make parkas and boots for their dolls.

Fathers and uncles carefully made miniature tools and hunting implements for their boys, who were also taught to carve. Carving developed their fine motor abilities, while at the same time teaching them vitally important survival skills. Central to Aleut teachings were safety and simple first-aid treatments to be used in their harsh yet beautiful northern environments.

An important healing plant was and still is the Arctic willow, *Salix arctica*. This valuable tree serves artistic as well as medicinal needs. Young children can easily break off the willow stems, bending and weaving them into dream catchers or hoops for simple target games and ring toss. In addition to making a good toothbrush, chewing a young willow twig offers simple pain relief and can reduce a fever. Throughout the Americas willows are primary healing plants.

One of the most fascinating items Inupiat fathers created for their little girls was the story knife. This was usually carved out of bone or ivory and ornately decorated. While telling a story she learned from her female relations, a girl used her knife to illustrate it, communicating with traditional symbols and also making up her own picture codes. She drew the symbols—simple stick figures and pictographs—in snow, sand, or mud, depending on the season. Each scene of the story was etched, discussed, and then swept clean, until the whole story had unfolded. The story knife was an early form of art therapy, a valuable tool for working out troubling concerns, calming fears, or reacting to curious dreams, all while playacting.

In addition to the usual course of Aleut teachings, certain children receive special instruction. *Angakoo* (shamans) are the sacred practitioners among the Inupiat. They are often doctors and medicine people. They usually begin to follow their pathway when they are very young. Although they lead relatively normal lives with siblings and other children, these chosen individuals also receive additional training in healing substances and accouterments, songs, prayers, and vision and dream awareness.

Salish Guardian Spirit Quest

In most societies you didn't just inherit spiritual power and guidance; you had to search for it. Sometimes the quest began early and entailed hardship. Among the Salish of the Northwest Coast, children as young as six or seven were sent out to "find a spirit," and the more spirits a child found, the greater his power or invulnerability.

The late Salish writer Mourning Dove, from the Colville Federated Tribes of eastern Washington, described in her autobiography how young children were sent out at night to undertake this search for a guardian spirit. In the beginning, they might be sent out to a spring or a creek for water. Bringing the water back to their parents or spiritual teacher proved that they had completed their designated journey. This exercise also helped children overcome their fear of the dark.

Each night the child was sent farther away. When the search covered a long distance, parents or grandparents gave the child the skin or bone of an animal to take with her. The child hoped she would receive a vision of the animal spirit imbued in the special article she carried while she slept at the assigned destination. Children were instructed not to run away from an apparition who chose to speak to them.

Storage basket design element, Alaska

These nightly expeditions taught children the importance of spiritual training and also instilled discipline and courage. They paved the way for training as shamans, which began in adolescence. But one doesn't have to be a shaman to have spirit guardians. At times of great need or crisis, belief in these spirits strengthens courage and a sense of well-being.

Hopi and Zuni Childhood Teachings

Among the Hopi and Zuni, healing rites are strongly linked to kachinas. These living manifestations of supernatural spirits are believed to descend from the sacred San Francisco peaks in northern Arizona to live in the villages during almost six months of every year. The Creator works through them to improve pueblo life. Kachinas are one of the oldest healing cults in North America; there are more than three hundred different kachina spirits, each represented by its own special society.

Hopi and Zuni childhood teachings from infancy to puberty school the child to become an aware, well-trained member of his clan and of a specific kachina society. Because the kachinas are so critical, more than one clan and both the maternal and paternal relatives are usually involved in the year-round tutoring of the child.

These tribes spend much of their year preparing for the kachinas' visit, creating the ceremonial materials, carving kachina dolls, and practicing the various dances, songs, and rituals they will perform during the kachina rites. Ceremonies address health and healing from a broad perspective, embracing everything from the community's need for rain and good crops to specific, individual health needs.

The kachina rites occur mainly between the winter solstice and the summer solstice, beginning in early December and ending sometime in July. During the ceremonies, the Hopi introduce their children to various kachinas and kachina manas (the female counterparts). They give them gifts of sacred food and other symbolic teachings, including lashings with a yucca whip administered by the whipper kachina, who keeps the crowd awake during the long rites, which sometimes last all night.

A high point for the children occurs when a loving uncle, disguised as a kachina, gives them one of the most popular gifts of early childhood—the kachina doll. Although children may play with these dolls, more often they are put on a shelf or pinned to the wall in the child's home. They serve as blessings, companions, and memory aids to the children as they become active members of their kachina clans.

As children approach puberty and adolescence, they reach another level of maturity. Now their training and education expand to more pointedly encompass the spiritual. This is when personal relations with the mysterious power that controls nature and all of life assume importance, and young people begin to make their sacred commitments. It is a time the Omaha describe as "old enough to know sorrow," since awareness of one's own individual life often comes through the inevitable contact with death.

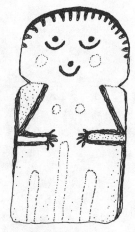

Putsgatihu, Hopi kachina doll representing Hahay'iwuuti, the mother of all kachinas, the first toy given to Hopi infants and often tied to the cradleboard

The Four Elements of Wellness:
Body, Mind, Spirit, and Nature

Traditionally, children born into American Indian cultures often grew up within a secure, multi-textured fabric that included their family, extended family, clan, band, village, and tribe. A child's physical and emotional development took place within this safety net. Learning about the Spirit World was a vital life lesson.

Mysteries surrounded and filled native life, and people sought explanations for the inexplicable abnormalities or accidents that occurred. For many, the idea of the Great Unknown or the Great Mystery—what we today call the Creator or God—accounted for these events. When someone in the family violated a taboo or spiritual tenet, or angered the Creator in some other way, there could be unfortunate consequences, such as the birth of a deformed child, a stillbirth, infant death, or a terminal disease.

Children also learned that mishaps might come about because of a mysterious action of the Creator or, occasionally, the whim of lesser trickster beings. The Great Unknown also had decisive influence over people's illness or wellness. Tribe members used prayers, rituals, and amulets to petition the Creator for protection.

Along with the body, mind, and spirit, nature or place is the fourth and often controlling element in the American Indian healing spectrum. Nature is part of Mother Earth and reflects the practical aspects of the surrounding environment, the here and now. It encompasses not only the natural world, but also a person's relationship to his family and village.

Because nature is an overarching force that embodies universal energies and is interwoven with life at every level, it can upset an individual's balance, or wellness, in awesome ways. When a person becomes ill in body, mind, or spirit, it is often the result of something she has done or experienced in her world, in nature. She may have been bewitched, or perhaps she insulted a neighbor. Whatever the cause, the balance has gone awry, and healing is an attempt to restore it.

Much of American Indian life is geared toward mindfully maintaining the fragile equilibrium of body, mind, spirit, and nature. From the earliest conscious stages of a child's life, this lesson was carefully woven into childhood teachings.

EARTH REMEDIES

Teach your children
what we have taught our children—
that the earth is our mother.
Whatever befalls the earth
befalls the sons and daughters of the earth.
If men spit upon the ground,
they spit upon themselves.

This we know.
The earth does not belong to us;
we belong to the earth.
This we know.
All things are connected
like the blood which unites one family.
All things are connected.

Whatever befalls the earth
befalls the sons and daughters of the earth.
We did not weave the web of life;
We are merely a strand in it.
Whatever we do to the web,
we do to ourselves.

—*Chief Seattle*

Flowering dogwood
Cornus Florida (fruit red)

In many tribes, children chosen as healers begin their preparation when they are quite young. The Mohegan, known as the Wolf People, are a branch of the Lenni Lenape (Delaware Indians) who migrated eastward and settled in what is now eastern Connecticut more than four centuries ago. Gladys Tantaquidgeon, a Mohegan Indian historian, was honored as her tribe's medicine woman in August 1992. Born in 1899, the oldest of four children, she was learning traditional folklore and herbal medicines from Mohegan medicine woman Emma Baker, her maternal grandmother Lydia Fielding, and elder Mercy Ann Nonesuch Mathews by the time she was five.

But knowledge about natural medicines is not limited to healers. Native children begin their study of healing substances very early, often by gathering herbs, bark, roots, fungi, minerals, and animal substances with their elders. Each season they master more. One thing they learn is that as important as what people collect is the respect with which they harvest the precious substances. Cecelia Mitchell, a Wolf Clan herbalist from Akwesasne, teaches that "medicines are like people and can play games on you and hide." You must also "have good thoughts when you go for medicines." And she suggests that you "take some and leave some, and only take what you need," remembering to give thanks to Mother Earth by leaving tobacco, cornmeal, or another small gift.

American Indian parents teach their children the beneficial and harmful properties of a variety of plants. One of the first things they share is how to make dentifrices or toothbrushes, chew sticks, and toothpicks from the fresh stems and twigs of numerous herbs, shrubs, and trees. Children also learn to make poultices to relieve toothaches and abscesses and to massage their gums or scrape their tongues.

Children quickly learn the safest, best botanicals to use in their area. The needles of most evergreens, especially the long-leaved pines, are especially choice because of their sweet-and-sour taste and high vitamin C content. These include the fresh green needles of the balsam fir, *Abies balsamae;* Fraser fir, *Abies fraseri;* Canadian hemlock, *Tsuga canadensis;* and white pine, *Pinus strobus.*

Additional native dentifrices are the highly astringent goldthread (canker root), *Coptis groenlandica;* the fresh twigs of American ash, *Fraxinus americana;* most maples, *Acer* spp.; most dogwoods, *Cornus* spp.; American mountain ash, *Sorbus americana;* sweetgum, *Liquidambar styraciflua;* sycamore, *Platanus occidentalis;* cucumber magnolia, *Magnolia acuminata;* sweet bay, *Magnolia virginiana;* redbud, *Cercis canadensis;* the willows, *Salix* spp.; beech, *Fagus grandifolia; Amelanchier* spp. (known as shadbush, shadblow, and Juneberry in the east, and Saskatoon berry in the west, among many other names); balsam poplar, *Populus balsamifera;* cottonwood, *Populus deltoides;* quaking aspen, *Populus tremuloides;* sweet birch, *Betula lenta;* and slippery elm, *Ulmus rubra.*

Other botanicals used as dentifrices in different regions include the fresh stems of most native mints, goldenrods, asters, sarsaparillas, yarrows, clovers, and wild grasses. If you want to try any of these botani-

Round-leaved, blue-berried dogwood
Cornus rugosa (fruit light blue)

cal toothbrushes, proceed with care. With some, overuse can cause the gums to recede. Less is best in most cases.

Early on, children also learn to identify the trees or shrubs they can use to treat simple ailments. For example, after running or playing in summer heat, pressing the soothing leaves of grape, beech, coltsfoot, sycamore, or maple on the temples or wrists cools the body and relieves headache pain.

Toxic plants that irritate the skin, such as stinging nettles, thistles, and poison ivy, are a hazard children frequently face when playing outdoors. Many of these plants are very useful: Stinging nettles and some thistles are important fiber plants, and many people also collect, steam, and eat stinging nettles. But because of their stinging hairs and alkaloids, they can irritate sensitive skin for more than twenty-four hours after contact.

Until children begin to recognize these harmful plants, they can get into them without realizing it. It's important to teach them how to recognize not only the toxic plants but also their antidotes, because simple topical treatments can help relieve the pain and misery.

Crushing the fresh-picked leaves of yellow dock or curly dock, *Rumex crispus;* the jewelweeds, *Impatiens* spp.; or sweet fern, *Comptonia peregrina,* and rubbing them on the skin can soothe an irritation, especially when caused by the urtic acid of stinging nettles. And although rhubarb leaves can be highly poisonous if eaten, you can use the juice from large raw rhubarb leaves to make a cooling poultice to place on the skin. This is another trusted antidote to stinging nettles.

The docks, jewelweeds, and sweet fern are also valuable in counteracting the irritating oil of poison ivy. They are most effective if you rub them on your child's skin shortly after an encounter with poison ivy. Once the poison ivy dermatitis erupts, these plants may help soothe it, but they won't clear it up.

Some children also experience unexplained rashes and skin irritations. If your child has a mild rash, you can dust it lightly with cornstarch or wash it gently with commercial witch hazel. Milder yet is the tea American Indians make from the leaves and twigs of witch hazel. You can even make this healing tea in winter by using the plant's twigs. These

Fox grape
Vitis labrusca

Frost grape, or river-bank grape
Vitis riparia

twigs also make reliable chewsticks for relief of gum irritations or other mouth problems.

Food sensitivities and other allergies sometimes begin in childhood. It is important to eliminate irritating food and environmental problems wherever you can and soothe the body's systems with gentle herbs, minerals, and vitamins. Often this can help to increase the body's tolerance to allergies.

Asthma is a particularly serious allergic response that can make breathing difficult. **Because asthma can be life-threatening, one should seek professional help in severe cases.** One of the more effective herbs for asthma is the native sundew, *Drosera rotundifolia,* which is antispasmodic and a relaxing expectorant. This tiny carnivorous plant of America's southern bogs, seeps, and marshes is a powerhouse of healing possibilities, especially when used in balanced formulas and tinctures.

Note: It's always best to purchase herbs from reputable sources if you don't have them growing organically on your own property. Wild herbs, although once a trusted resource for our ancestors, are no longer highly recommended. Many valued medicinal herbs, such as sundew, are on state or national threatened or endangered species lists. Others can be systemically poisoned by environmental toxins that are often invisible.

Many beneficial complementary treatments, including the recipes below, draw on native wisdom without presuming to take the place of mainstream medicine. Whenever in doubt, consult your health care provider.

Curly dock
Rumex crispus

1 cup calendula blossoms, freshly crushed

1 tablespoon slippery elm bark, freshly ground

1 teaspoon ginger root, freshly chopped

2 cups water

Corn or sunflower seed oil

1 ounce fine beeswax

1 tablespoon pure honey

$^1/_4$ ounce vitamin E oil

SLIPPERY ELM HEALING SALVE

Calendula blossoms and slippery elm bark have a soothing, curative effect on the skin, as well as fungicidal benefits. A salve provides a protective coating for the skin; it is not readily absorbed. This one is especially useful for chapped or extremely irritated or sensitive skin. You can use it for sunburn, chapped lips, bad diaper or heat rash, or even ringworm.

First make a decoction, and then strain it and simmer it a while longer with additional ingredients to complete the salve.

Slippery elm
Ulmus rubica

Simmer first four ingredients in a small pot for half an hour, stirring occasionally to blend thoroughly. Strain off the liquid and measure. Return the liquid to a clean pot and add an equal amount of corn or sunflower seed oil. Simmer for about 3 hours on low heat. Check, stirring occasionally, to keep from burning. **Note: Always be careful not to boil or burn; this will make the product too harsh. Results are far better when simmered.**

Add beeswax, honey, and vitamin E oil. Stir constantly and remove from heat when all of the beeswax melts. Whip with a wire whip or sturdy spoon until almost cool and thoroughly blended. Pour immediately into small containers before it hardens.

When cool, gently rub on dry, affected skin areas several times a day while symptoms persist.

VARIATION: You can change this recipe to make a deeper, penetrating herbal emollient cream or oil, which will be absorbed and convey the herbs and minerals deeper into the skin. To do this, omit the beeswax and shorten the simmering time to about 1½ hours.

Purple bergamot
Monarda fistulosa

HUMMINGBIRD DIGESTIVE TEA

Wild bergamot, also called bee balm, is a favorite flower for hummingbirds. A tea made from bee balm and marshmallow has a soothing effect on the throat and stomach. It can relieve gas and aid digestion. It is good at any age, but mild enough to be given to children.

1 tablespoon dried bee balm leaves, crushed
1 teaspoon dried marshmallow root, cut fine or powdered

Place ingredients in a tea ball or cheesecloth bag in an 8-ounce teapot. Pour boiling water over them to fill the pot. Cover and steep for 5 to 10 minutes.

Pour ½ cup in a small glass and sweeten with a teaspoon of honey or maple syrup. Drink 4 ounces just before each meal.

Red bee balm, Oswego tea
Monarda didyata

You can easily tincture common plants in vinegar solutions, which work better on young skin because they are milder than those made with alcohol. These tinctures can help soothe a variety of everyday problems from insect bites to rashes.

Our common jewelweed has fungicidal value, making it useful for treating ringworm and other fungal skin infections. It is also a valuable antidote for poison ivy, especially if you rub it on the skin as soon as possible after contact with urushiol, the irritating oil of poison ivy. It is more effective if you apply it when it is cool. You may also substitute yellow dock leaves and roots for the jewelweed.

You can add this tincture to a foot or tub bath to cool and soothe heat rash, sunburn, chickenpox, and other skin irritations. It also helps athlete's foot, tired feet, or sprains.

Because this tincture is made without preservatives or alcohol, it does not have a long shelf life. After about six months or so, discard it and make a fresh supply. It will last a bit longer if you keep it refrigerated or in a cool place. Remember to make a fresh batch to last through the winter before the first killing autumn frost.

Fill a sterile 8-ounce jar with freshly picked, clean jewelweed plants (blossoms, leaves, stems—everything but the roots). Press the plant material down until the jar is full. Cover the plants with good apple cider vinegar or white vinegar. Cover tightly and shake gently. Label and date the jar. You can use this tincture immediately, but it is better to let it rest in a dark, cool place for a week to ten days. After straining, it is ready for use.

Jewelweed
Impatiens capensis

SASSAFRAS SQUISH TOPICAL INSECT REPELLENT

This recipe enhances the insecticidal properties of sassafras, a common native plant. *Sassafras* is an Algonquian word meaning "green twig." Sassafras twigs used as chew sticks revive the mouth and massage the gums; they also make delicious toothbrushes.

Since this insecticide is made without preservatives, it is best to make it frequently in small amounts and use it up. If refrigerated, it will last three days to a week. Discard it if it appears moldy.

Crush 6 fresh sassafras leaves in a small clean bowl with a charcoal tablet. (These are available at health food stores. **Do not use charcoal briquettes.**) If you want, you can substitute a small, clean piece of charred wood from the fireplace for the charcoal. Bind the ingredients together with one to two tablespoons of vegetable oil.

Dot the mixture on your forehead, nose, and around the mouth and ears and rub gently. Allow it to sit on the skin. This natural, homemade insecticide should be reapplied frequently. The ingredients are nonstaining and will wash out readily if they get onto your clothes.

VARIATION: Substitute the leaves of our native bee balm, jewelweed, sweet fern, or the garden mints, such as peppermint and spearmint.

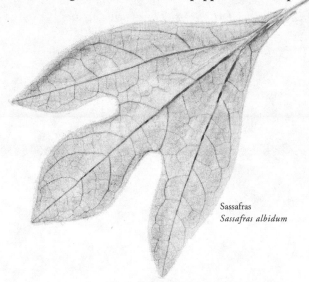

Sassafras
Sassafras albidum

CHAPTER THREE

Puberty

CHANGING WOMAN

〜〜〜〜〜〜〜〜〜〜〜〜〜〜〜〜〜〜〜〜

My mom and dad wanted me to have this ceremony.

They told me that I would have a blessing and a good

life. And they told me, "After you have this dance, you're

not a child anymore. You must put away all your

playthings." And I thought, How can this be?

I'm still young. But that's how you feel after

the dance is over. You're not a child anymore.

—PANSY CASSADORE, SAN CARLOS APACHE

〜〜〜〜〜〜〜〜〜〜〜〜〜〜〜〜〜〜〜〜

High-bush cranberry,
or crampbark
Viburnum opulus

Wild yam
Dioscorea villosa

For people around the world, puberty is a critical life-changing period, and American Indians are no exception. The Salish writer Mourning Dove's humorous description rings only too true for most parents with a child between the ages of eleven and fifteen: "A boy reached this age when his voice began to change and he got lazy, preferring to sleep late in the mornings and yawning through the day. Then parents would exchange knowing glances with each other and remark, '*Su-le-whoo-mah*' (puberty)."

Puberty and the onset of fertility signals the beginning of adulthood. Many American Indian families anticipated this coming of age by having their children undertake a rugged regimen to build their stamina, ensure a healthy long life, and prepare them for the physical challenges of puberty rites. In some tribes, parents had their sons and daughters rise before dawn and assume responsibility for more of the family's chores.

Among others, like the Salish, young people went into isolation for a period at the beginning of puberty. They had to fast and bathe in cold water each morning at the first streak of dawn, drying off with boughs. They repeated this rigorous cleansing routine later on in life when they did vision quests. If the young man or woman planned to follow a healer's path and train with an elder who was a medicine person, cleansing preparations were especially strict.

In many tribes, boys and girls took up endurance running, which is a highly prized native talent. One of America's best athletes this century was Jim Thorpe, a Sac (Sauk) Indian born in 1888 in Oklahoma. The Sac and Fox Indians of the Mississippi River regions in Iowa are also known as the Mesquakie, or Red Earth People.

Named Bright Path by his mother, Jim Thorpe had exceptional athletic talents that were well honed in childhood. He won gold medals in the pentathlon and the decathlon in the 1912 Olympics in Stockholm, Swe-

Wild yam
Dioscorea villosa

High-bush cranberry, or crampbark
Viburnum opulus

The Importance of the Breath

Besides building endurance, running is a valuable way for children to develop greater lung capacity and improve their breathing. We know today that good respiratory fitness enhances overall body tone and vitality. Through running, children learn to balance inhaling and exhaling and to empty their lungs before they take in more breath.

Besides, the breath is associated with the Creator; it represents the soul or life force. Breath adds the Creator's energies to healing rituals. Many American Indian medicine people know the importance of breathing over or on medicines just before they give them to a patient. Some Indian medicine people even use a medicine pipe or blowing (bubbling) tube to breathe down into medicinal teas and add healing strength.

To treat respiratory problems, many tribes used the roots, leaves, and seeds of three species of wild prairie parsley, *Lomatium foeniculaceum, L. dissectum,* and *L. triternatum.* The Pawnee called this *pezhe bthaska,* meaning "the flat herb"; across the Great Basin region and along the Northwest Coast these wild perennials were called "the big medicine."

Indians in many tribes used these plant parts internally and externally. Blackfeet long-distance runners chewed the seeds to avoid respiratory problems and side cramps. People in other tribes made them into therapeutic teas and inhaled the warm steam for respiratory relief. Medicine people chewed the root, which they blew through an eagle bone tube onto the patient's injury. Herbalists continue to use wild prairie parsley roots in tinctures, formulas, lotions, and creams, especially to treat respiratory problems.

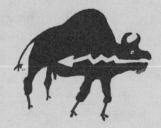

Bellowing buffalo bull showing breath (life) line

den, and he also played briefly with the New York Giants baseball team. He continues to be an honored role model.

When children have handicaps or other problems that make it difficult for them to participate in endurance training or similar activities, the tribe cultivates their other capabilities. Some American Indian elders recall how, as sickly children, their tribe relieved them from normal duties. Instead, they spent their time with the grandmothers and grandfathers learning to sew, weave, make pottery, or gather and prepare medicines. They found their strengths and life-shaping abilities in these early practices.

In American Indian cultures, when the changes of puberty become apparent, they are not hidden or viewed with embarrassment, as they so often are in our society. Native tribes openly recognize and esteem this critical transition in a wide variety of ceremonies and practices. Although this is an important time, it is also an age that frequently is marked by hypersensitivity, confusion, depression, and anger. Careful planning and sensitive attention to a child's everyday needs are the hallmark of many puberty rites, whether they are celebrated privately with family or in a large community gathering.

These rites of passage are reassuring and positive; their primary purpose is to ensure a long, healthy life for the young men and women who are celebrated. The tribe rejoices in their approaching fertility, strengthening their sense of identity and affirming their importance to society. The rituals also reiterate the value of making a commitment to leading a good life and ensuring the continuity of tribal traditions.

Some children do not go through puberty rites. Sometimes it's because the traditions have been broken by political changes, economic distress, and changing family patterns. Others simply cannot afford the time or cost of such major observances. But many families, clans, bands, and tribal groups still celebrate their fine old traditions, and growing numbers of native people are rediscovering these ceremonies.

And then they danced me. All that month they danced me, until the moon got back to the place where it had been at first. It is a big time when a girl comes of age; a happy time. All the people in the village knew that I had been to the Little House for the first time, so they came to our house and the singer for the maidens came first of all.

—Maria Chona, a Papago woman, recalling her puberty ceremony

Girls and the Menarche

For young women, coming of age begins with their menarche, the first menstrual flow. People living in close harmony with the changing seasons, moon phases, and heavenly signs were especially sensitive to the "moon time's" governance of female rhythms and energies. Many cultures felt the

Havasupai Origin of Menstruation

Coyote is an enigmatic character who appears again and again in many tribes' stories. He is invariably involved in making things happen, whether mischief or magic. Coyote stories leave a lot unexplained; that is part of his mystery. But the stories are used to explain things that are otherwise unaccountable.

This story comes from the Havasupai, whose homelands are around the rim of the Grand Canyon in the desert Southwest.

Squirrel and his daughter and Coyote lived together. The squirrel was a little older than Coyote; he was Coyote's uncle. Squirrel went hunting and brought in a deer. While Coyote was skinning it he put his finger in the blood and flipped it on the inside of the girl's thigh. Coyote said to her, "Sister, you're menstruating. You can't eat the meat for four days." When he said that, the girl didn't believe him. Finally she grew angry; Coyote knew about menstruating, the girl didn't.

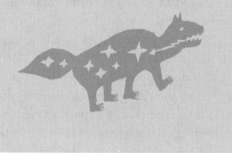

close, obvious harmony between the moon's monthly twenty-eight-day cycle and a woman's monthly cycle. This connection accounts for the contemporary term "she's on her moon," which refers to a woman's menses.

Diegueño Indians, like many other tribes, believed that the moon controlled men's cycles and moods, too. One of their origin stories describes how the moon was sent up into the Sky World to watch over the people and regulate all things. The moon was responsible for women's menses, and men's strength grew or diminished with its waxing and waning.

Countless American Indian stories explain the origins of the menarche, giving great power and respect to this phase of life. The tales also elevate the mundane into the realms of the mystical and holy.

Along with these often fanciful stories come the origins of certain taboos. During her menstrual period, a woman is considered too powerful to come into the sweat lodge, dance during many rituals, handle certain ceremonial foods, gather healing herbs, or clean the meat of wild game. And at the time of their first menses, young American Indian women have special powers of healing or even more esoteric shamanistic abilities.

Personal, family, and village ceremonies note this vital turning point in a young girl's life. It is a nearly mystical time of celebrations, prayers, and miraculous healing.

Puberty Rites of the Navajo and the Apache

Two major tribes in the Southwest, the Apache and the Navajo, continue to perform their traditional puberty rites today. Their ceremonies, the Navajo *kinaalda,* or Changing Woman and Lightning Way Ceremony, and the Apache Sunrise Ceremony, are similar. In these tribes, puberty rites date back to the beginnings of time; they are part of their origin stories. Their sacred rituals acknowledge the significance of dawning womanhood in each girl at menarche and make the whole process holy.

Among the Navajo, it was Changing Woman (Esdzaanadleehe), one of the Holy People instrumental in creating the tribe, who had the first *kinaalda.* The *kinaalda* began so that women would be fruitful, enabling humans to multiply. According to legend, the first *kinaalda* happened to Changing Woman at the rim of the Emergence Place in First Woman's home. There the Holy People sang her into the critical new phase of her life. Among the Apache, Changing Woman's counterpart is White Painted Woman, who survived a great flood to become the first Apache and the progenitor of all humans.

Traditionally, these Apache and Navajo rites last four days. They entail months of preparation, hard work, and expense on the part of the girl's family. To celebrate her emerging puberty and to bless her fertility, the tribe honors each girl, instructs her, and dances her into womanhood. Her body is pressed and molded, almost as clay is shaped, enabling her to be beautiful, healthy, and fecund in the likeness of White Painted Woman or Changing Woman. Group participation, socializing, dancing, and feasting fill the days and nights.

Happily may I walk.
Happily, with abundant
  dark clouds, may I walk.
Happily, with abundant
  showers, may I walk.
Happily, with abundant
  plants, may I walk.
Happily, on a trail of
  pollen, may I walk.
Happily may I walk.
Being as it used to be long
  ago, may I walk.

May it be beautiful
  before me.
May it be beautiful
  behind me.
May it be beautiful
  below me.
May it be beautiful
  above me.
May it be beautiful all
  around me.
In beauty it is finished.
In beauty it is finished.

—From the Navajo
  Beauty Way

The Apache Sunrise Ceremony is highly dramatic and thrilling to see. During these four intense days, the young girls become White Painted Woman and take on her healing powers. The Ga'an, powerful spirits who protect the Apache people, come down from their home in the mountains to dance. They are also known as the Crown Dancers or Mountain Gods. As they move, these sacred dancers use body adornments, bells, dance staffs, music, and voices to symbolize the sounds of nature. Because they represent the earth, fertility, and the universe, they are said to control the natural forces that the community depends on for its way of life. Some believe people can be healed just by seeing the dances of the Mountain Gods.

This is a highly charged and festive time, but it is physically, emotionally, and spiritually strenuous for the girl. Endurance is key, for she has to dance for four days, guided and ritually massaged by an elder woman. Every day she runs to each of the four directions, and the entire group attending the rites runs along with her. At night, the Ga'an dance with her, casting awesome shadows. People bless her with sacred cattail pollen; in turn they ask her to bless and heal them while she embodies the power of Changing Woman. Early in the morning of the last day, the girl's body is painted with clay and the assembled guests dance behind her as the medicine people chant a song cycle. At last she is a woman.

These rites are cornerstones in a young woman's development. Along with her memories, a woman retains concrete mementos from the ceremonies for the rest of her life. For example, as a girl becomes Changing Woman, she dances with a special feather-topped cane that absorbs the power of the ritual. She keeps this cane throughout her life and may use it as a walking stick when she is an old woman. Besides their importance to individual girls, these rituals, which survived the tremendous upheaval, disruption, and death the Apache people suffered during the westward expansion, are also symbols of extraordinary healing for the entire tribe.

Today many Apache people return to their reservation over the Fourth of July holiday for joint puberty rites honoring a number of girls. Those who can afford it have weavings, baskets, and other regalia made for the occasion. They give special gifts to the medicine people and elders performing the ceremony. The first two days of the rituals are private. Afterward relatives and friends participate, both to lend their support to the

Corn Bug Girl on the Moon

young girl and to reaffirm and strengthen their own commitment to Apache traditions. Outside visitors and tourists are also welcome during these days.

The Sioux Sing the Girl Over

The rituals marking a girl's impending womanhood are not all as colorful or dramatic as those of the Apache and the Navajo. Some tribes mark the event privately, recognizing and congratulating the young woman and enfolding her in a supportive group.

With these ceremonies, people recognize that menarche can be an emotional, exhausting time for a young woman. Her body and mind are changing in significant ways, and so is her world. As she becomes a woman, she is subject to new societal pressures and taboos. While family support is always vital, it is especially valuable now.

The Sioux are fourteen tribes whose homelands stretch across the northern Plains from the Great Lakes to the foothills of the Rockies, but they are centered in the Dakotas. Their way of life blended western woodland and prairie traditions into their own distinctive culture. The name they called themselves meant "the Allies," but their enemies called them the Sioux. We know them today as the Dakota, Lakota, Yankton, and Yanktonai.

Family and kinfolk celebrate young Sioux women at the time of their menarche with the Sing the Girl Over. This is usually a small gathering, although it can be a larger group, of sympathetic people who converge at the family's request to sing the young woman over her first period. With their special song cycles, the group takes note of her natural body changes and welcomes her new status in the family, clan, and tribe. If family circumstances allow it, there is also a feast.

Teaching the Taboos

In most native cultures, a pubescent boy or girl is considered powerful, even holy. During this period in their lives it's critical, for their own health and that of the tribe, that they learn and begin to observe certain essential taboos.

O our Father, the Sky,
  hear us
and make us strong.
O our Mother, the Earth,
  hear us
and give us support.
O Spirit of the East,
send us your wisdom.
O Spirit of the South,
may we tread your
  path of life.
O Spirit of the West,
may we always be ready
  for the long journey.
O Spirit of the North,
  purify us
with your cleansing winds.

—*Sioux prayer*

Changing Woman

The rich storytelling traditions of the Navajo include detailed accounts that trace the evolution of the First Holy People, the First Cradleboard, the sacred colors, and the creation of ongoing life. Telling and retelling these sacred stories and origin myths perpetuates valuable truths of Navajo life and guards their traditions.

Central to Navajo beliefs is Changing Woman, who was created by the sacred union of Earth Woman and Sky Man in the earliest time. Earth Woman symbolizes beauty, and the cerebral Sky Man stands for the spiritual life. Connected by a rainbow, Earth Woman and Sky Man often appear in traditional sand paintings used for healing.

Changing Woman was born following the mystic coupling of Earth Woman and Sky Man atop sacred Spruce Mountain. Because she is without faults, she shows us, the earth-surface-walkers, the potential we possess if we follow the Beauty Way and live a life of balance and harmony.

Changing Woman is immortal. She incarnates the cycles of Navajo life, the rhythm of day and night, the seasons and the stages of life. Wearing a dress richly detailed with white shells, she is the youthful White Shell Woman of dawn. She is also the mature Turquoise Woman, and later the matronly Abalone Woman. Finally Changing Woman becomes the matriarch of winter, Black Jet Woman.

Changing Woman symbolizes benevolent power. She created the animals, birds, and corn to provide life for the Navajo people. Along with Sun Bearer, she represents the balance of energies and qualities essential to Navajo life. These male and female forces are frequently represented on the talking prayer sticks, sometimes plumed with wild turkey feathers, used in many Navajo rituals.

Because women were supposed to have awesome power when they menstruated, every month they were subject to taboos regarding food, hunting, and healing. They could not touch or prepare foods for the menfolk or other family members. In addition, in many tribes women could not eat the meat of certain game animals or drink cold water.

Since the idea of flowing blood was disturbing, many tribes had menstrual tipis, moon lodges, or brush arbors, small huts where women secluded themselves during their menses, especially the three to five days of their heaviest flow. They were usually located downstream from the camp so as not to pollute the water used for cooking and drinking. The purpose of this isolation was to keep the menstruating woman's power contained so that no one would be inadvertently hurt.

For many Indian women this unique treatment was a positive time of self-discipline during which they learned more about the responsibilities of womanhood, taboos, and the promise of motherhood. They often valued their confinement, enjoying special foods or fasting, games, singing, and laughing. Older women would speak to their younger women friends and relatives about sexuality, emotions, and physical changes they were experiencing.

Menarche rites in some tribes focused on teaching a young woman the many rules and responsibilities that accompanied her new status. Among some, like the Paiute, these observances went on in private or even in isolation.

The farming and mining lease operations of ten Southern Paiute groups dot the primal landscape of their homelands, which lie across the northern areas of the Southwest and the vast Great Basin regions of Arizona, Utah, and Nevada. One of their oldest, most sacred practices is the menarche ritual. (See Chapter 6 for the rite-of-passage ritual performed for a couple after the birth of their first child, the symbolic counterpart of this Paiute ritual.)

At the time of her first menstruation, a young Paiute woman was isolated for four days in a separate room or area of her family's home, where her male and female elders came to teach her. During this time she could not touch or scratch her face and hair with her hands; instead she used a special stick. She could not drink cold liquids or eat any animal foods. Each day she had to run to the east at sunrise and to the west at sundown.

On the morning of the fifth day, the concluding rituals took place. She was bathed in cold water, massaged, and dressed in clean clothes. Her cheeks were painted with red ochre or white clay. She ate rabbit or sheep liver wrapped in cedar and bitter herbs, spitting some of this into the fire. The ends of her hair were cut. She was created anew, ready for adulthood.

The Papago, another southwestern tribe, marked this event in similar ways. Because she was considered dangerous, a young Papago woman withdrew for the first four days of her first period. She usually went to a separate outer dwelling, the Little House, a small brush house behind her family's living quarters. She ate separately from her family and had to refrain from eating salt and meat. Like the Paiute women, as well as women in other tribes, taboos forbade her from touching her face and hair, except with a scratching stick, to prevent harm.

When she came out of isolation, the girl was washed and her long hair was cut shorter, perhaps shoulder length, for practical purposes. Chosen elders danced with her and instructed her, providing reassurance and giving her special strength, awareness, and respect. The observances continued during her first month of womanhood, when she worked hard, slept little, and gave gifts to the family members and friends who accompanied her through her coming of age.

At the month's end, the medicine man ritually cleansed the young Papago woman and gave her an important gift: her new name, which he had gotten from a dream. Most American Indians believe that one's name is associated with personal power. Among many tribes, it was not unusual for an individual's birth name to be changed at puberty as a way to fully confirm and recognize her new adult identity in the tribal group. And it was frequently the medicine people who bestowed these new names.

In some tribes, young women marked the onset of menstruation alone, with practices we might consider harsh or frightening today. Among the Salish, when a young woman's first period began she was considered contaminated. She had to go into isolation and fast for ten days, observing a number of taboos. She could pick berries and roots, but she was not allowed to pick herbs or make love potions. And she was supposed to stay away from the camp, the sweat lodge, and hunting areas during this time. If she did go near the camp, she couldn't go behind a tipi or step near the head of a bed. If she went close to someone who was already ill, she could bring on his death.

The Salish recognized the connection between puberty, sexuality, and fertility. The young woman was supposed to spend her time in isolation praying about motherhood. When she returned, she was purified in several sweat baths and dressed in a complete change of clothing. Her discarded clothes, tied in a bundle, were put in the fork of a tree near the menstrual tipi. She began to wear a virgin's cape so men couldn't see her body, and she remained with her parents, rigidly chaperoned.

Although some might dismiss these rituals as old-fashioned or even sexist, many of these American Indian practices and concepts translate into contemporary life. Out of some of these ancient taboos—like avoiding salt and meat—comes practical advice for avoiding premenstrual syndrome (PMS) and reducing the cramping and heavy flow some young women experience with their periods.

And some of these ancient American Indian taboos are bridges to modern health practices in other cultures. Among many Middle Eastern peoples, abstinence from salt, meat, and meat fats is considered important for religious purity as well as for good health; the same is true in many African cultures.

Continuing the Traditions

In addition to learning about taboos, puberty is an important time to teach young girls and boys more about personal responsibility. The tribe challenges youngsters to learn both practical and abstract concepts and to take up the responsibility to pass these traditions on to future generations.

Knowledge is passed on in a variety of ways. Sometimes it occurs informally, through the mundane chores of everyday life. On some occasions teaching is secret and privileged, and at other times it occurs publicly in ceremonies, rites, and rituals. The custom of storytelling, begun in childhood, continues during puberty with morality tales designed to illustrate correct behavior. Practical talks and prayers confide the wisdom of healing herbs and medicinal practices that will help each individual throughout her life.

Puberty rites are central to wellness and balancing for many tribes. Their focus is to keep young men and women strongly connected to their traditions, and to give them a solid personal sense of who they are. This is especially vital for small tribes, who feel they have lost ground in the modern world.

Years ago California, because of the lushness of its environments and its proximity to the sea, was densely settled by numerous American Indian tribes. But these tribes suffered some of the worst pressures from missionaries and settlers. Thousands were murdered and their tribal infrastructures were shattered.

Despite this horrific history, the Luiseño, Mission Indians of southern California, have continued their custom known as the Girls' and Boys' Sand Painting and Puberty Ceremony. In this ritual, a respected elder speaks to maturing boys and girls gathered around a special sand painting, which encircles and fills a slightly raised earth mound and represents their world. The elder uses the sand painting to illustrate how important it is for these young people to maintain the tribe's sacred ways.

After this joint ceremony, the boys and girls are celebrated separately.

Everything we do in a way has to be witnessed by other people. You pass on a particular ritual ceremony to other people and we teach it to our children.

—*Lakota Elder*
Lloyd One Star

Both the Luiseño and Diegueño Indians call their girls ceremony "the Roasting of the Girls." It is believed to ensure a long, productive life. Successive days of feasting, dancing, giveaways, and special talks and music draw together disparate family groups and their relatives.

These rituals go beyond initiating young men and women into adulthood. They are healing ceremonies that bring about strengthening of the land, the people, and forgiveness.

Dreams and Visions

Visions and dreams have always been considered sacred paths to valuable knowledge and direct links with God, the higher powers, and the supernatural. Although they can happen spontaneously at any time and place, the practice of deliberately seeking visions, especially ones of life-shaping magnitude, often begins during puberty.

Even before they reach this age, many young American Indian men and women know about seeking visions and have begun training to do it. But it is at puberty that they are considered ready to undertake their first vision quest—a prescribed period of time when an individual prepares and then journeys alone to a remote spot to fast, pray, and seek a vision.

It's rare for young women to experience a vision quest at puberty. At this stage of life, monthly cycles of fertility and menstruation are the most powerful influences over their ritual lives. But for young men, there are many ceremonies, such as the Sioux Boys' Vision Quest, that mark this important step on their path to adulthood. Like the rites surrounding women's menses, men's vision quests are associated with the need to exercise considerable discipline in response to notable bodily changes and increasing personal power.

At a time when many young people are figuring out who they really are, a vision quest can provide amazing gifts of clarity. But it is also a grueling challenge and a personal test of courage, strength, and humility. Traditionally, an elder mentor, perhaps an uncle or chosen medicine man, tutors and prepares the boy for this ordeal and privilege. The mentor explains the vital importance of the quest and afterward helps the boy understand his visions.

Endurance training and spending nights camping out alone with little or no food help to prepare each youth for the rigors of his spiritual journey. As the time for the quest approaches, rituals of purification, such as fasting and smudging—the burning of one or more sacred substances and bathing in their smoke—take place, accompanied by special prayers.

Then the boy goes off by himself to seek a vision. He spends four or five days and nights fasting, alone with his thoughts, on a windswept butte or within a shallow pit. He learns to deal with fear and find out about his own personal strengths. Each boy also looks for power and meaning in the natural world. The vision quest frequently brings on life-changing visions and dreams that provide glimpses into mystical and spiritual realms beyond his ordinary experiences.

A vision quest draws a person deeper inside himself and at the same time allows him to look at himself from outside. So much does a person learn in the process that in many tribes it is thought to be essential to the proper evolution of a healthy life path. Pete Catches, a noted Lakota medicine man, once said, "I do believe every young Indian, about high school age, should do a *hanblecheyapi* [vision quest] to get direction in life, to know what life is all about."

McKee Springs petroglyph

The Sweat Lodge

Even at puberty, young men and women cannot yet fully partake of the sweat lodge purification rites, which are still considered too powerful for them. Full use of the sweat lodge begins later, during adolescence. But at this age the tribe introduces young men and women to the privilege in limited ways, giving them, for instance, the honor of helping an uncle, father, or aunt tend the sweat lodge for other tribe members.

The sweat lodge is a small domed structure. It usually stands alone at some distance from the dwellings and, where possible, near water. Its frame is formed by bent saplings lashed together. In some regions the sweat lodge is covered with grass mats, bundles of brush, reeds, or large sheets of tree bark. The doorway opens to the east and there is a small smoke hole in the center of the top. Large pieces of animal skins, canvas, or old quilts cover the framework when it is not in use.

Participants take a steam bath in the sweat lodge, reciting prayers and sprinkling sacred herbs over the steaming rocks or into the fire outside. Afterward they bathe in cold water. They do this even in winter, finding it therapeutic to break a hole through the ice and take a brisk dip in a frigid river or lake following the sweat bath.

The sweat lodge and its purification ceremonies are sacred among all tribes. Like the Scandinavian sauna and its other northern European counterparts, the sweat lodge is considered to be a fine technique for purifying and cleansing the body. But among American Indians, the sweat lodge is a deep, personal, holy experience, essential to staying well and in balance.

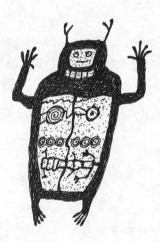

Deer shaman; Rio Grande Valley petroglyph

White floating clouds,
Clouds like the plains,
Come and water the earth
That she may be fruitful.
Moon, lion of the north,
Bear of the west,
Badger of the south,
Wolf of the east,
Eagle of the heavens,
Shrew of the earth,
Elder war hero,
Intercede with the cloud people for us
That they may water the earth.
—*Sia prayer*

Many girls and boys passed easily through the growth spurts and
other body changes of puberty. But for those who had a more difficult
time, a host of native botanicals provided relief. Their common names—
fever bush or cramp bark—signified discrete herbs in different regions,
but they accurately reflected their uses. Shadblow bark *(Amelanchier*
spp.), along with cramp bark *(Viburnum opulus),* slippery elm bark *(Ul-*
mus fulva), and willow bark *(Salix* spp.), have long
been reliable analgesics.

Many of these time-honored botanicals are part
of our rich American Indian medicinal heritage and
are still worth our attention. They can be used for
pain relief, especially for menstrual cramps, as well as
for PMS, indigestion, and headache.

A wide range of herbs can be used to relieve
bloating, cramps, and other menstrual symptoms.
American pennyroyal, *Hedeoma pulegioides,* either fresh
or dried, was steeped to make a valuable tea and used—in
limited amounts—to ease pain. Although they are different,

Slippery elm
Ulmus rubica

our contemporary herbal uses for pennyroyal abound. It is a fine insecticide, fungicide, household fumigant, and tick repellent. **Caution: Pregnant women should not handle or use pennyroyal since it is a strong abortifacient.**

Algonquian women in the Northeast made teas with the leaves, twigs, and ripe red berries of spicebush, *Lindera benzoin* (also known as fever bush), to relieve cramps; they also used it to reduce fever. And Plains Indian women made infusions from various wild sage roots and leaves to control heavy menstrual flow and regulate their menses. **Caution: Sage should be used carefully because it can act as an abortifacient. It may also cause respiratory problems in sensitive individuals.**

American Indians throughout the country have long esteemed corn silk tea as a gentle diuretic and kidney tonic to be taken for several days just before the menses. It is still used today.

Women in many tribes employed massage to relieve menstrual cramps and bloating. In some cases they would sprinkle a pinch of sage, tobacco, or sacred pollen onto the troublesome area, and accompany a gentle massage with quiet songs or prayers. From the Eastern Cherokee to the Western Pawnee, women also used the blossoms and oils of various perennial herbs, such as goldenrod, yarrow, and evening primrose, along with abdominal or total body massage. Contemporary herbalists continue to make and use products from these herbs, especially evening primrose oil, which is often recommended as a treatment for PMS.

Spicebush
Lindera benzoin

Early Sanitary Pads

We may prefer our modern conveniences, but the resourcefulness and ingenuity American Indian women displayed in finding sanitary protection and padding during their menses is fascinating. What women used varied from region to region; many natural substances with antiseptic virtues as well as purifying fragrances were readily available. Sphagnum mosses and other thick, clumping mosses were abundant in some areas, and women used and reused them, washing them out and drying them in the sun. In a similar fashion, they also used shredded, softened cedar bark, sometimes placing ripe cattail fluff inside a wad of shredded bark. In the West, where sage abounds, women used peeled sage bark and leaves or softened grasses wadded inside strips of tanned animal skins or bound within young corn husks.

Hair and skin care take on added importance during the physical and emotional changes of puberty. American Indians have always used soapweed roots and fibers to wash their hair and get a rich, glossy shine, as well as to keep their skin healthy. Many different plants around the country are called "soapweed," but they all usually contain compounds called saponins, which produce a soapy lather when pounded or rubbed in water. Some of these are:

Amole roots, *Agave schottii*
California soap plant roots and leaves, *Chenopodium californicum*
California soaproot roots, *Chlorogalum pomeridianum*
Guaiac leaves, *Guaiacum officinale*
Papaya leaves, *Carica papaya* and other species
Quillai bark, *Quillaja saponaria*
Red campion roots and leaves, *Lychnis dioica*
Saltbush roots, *Atriplex californica*
Soapberry berries and leaves, *Sapindus saponaria*
Soap pod roots and pods, *Acacia concinna*
Soap tree roots and leaves, *Yucca elata*
Soapwort roots, leaves, and blossoms, *Saponaria officinalis*
Spanish bayonet roots, *Yucca baccata*
Wild gourd fruits, *Cucurbita foetidissima*

The following remedies provide helpful relief for some of the body's needs during puberty. Some herbal medicines have many personalities and can be as beneficial inside our bodies as outside. Many are especially fine when rubbed on troubled skin rashes or massaged into sore muscles or aching backs.

**1 rounded tablespoon dried
crampbark or black haw
bark**

8 ounces boiling water

This tea is a multipurpose, unisex remedy, since it is as good sipped as it is gently rubbed on the body. Young women can relieve menstrual cramps by sipping this gentle decoction of the bark of crampbark, *Viburnum opulus,* or black haw, *Viburnum prunifolium,* all day while their symptoms persist. Native athletes use this same decoction as a muscle relaxant. The Catawba, Penobscot, Meskwaki, and Menominee use these shrub and root bark medicines to treat cramps, colic, swollen glands, and diarrhea. Many other tribes have similar uses for these two viburnums.

Although it can be gathered at other times, late spring and summer—while these deciduous shrubs are flowering—is the best time to gather the bark. This is the easiest time to identify the shrubs, as well as their time of greatest potency.

Measure the dried bark into the bottom of an 8-ounce teapot. Pour boiling water over it. Cover and steep for 10 minutes. Strain this into a cup and sip as needed throughout the day.

VARIATIONS: You can steep this decoction for a longer time if you want to use it as a lotion or a poultice on sore muscles or other areas where you have aches or pains.

For stronger relief, you can also make a tincture with either one or both of these medicinal barks (see page 240), using vodka or vinegar. A vinegar tincture is excellent when used externally as a liniment. And several drops of the tincture blended into $1/4$ cup of vegetable oil, such as corn or sunflower seed oil, makes a good massage oil for abdominal cramps, legs, and feet.

High-bush cranberry, or crampbark
Viburnum opulus

MAYAN CRAMP RELIEF TEA

The root of wild yam, *Dioscorea villosa,* has long been used by native peoples in Central and North America to treat painful menses. The Maya and Aztec Indians also used this medicinal plant for pain relief. Wild yam can act as a diuretic, and teas and tinctures made from it are also effective treatments for indigestion.

Measure the roots into the bottom of an 8-ounce pot. Pour boiling water over them. Cover and steep for 5 to 10 minutes. Strain this into a cup and sip it throughout the day to ease cramps.

1 tablespoon dried chopped roots of wild yam
8 ounces boiling water

Wild yam
Dioscorea villosa

RESTORATIVE BATHS AND SKIN WASHES

You can add healing herbs to a hot bath to relax and soothe irritated skin and sore muscles or just to improve general skin tone and comfort. A generous handful of fresh chickweed, *Stellaria media,* crushed and tied in a cotton cloth and immersed in a hot bathtub provides relief for eczema and will even ease the irritation caused by stinging nettles.

The summer blossoms of calendula, *Calendula officinalis,* are soothing for eczema and acne. Allow yourself to soak for 15 to 20 minutes in a bath of hot water in which you've immersed a generous handful of fresh blossoms, crushed and tied in a cotton cloth.

Calendula flowers are also used in tinctures, creams, and burn ointments (see pages 240, 244, and 245).

IRON-RICH ENERGY FOOD

Young people may need extra iron in their diets to help them through the physical changes of puberty. This is especially true for young women, who lose iron during menstruation.

Stinging nettle
Urtica dioica

Nettle, *Urtica dioica,* is a delicious iron-rich potherb. Additional iron-rich plants are yellow dock, skullcap, ginseng, chickweed, hops, burdock, mullein, sarsaparilla, rosemary, and peppermint. They can all be used similarly, on their own or in combinations of your choosing.

To eliminate nettles' stinging properties, clip the top four to six inches of young nettle tops and fill a small pot with the leaves. Pour $1/2$ cup water over them, cover, and place on medium-low heat. Bring to a slow boil and immediately reduce heat to a simmer for four or five minutes. At this point, you have several choices. You can eat the nettles like spinach and drink the iron-rich broth. Native peoples from the Adirondacks to the Andes have long enjoyed this infusion as a daily tonic.

Creamy nettle soup is another option. When you remove the pot from the heat, simply puree the contents in a blender with $1/2$ cup each of steamed carrots and onions.

Hops
Humulus lupulus

YUCCA ROOT AND CORNMEAL FACIAL MASK

1 tablespoon pounded or beaten yucca roots (you can do this in a home blender)
1 teaspoon fine cornmeal
water

Yucca root shampoo mixed with fine cornmeal makes a cleansing, healing skin wash that helps to feed and tone the skin, and is especially good for clearing up facial blemishes.

This cleansing formula and the variations listed are based upon early American Indian practices. They are very active, organic treatments. Your skin may start tingling immediately after application. The first several times you try this cleansing facial mask you may want to leave it on your skin for only five minutes.

Mix ingredients together and work into a paste; add water if it seems too dry.

Gently pat the mixture all over your face and especially on trouble spots, making a mask. You can even put some under your chin and on areas of your neck that need attention. Rest for 10 to 15 minutes, if possible. Then gently wash off all of the herbal mask with cool water to close the skin pores. Pat your skin dry, or allow to air-dry.

VARIATIONS: Instead of the yucca, substitute 1 tablespoon fresh pureed cucumber, 1 tablespoon chilled plain yogurt, and 1 teaspoon raw honey. Mix with 1 teaspoon of fine cornmeal. Blend well and follow the directions above for making a mask. When they are in season, use strawberries instead of the cucumber. In any of these recipes, you can use oatmeal instead of cornmeal to achieve similar benefits.

Wild cucumber
Echinocystis lobata

O Earthmother from whom we grow,
sandy gravel into whom our roots branch wood
and sap deep down,
bless us in our night-sleep, in our death and decay
Bless us, dark earth as we give back
that which we have received
as we make a forest of blessing
a ridge of blessing
for the future to grow upon.
          —*A Chinook prayer*

CHAPTER FOUR

Adolescence

"THE LITTLE BROTHER OF WAR"

White oak
Quercus alba

✦✦✦✦✦✦✦✦✦✦✦✦✦✦✦✦✦✦✦✦✦✦✦✦✦✦

Because of running I learned how to

pursue excellence, accepting only defeat, not failure.

It has ultimately led me to victories in my positive desires.

God gave me the ability with the rest up to me.

We compete against ourselves to the greatest extent we're

capable of. We have to believe, believe, believe.

—LAKOTA ATHLETE BILLY MILLS, WHO WON AN
OLYMPIC GOLD MEDAL IN TOKYO IN 1964

✦✦✦✦✦✦✦✦✦✦✦✦✦✦✦✦✦✦✦✦✦✦✦✦✦✦

White oak
Quercus alba

Games and races are an essential part of the highly energetic and impressionable phase of life known as adolescence. Through participation in sports, young people strengthen and push their bodies, test personal limits, and learn to know themselves in new ways. And sports can be used to heal psychological problems such as anger. During games, young men and women express their aggressive impulses in a controlled fashion, preventing more flagrant and possibly dangerous behavior.

Besides teaching valuable lessons about competition and cooperation, games illustrate that the process or journey toward a goal is more important than any singular achievement. Developing the power of concentration, strategic thinking, and the spirit of team play are as important as individual skill and prowess.

And games are tied to healing and balance. Native people value games of skill and chance as a way to avoid too much seriousness, which can unbalance an individual as well as a community. Humorous, enjoyable games have always served to make life endurable, especially in the past, when early American Indian life was filled with sorrow, separation, starvation, illness, and death. Sometimes a simple game of ball took on a mystical complexion.

Many native games began in religious rites and ceremonial celebrations. Over time they evolved into popular sports like footraces, running games, stickball, lacrosse, and some of the earliest ball games. Many of these games are still wildly popular and are played, with wide variations, across the continent.

Perhaps the most universal of all Indian sports are footraces. A longstanding tradition among many tribes, their origins and purposes are sacred and connected to healing. Often running in a footrace involves giving your best skills and energy to the Creator on behalf of someone else. Speed and distance covered are secondary.

White oak
Quercus alba

American Indian runners of international repute, famed for their running abilities, have emerged from these age-old customs. Men such as Jim Thorpe, the noted Osage Olympic medalist, and Billy Mills, whose words open this chapter, stimulate pride and motivation among Indian youth.

But running isn't only for champions. For both boys and girls it is a way to channel energy, a source of physical fitness, and a connection to the universe. Many American Indians reflect back on the sheer joy of running and competing as a memorable part of their youth. Late in his life, suffering from diabetes, which made walking and other movement difficult, Richard Chrisjon, the late Oneida artist and head of a respected family of traditional artists, poignantly reflected on his boyhood. Describing how he and groups of adolescent boys and girls visited friends by running from one Iroquois village to the next and on to the next, he recalled, "We would cover many miles without even thinking about it." Their exhilaration and their prowess grew out of the natural energies of adolescence.

But it's important to shape more than individual physical abilities. The family and tribe, as well as many rituals, focus on helping young men and women develop a sense of wholeness—personally, socially, and spiritually—and of finding a secure place within the context of their tribal traditions.

Gambling and Hand Games

Games of chance have a long history, although gambling today is a contested issue among American Indians. For children, adults' games of chance are part of their birthright; they grow up watching them and playing their own childlike imitations. Although they look like play, games are serious business, a deeply respected part of sacred traditions that goes back, among some tribes, to their origination stories.

For example, among some Cherokee, Creek, Pueblo, and Plains cultures, individuals threw sticks or bones, like the modern-day equivalent of tossing dice. But this simple game had a deeper meaning because reading the sticks or bones was a way to divine an illness. As children grew into adolescence and were ready to play the games, they developed a greater understanding of their significance.

Because of their sacred heritage, many games can only be played during rites at certain times of the year. The Iroquois bowl game, *gus-ka'-eh*, symbolizes the struggle between the original Twin Boys born to Sky Woman. The twins represent good and evil in the Iroquois creation legend. *Gus-ka'-eh* is the contest between the creative and the destructive. It reminds the Iroquois to maintain balance within the life-giving forces of nature and to honor the Creator with pleasure.

The game was first played with five to seven dice made from the woody pits of wild plums, which were tossed in a maple burl bowl. The rhythmic noise caused by tapping the hardwood bowl with the small wooden dice inside it was often accompanied by the chant *"hubbub,"* and this became the name of the bowl game in some regions. (This is also the origin of our American term *hubbub.)* Today Iroquois women play the sacred bowl game only during their Midwinter Ceremonies, which celebrate the end of one cycle in nature and the beginning of the new year and another cycle of Iroquois life.

The Navajo moccasin game is also played only in winter. It is accompanied by songs that were given to the people by the first animals, who played this game in earliest times. The Navajo believe that the animals received their natural colors and unique characteristics while playing the original moccasin game. The division of time into night and day also occurred at that time. American Indian adolescents growing up with these traditions learn how competition, games, and beliefs are laced together.

Hand games are traditional sleight-of-hand games that have long been popular among many tribes throughout North America. They are typically games of concealment that involve two teams of hiders, singers, and guessers. Usually played late in the evening after a full day of powwow or social dancing, some hand games don't begin until midnight. As teams square off against each other, their animated drumming, singing, hiding, and cheering can go on until morning. A team scores points by bluffing the opposition's guesser, or, on the other side, by the guesser's success. Hand games develop various skills and bond people together in friendly competition.

The Cherokee Stickball Games

Deep in the lush southeastern homelands where the Cherokee culture has flourished for thousands of years arose the stickball games, which symbolize the constant struggle between the opposing forces in people and their universe. The Cherokee, who have formulas and chants for every major occasion, had a particular chant for this game, where they invoked *watatuga,* a small species of dragonfly, and the bat. According to legend, the bat won the first great ball game for the birds, who were playing against the four-legged animals to settle a dispute in that long-ago time. Because the bat and dragonfly had superior skimming and dodging abilities, they nimbly outmaneuvered all their opponents.

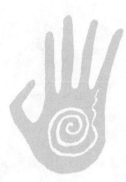

Many tribes have games that test endurance but these contests have always been much more than macho tests of skill and strength: The stickball game began as a sacred ritual reenactment of myth to remind the Cherokee of their origins. In earlier times, young men underwent a rigorous regimen, including periods of fasting and abstinence from sex and salt and other foods, to prepare for the stickball games. Their coach or shaman administered ritual scratching with sharp four- and seven-pronged instruments. This sacred tattooing was designed to bring them strength and good fortune as well as to recognize their abilities as they trained to build rugged endurance.

Besides those actually playing the game, other adolescents often filled key support roles. Historically, members of the seven Cherokee clans, led by their Clan Mothers, chanted and danced for the players' success, while drummers and other musicians kept the energizing rhythms throbbing loudly, calling everyone to the ball games.

Special songs and dances traditionally preceded and followed the ceremonial stickball games of the southeastern Cherokee, Creek, Choctaw, and Seminole. These are not usually performed during today's more competitive stickball games. To keep their power protected, certain ancient sacred curing and ceremonial songs are rarely, if ever, shared in open, mixed performances.

Today, the stickball games draw big crowds, especially during the Eastern Cherokee Fall Festival in October in Cherokee, North Carolina. Now, as in the past, the players use long sticks that curve upward and, inspired by spiderwebs, bend into rounded heads with netted pockets to catch and hold the ball. In this game, which is akin to lacrosse, the ballplayers battle furiously to score goals and best their opponents. Cheered by crowds of supporters—sometimes whole villages—the two teams strain to play their very best in contests that rival our modern Super Bowls.

While some of the traditional meaning of the stickball games has been lost to modern concepts of bravado and recognition of physical prowess, the games have not strayed too far from their origins. The Cherokee and other tribes acknowledge that the good and the bad often coexist, and they play their games in order to overcome the negative with the positive. Many people find that coming together to perform the rites of the stickball games helps them reconnect with their roots and restore their balance.

Lacrosse: The Little Brother of War

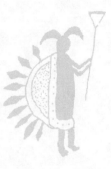

While many American Indian stickball games continue in recognizable form today, some, like lacrosse, can be found in schools across the country and have gained international acceptance. An ancient stickball game of the northeastern Indians, lacrosse is a tumultuous cross between field hockey and soccer, in which two teams of ten players vigorously play back and forth across the field to knock or carry a small ball into their opponents' netted goals. Each player carries a lacrosse racquet, which is a straight stick with a curved, webbed pocket at the head for catching, carrying, or throwing the ball.

Many tribes across the Northeast had their own unique versions of this game. There were a variety of names for it in different tribal languages, but the French missionaries and travelers who first watched the game named it *lacrosse* for its characteristic stick, or *crosse*.

Among Indian youth, lacrosse competition was a fine training program. Neighboring tribes' ball teams would often play against each other. Early observers noticed that Indian lacrosse games seemed little short of war, and indeed, some peoples played lacrosse as a means of settling disputes between their tribes, instead of using the more dangerous implements of war. The powerful Iroquois Confederacy, which established their League of Six Nations to consolidate their awesome strengths and settle internecine disputes as well as to exert influence over their neighbors, held the playing of lacrosse in such high esteem that it was called the "Little Brother of War."

Lacrosse could be played upon the request of any individual within the community. Because it was used to settle disputes and bind communities together, lacrosse was considered a medicinal game and a spiritual gift from the Creator. Individuals who played lacrosse underwent special instruction, including learning how to use traditional medicines gathered from the forests.

The Iroquois considered themselves fine lacrosse players, and today their teams are still hard to beat. The Iroquois National Lacrosse Team from New York State has developed a considerable international following during recent years, a result of the way they select, nurture, and train young Iroquois athletes for competition. And the National Indian Athletic Association coordinates and promotes youth clinics and national championships across the country, serving as a resource for Indian sports activities. Underlying their success in lacrosse, as with the hoop-and-stick games of other tribes, is the understanding that maximum performance and passionate sportsmanship are as important as winning.

Ancient Indian games such as lacrosse have their own songs and chants, which are akin to the cheerleading at modern American sports like baseball, football, and basketball. These special energies weave the audience into the games with enthusiasm and passion. Modern players often give their best energies and performances for those who cannot play. Even people who are wheelchair-bound or otherwise incapacitated, or who never wished to be a ballplayer, are drawn into the action and become part of the game.

The Wampanoag Fire Ball Game

"We're deeply involved in the spirits of all forms of life, not just human life," says John Peters, also called Slow Turtle, the Wampanoag supreme medicine man in Boston, Massachusetts. Wellness, the state of maintaining vigorous good health, and healing, the act of returning to wellness, require perceptive work on many levels.

Athletic activities are a productive and enjoyable outlet for adolescent energies. They teach valuable lessons about team building and cooperation as they bolster strength and self-esteem. But in American Indian games there is another, deeper level. Running, endurance games, and footraces are interwoven with healing rituals to enhance the power of medicines and other healing practices. For example, while a medicine person treats an ill parent or grandparent, a youngster might offer to run a marathon or enter another type of event to give his strength to the Creator and help his loved one fight the illness. The Wampanoag fire ball game, an astonishing contest of field soccer using a flaming ball, is just such an event.

The ancestral homelands of eastern Massachusetts, Cape Cod, Martha's Vineyard, Nantucket, and Elizabeth Island resonate with countless Wampanoag Indian legacies. Archaeological evidence suggests that ancestors of today's Wampanoag people have inhabited these regions of southern New England for more than twelve thousand years. Known as whaling people, the Wampanoag's maritime knowledge and skills enabled early whalers to prosper several hundred years ago, and many Wampanoag retain their nautical passions today. It was the Wampanoags who shared their harvests with the Pilgrims in the early 1620s, after showing them the techniques for planting and harvesting corn, squash, and beans, and for gathering various native foods and hunting wild game.

Wampanoag celebrations and food traditions continue year round, but their annual powwow, held over the Fourth of July weekend in Mashpee, near the southeast coast of Cape Cod, is especially vital. Thousands of native people and summer visitors gather here from all over North America to enjoy the dances, foods, fine crafts, and festivities. The centerpiece of the powwow is the great fire ball game, a haunting spectacle that is played only once a year, on the Saturday night of this major weekend.

Fire ball is a traditional medicine game, dating back hundreds of years. It is played by men, especially young men, who have chosen to give their strength and participation for a sick relative or friend in need of healing. Played with a flaming ball wound with deerskin strips and soaked for days in whale oil so that it will burn steadily, brightly, and intensely, it is like a primal type of soccer, only much freer and more dangerous. Like a comet in the night, the burning fire ball flies across the dark grassy field, with the players chasing, kicking, and slapping it. Great healing energies reside in this highly charged display of manhood and bravado: The bruises, wounds, and burns suffered during this strenuous game are believed to minimize or relieve a loved one's illness.

Passionate games such as fire ball have a spectacular and sometimes unsettling effect on all who gather to witness them. Encountering the wounded and bandaged players in the days that follow is evidence that sacrifice is not easy or pleasant. Perhaps there are parallels in the honor and pain of those who choose to donate a kidney or bone marrow to a loved one.

Games and athletic events are an important way to channel adolescents' energies, but there are others. Among many tribes, membership in any of a host of groups—warrior societies, kachina cults, and medicine societies, among others—trained young people in religious practices and a variety of crafts while binding them closely into the tribal community. A number of these groups still exist today.

Warrior Societies

During adolescence, the last step on the way to adulthood, developing a sense of who you are and testing your limits, without endangering your physical or emotional well-being, is key. During the 1800s a complex, flourishing system of warrior societies, especially among the more than twenty tribes of Plains Indians, taught young people not only endurance and pride in their abilities, but personal discipline and a code of ethics to help them in battle as well as in peacetime pursuits.

These societies played a critical role on the battlefield. As warriors, their members learned to understand their strengths and weaknesses and to exercise self-discipline by avoiding excessive displays of anger. Above all, a society member was expected to be brave. The most courageous were officers, who were expected to flout danger deliberately, leading battles and never retreating.

The groups also had power and authority within their own communities. When called upon by the headman of the village, the various societies took turns guarding the camp. Their distinctive tipis, lodges, bundles, and shields showed who was on duty. Young boys emulated their older peers, forming imitation warrior societies, and when a serious emergency occurred, much was expected of them, too.

Tattoos and Body Piercing

Perhaps more than at any other point in their lives, adolescents try to make striking statements about who they are. These days, they seem to be taking it to extremes, with extensive body piercing, hair coloring, and tattoos. But some of their actions have a remarkable resonance with practices followed by American Indian adolescents for centuries.

Tattoos were often status symbols in earlier times, and they said particular things about those who had them. From the Arctic Native peoples to the Eastern Algonquians, body painting, piercing, and tattooing signaled special status. Small shoulder tattoos for boys and girls reaching puberty might be further enhanced with facial tattoos at the time of marriage. Red ochre was carefully rubbed into some tattoos, while other groups preferred black or blue pigments.

Not all tribes favored tattoos or body piercing, yet those who did were noteworthy. Lip labrets (bone or ivory adornments worn in the lip) were favored by some of the northern Athabascan peoples, both men and women. Along the West Coast and across the high plateau regions, various tribal women sported chin tattoos as beauty marks.

Both men and women wore earrings. Choctaw men took this art to the highest level by using multiple piercings all the way up the ear, as pictured by early Indian painters. Prehistoric burial goods reveal spectacular earrings of semiprecious stones, pearls, bone, ivory, and copper worn in various North American regions, especially among the Mound Builders cultures.

Although they were called warrior societies, these groups possessed other powers, too; many had extremely potent medicine bundles. Members opened them only occasionally, during traditional rites held to renew and bless them and other implements of hunting or war.

Warrior societies took their names from animals typically found in the tribe's ecosystem, such as the kit fox or the bear, which were highly esteemed for their strength. They came into existence as the result of a tribal leader's dream or vision, which often specified a "charmed" maximum number of members. Some groups admitted new recruits only when the society sustained losses through battle or death.

In some tribes, a young man progressed through a series of clubs as he grew older, each with its own training and initiation rites. For example, among the Hidatsa, the youngest warriors—the adolescents—belonged to the Kit Fox Society. These young men trained the way that kit foxes do in their den, fledging and then emerging into society. Often tribal elders determined which boys could be initiated; in some cases young men had to buy or barter their way in. Such exclusive and hard-won membership was dearly held and staunchly defended.

These elite societies were a high-water mark in the realm of social customs. Each had its own unique shields and other paraphernalia, as well as a tipi or ceremonial lodge, painted with the symbols and colors given to the founder in his original vision. Society members also wore distinctive costumes. For example, the Oglala Sioux Kit Fox wore kit-fox-skin necklaces, a forehead band decorated with kit-fox jawbones, a crown of crow tail feathers, and two erect eagle feathers at the back of their heads. The regalia was so distinctive that someone's society and rank could be read at a distance in battle or during trading missions and other peacetime pursuits. Enhanced by their spectacular costumes, warrior society dances were legendary, but because of their secret and religious aspects, only a few white people were ever allowed to see them.

The Warriors of High Steel

The warrior ethic continues to flow through native society in many ways, even for people who are not members of warrior societies. One of the more dramatic illustrations is the men and women who walk high steel, contributing their skill, courage at great heights, and amazing sense of balance to the building of America's bridges and skyscrapers. Young American Indians view their feats with tremendous pride, as recalled in the words of the steel warriors themselves:

Working on structural steel carried prestige. Ironworkers were role models for us kids on the reservation. You'd see the way these men walked on the iron. They were good. They seemed to be the ones who had the most guts, and everyone wanted to be like them. . . . I guess we did feel like modern warriors way up there on the high steel.

—David Richmond, Snipe Clan, Akwesasne Mohawk,
former steel warrior and Vietnam veteran

Working steel was challenging. It was a chance to prove yourself. In my day, you would get up so high and there would only be Indians working. No one else wanted to climb that high. It made you feel good.

—Donald Richmond, Akwesasne Mohawk,
healer and former steel warrior

Many of the concrete functions of the warrior societies are now gone, but the raison d'être for these and similar groups remains highly relevant. For young American Indians in seemingly hopeless situations, warrior societies still provide an outlet for athletic abilities and traditional passions that can counter the looming specters of teen suicide, alcoholism, and drug addiction. The Kit Fox Society and others like it foster the warrior spirit, giving a sense of personal worth to the young people upon whom society depends for future leadership. They provide a secure place where an adolescent can reinvent himself in the context of a closely knit, supportive peer group, at the same time channeling potentially dangerous adolescent macho energy into safe outlets. Society memberships are cherished, and they closely wed young people to their community.

Although membership in some warrior societies is limited, other groups can be accessed freely through dreams or visions. Mystic animal cults, open to men and sometimes to women, maintain that their supernatural power comes from a certain animal in a vision. These cults have their own regalia, associated with the animal for which the cult is named. The Bear Cult, which survives today as a leading healing society, is a prime example. Among the Pueblo as well as certain northeastern and southeastern tribes, the bear is a nearly universal symbol of medicine, and members of the Bear Cult are known for doctoring the sick.

Dreams, Visions, and Healing

Adolescent men and women sometimes have dreams and visions that direct them to dedicate their lives to healing, shamanism, or another spiritual calling. In many tribes training for these sacred commitments, including initiations into medicine societies, begins in earnest during this stage of life.

As we mentioned in Chapter 2, young Salish children were sent out at night to seek guardian spirits. According to their tradition, lost spirits hovered in the air, waiting for the right children to find them. The sweat lodge spirit was the most powerful one they could find. This early training strengthened them, so they were unafraid of ghosts or the dark. By the time they were adolescents, certain children became receptive to supernatural events that might come through their dreams or in visions, paving the way for them

The Sweat Lodge

The Sweat Lodge Spirit is part of the Great Spirit/Creator itself. Some believe that the Great Spirit changed his mate into the conical, ribbed sweat lodge, which no other guiding spirit can ever overpower.

The sweat lodge embodies the concept of the circle, sacred in all American Indian cultures and in many others around the world. American Indians see life from thousands of individual points of view, and yet they all honor the circle, often picturing it in artwork, regalia, sacred and secular accouterments, dances, and lodgings. Numerous large prehistoric medicine wheels constructed all across the high plains in North America still hold immense sacred power for native peoples. The circle is part of their basic beliefs, symbolizing the interconnectedness of all living things with each other and the Creator, as well as the connection between life and death.

The sweat lodge structure symbolizes the combined strengths of five special powers: earth for support, stones for stamina, fire for heat, water for cleansing, and wood for ribs and heat. The entrance faces east toward the rising sun, and from this a path leads to the outer fire. Here rocks are roasted before they are carried into the sweat lodge, where they are sprinkled with water to create the steam.

As an individual sits within the dark, often cramped, hot womb of the squat sweat lodge, facing the center pile of steaming rocks, and making offerings of prayers, tobacco, and healing herbs to the Creator, ancient traditions enfold her. Cleansing, physical purification, and spiritual strengthening are the key benefits from sweat lodge rites, but they can be a deep or even holy experience.

The sweat lodge contains too much power for children, so it is only during adolescence that both men and women begin to have an actual, regular connection to it. Even then, it may only be occasional, depending on the tribe's customs and the availability of the sweat lodge. Within some native traditions, the sweat lodge rites are primarily the province of the males, since it is believed that women have their monthly purification with their menses. In any case, the two sexes use the sweat lodge separately, often directed by an elder in the tribe. And men and women use different prayers, songs, and appeals to the Creator for their own special needs.

Although the sweat lodge is an ancient practice, many contemporary American Indian men and women continue the custom, believing that it purifies and strengthens them. For young people, the sweat lodge is especially useful, helping them stay centered and connected to their life path, regardless of what it is.

to begin training as shamans. These young people were specially tutored; they were taught to welcome the apparitions rather than to fear them.

Tribe members believed that these young men and women had the ability to cure the sick or to foresee things—mishaps, sickness, death in the family—that might happen to others. Because guardian spirits often warned them of dire events while they were asleep, these shamans-to-be had the power to prevent accidents from occurring. And the spirits also specified what to do to cure sickness.

In many tribes, adolescents had dreams or visions that laid the groundwork for healing or other secret societies. Indian legends abound where a young man or woman's dream carries detailed lessons or ceremonies that are essential to the well-being of an entire tribe.

Each of the Iroquois secret societies has its own story explaining its origins; in many cases the society's founder was an adventurous youth or an outcast orphan who met with supernatural assistance. In these long, complex tales, a dream conveyed warnings and valuable secrets, along with the rituals necessary to safeguard the tribe. Once established, these serious and sacred societies were governed by respected adults within each longhouse.

For example, the rituals for the complex and highly important Seneca society known as the Pygmy Society or the Little People were given by an old man to a boy, as told by Tonawanda Seneca author and artist Jesse J. Cornplanter in *Legends of the Longhouse:*

> We will rejoice with our own ceremony, which will also be yours from now on. This ceremony is called "Dark Dance" and really belongs to us, you must observe everything that takes place and remember everything so you can carry it back to your people, which will bring them good luck. They in turn will remember us and our relation by getting up the ceremony for our enjoyment. So I command you to watch now.

The Dark Dance Ceremony of the Little People has been handed down for centuries. The Pygmy Society's ceremonies always open with a welcoming speech and a prayer to the Creator. Using the water drum and the horn rattle for keeping time, people in this powerful group sing for all the medicine charms and all the magic animals, who are also members of the society. The members perform the rituals, which consist of 102

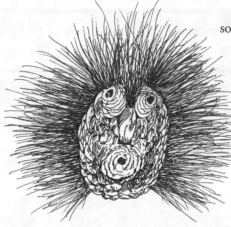

Iroquois dream-guessing mask

songs, in darkness to encourage the spirit members to come and join in the singing; at times their voices can be heard. Nonmembers troubled by certain disorders or other signs associated with the Little People can become members of the Pygmy Society by asking for their services. Traditional Indians respect the "little folk" and seek their goodwill.

The Haudenosaunee, or "People of the Longhouse," as the Iroquois call themselves, have always respected dreams as important communications from supernatural beings. During adolescence, people begin to participate in Dream Guessing Rites, which probe the many levels of a dream to decipher its instructions and occasional forewarnings.

Dream Guessing Rites are an essential part of the annual Iroquois Midwinter Ceremonies, which begin on the fifth day after the new moon following the winter solstice, usually in January. Dream Guessing helps heal people who are troubled by disturbing dreams. An individual wearing the Dream Guessing Mask, a spectacular bushy face mask carefully crafted of dried corn husks, discovers the subject of the dream, and in so doing uncovers the problem and provides relief to the dreamer. Later, the guesser produces a miniature representing the dream and presents it to the dreamer to be kept as a good-luck charm.

Hopi and Zuni
Kachina Rites and Initiations

Although a select few may be specially singled out to be shamans, seers, or members of secret societies, most young men and women take on their customary communal spiritual responsibilities during adolescence. At the age of twelve or thirteen Hopi and Zuni children assume adult roles in their kachina societies. This is a major turning point in their young lives, comparable to a bar or bat mitzvah among Jewish people and confirmation among some Christian denominations.

Although the more than three hundred supernatural beings known as kachinas are only present in the village for half of the year, training in their rites goes on year round, beginning in early childhood. It is intricately linked to continuing the Hopi way (as well as the Zuni and other Pueblo

The Seven Star Dancers

At dusk during the Iroquois Midwinter Ceremonies, the Pleiades are flickering directly overhead in the cold winter sky. This conspicuous cluster of seven bright stars and one fainter one is significant in Iroquois cosmology, as well as in the beliefs of many tribes across the continent. As illustrated by this Iroquois legend, it is associated with adolescence.

Long ago in an earlier sacred time, in an Iroquois longhouse settlement near the great river, many families worked together gathering the forest and garden foods during late summer. Eight boys who were very close friends went off together each evening after their work was done to dance and drum. They had grown up together and were almost like brothers in their passion for sharing time together. They wanted to form their own medicine society, similar to the ones their elders belonged to, and they worked to fashion an Iroquois water drum, elm bark rattles, and a snapping turtle rattle. Meeting in their remote clearing on a hill away from the village, no one could hear them, nor did anyone realize what they were doing. If the adults had been aware of the boys' seriousness, they might have cautioned them not to copy the sacred ceremonies.

Winter set in and most evenings the boys continued to meet together in their secret clearing. They drummed and sang and danced, and talked of taking a journey together. They asked their parents for extra food to bring on these evening encounters, but winter rations were slim and no food could be spared beyond the essential one meal a day.

The eight boys continued to dance and sing with growing strength, although they grew increasingly slim and light. One cold, clear winter night the sound of their music grew so powerful it reached the village, and the people became alarmed. The growing boys had been given freedom and encouragement to gather and develop their skills, but now they sounded supernatural. The parents and others from the village made their way to the distant campfire on the hill where the music was throbbing. They were amazed to see the boys dancing skyward, high above the flames of their campfire, circling and climbing ever higher into the Sky World. They called out to them, but the boys could not hear them. The smallest boy paused to look back, and he became a shooting star. The remaining seven boys danced ever higher into the dome of the sky, where they continue to dance today, circling the Sky World.

The Iroquois know that the Dancers—which we call the Pleiades—return again each year to mark the celebration of the sacred Midwinter Ceremonies.

traditions) of maintaining personal balance and healing. Young men and women must learn everything they can about medicinal plants, from identifying and harvesting them to nurturing their living spirits as they are used in healing practices and medicinal formulas. Within each cult, individual families are responsible for the myriad details of making the masks, weaving the garments, and painting and carving other paraphernalia that will be used when the rites are performed.

For months, as the time draws near, fathers, uncles, and other relatives who help to initiate the adolescents prepare the regalia for these rites. They work in the *kiva,* an underground sanctuary that is the ceremonial chamber where kachina societies retire for their secret healing rites. Preparation of ceremonial accouterments for all major events, even those that culminate aboveground, goes on in the *kiva.* The power of these inner wombs, located beneath the central plazas of ancient Pueblo Indian villages, invests enormous energy in the all-important adolescent initiation rites.

In traditional pueblos, many of the particulars of the adolescent initiation rites are private and take place in the secrecy of the *kiva.* Afterward the young men and women are full-fledged members of their kachina cults, eligible to wear the regalia and dance when the kachina rites are performed during the year.

In the recent past, continuing this essential training when children leave their pueblos for schooling has been a thorny problem. Indeed, the loosening of the connection between American Indian children and their traditional roots has wreaked havoc among many adolescents of all tribes. Some young men and women make the transition to adulthood smoothly, but for others this is a difficult time. American Indian teenagers are especially plagued by grinding poverty, low self-esteem, alcohol and substance abuse, suicide, and other problems of the disenfranchised.

Today a spiritual revival is under way. Many tribes are working strenuously to reestablish time-honored practices, especially their puberty rites and traditional gatherings called "socials," in order to strengthen their family fabric and save their teenagers from slipping into harmful habits. And there is a national effort to target troubled American Indian teens on many reservations across the country. Thirteen diverse programs, including an Inupiat kayak expedition near Nome, Alaska, an Apache multimedia campaign against alcohol and drugs in the White Mountains of Arizona, and the Cheyenne River Sioux Camp Wolakota Yukini, in Eagle

Butte, South Dakota, work to instill traditional values and prevent problems among their youngsters. Gregg Bourland, chairman of the Cheyenne River Sioux Tribe, considers their traditional summer camp to be a "rebirth of the great Sioux Nation."

Tribal elders see these programs as a time to heal as they work to develop brighter futures for their youth. But for adolescents suffering from alcohol or substance abuse, stronger measures, such as a curing ceremony, may be necessary.

Pollen Boy on the Sun and Corn Bug Girl on the Moon

Sand paintings are used by most tribes throughout the desert Southwest and in a few other regions, such as the West Coast. In these intricately beautiful dry paintings, every primary color is derived from natural minerals, pulverized stone and semiprecious gems, charcoal, pollen, or fine cornmeal. Sand paintings focus unusual curing energies within their specific designs.

The Navajo have developed the greatest array of sand paintings, well over a thousand different designs. Each one represents some aspect of Navajo mythology or cosmology constructed to restore the patient to balance.

Sand painters use delicate handmade lines of color to trace the shapes of sacred feathers, clouds, medicine bundles, *yeis* (gods and creation figures), plants, and standing rainbows exactly as they are directed by the Navajo singer, or *hataalii,* in charge of each "sing," or ceremony necessary to create the cure. These are also called "chants" or "ways." The Navajo singer is a priest-practitioner who knows the chants or song ceremonials for specific cures. No one singer knows all of these complex chantways. Each concentrates on knowing and remembering the ones within his own areas of expertise.

The Navajo word for sand painting, *iikaah,* means "place where the Holy People come and go," as great supernatural powers are present during these ceremonies. "Only the medicine man knows how long the healing will take, which herbs to use, which sand paintings and songs to do," says Navajo sand painter Mitchell Silas.

The sand painting must be created between sunrise and sunset in one

Earth's feet have become
   my feet
by means of these I shall
   live on,
Earth's body has become
   my body
by means of this I shall
   live on.

—*From a Navajo
Blessing Way song*

day, and is usually made on the prepared, blessed earthen floor of a Navajo hogan, the traditional eight-sided home. Large, complex sand paintings can require four or more skilled sand painters working throughout the day to finish an intricate design that may be twenty feet in diameter. Most are much smaller and can be made by one sand painter. When it is ready, the patient is seated on the sand painting and parts of it are placed on his body in order to infuse him with the deities and their sacred landscapes. In this way, the patient is given their power and curing energies. Any evil, illness, or imbalance affecting the patient is absorbed by the sand painting during the ceremonies, so at the end the entire sand painting must be gathered up, carried away, and, often, ceremonially buried.

One of many powerful curing designs for adolescents undergoing problems with substance or alcohol cravings or other particular disabilities is the Pollen Boy on the Sun for boys and its counterpart for girls, Corn Bug Girl on the Moon. This sand painting pictures a pollen deity drawn in pollen at the center of a red sun or on a black buffalo face, symbolizing strength, protection, and the four winds on earth. Buffalo horns surrounded by eagle feathers signify wisdom, justice, and law. Radiating out from this in the four sacred directions are the four sacred plants: corn, beans, squash, and tobacco. Each stylized plant is a different color, again symbolizing the four directions: white is east, yellow is west, black (a male color) is north, and blue (female) is south. Red usually represents sunshine.

Great care, concentration, and time are involved in these chants, which can be quite costly. The Navajo singer(s) and sand painter(s) must be well paid. Abundant food must be provided for the many family members and friends who gather for the healing ceremonies, which may last from one to nine days. Many social activities also swirl about these gatherings because the people attending the healing rites feel blessed and energized by them.

Coyote Stories

Coyote has long been associated with American Indian stories, games, dances, and shamanism—healing is often helped or worked by someone with his special powers—all across America. Coyote is a changeling, a shape-shifter, a clown, and most of all a survivor. Some say that Coyote is everywhere, watching and waiting.

Coyote Places the Stars

In the beginning of Creation Time, Gluscap [the Creator] was busy filling the night sky with beauty, in order to balance the separate realities of day and night. He had gathered a huge leather bag full of "morning stars," valuable medicine plants that we know today as stargrass, *Aletris farinosa*, and Canada mayflowers, *Maianthemum canadense*. With his long walking stick he carefully placed each magical star bloom high up in the new sky, arranging them in bright pattern designs we know today as the Great Celestial Bear [Big Dipper], the Little Bear [Little Dipper], the Seven Star Dancers [Pleiades], the Great Star Road [Milky Way], and others.

Gluscap placed many star patterns carefully, like fine beadwork on black buckskin. He worked long and hard setting everything just right. When he grew tired, he looked for a great patch of soft green moss beneath a giant oak tree to lie down and rest, planning to finish placing the stars in the evening sky, when he could see better how to arrange these heavenly designs. Laying his heavy star bag down beside him, he drifted into deep sleep and dreamed of beautiful designs.

Along came Coyote. As always, he was thinking about food. He looked at Gluscap, sound asleep, and carefully nosed about his leather bag to see if there was something good to eat inside. When he saw the star flowers, he wanted to help Gluscap place them in the heavens, especially in coyote patterns. So he carefully grabbed the bag in his teeth and ran off with it. But being Coyote, he tripped over a great rock and the bag ripped wide open. Suddenly the blossoms flashed up into the sky, spreading across it every which way.

Gluscap awoke from his nap with a start. He looked up to see his stars flickering all across the Sky World. When he looked down at his empty, ripped bag and saw Coyote sitting there looking forlorn, he said: "Oh! Coyote! Look what you have done! There is such a mess across the heavens, where I planned to place star patterns like jewels and beautiful beads."

Poor Coyote. As he looked up, shame filled his heart and tears filled his eyes. He was embarrassed and he began to howl mournfully. He cried and yipped pitifully into the dead of night. Perhaps you have heard coyotes crying or howling in the night. They cry for many reasons; this is one.

Gluscap took pity on Coyote and eventually forgave him. But the stars remain scattered all across the night sky, except for a few prominent constellations in their midst, reminding us of Coyote's clumsy interference. You may still hear coyotes howling mournfully at the night sky, singing out their regrets for the foolishness of their distant ancestor so long ago. And so it is.

Coyotes are also good and caring parents. They often raise big litters of pups. Native families often felt a kinship with these animals, who group themselves in tribes or packs of their own.

Coyote stories entertain and teach throughout childhood, but they are particularly useful at this stage of life. In many tales, Coyote is part of creation. He accomplishes great things, but he often does them foolishly. And frequently he acts impulsively, regretting his behavior afterward. These are important lessons for adolescents who are in a hurry to grow up and be important.

Coyote stories are so powerful that they should be told only in the winter, after the snakes "have gone to ground" to rest for the coldest months, and "between thunders." Each region of the country has a unique natural sequence for these environmental phenomena. In the Northeast, snakes usually hibernate between mid-November and mid-April, and this usually, but not always, coincides with the last thunderclaps of autumn and the first thunder rolls of spring. For the Iroquois and Wampanoag peoples in the Northeast, the timing of seasonal stories is also affected by the fireflies, who are shape-shifters too, often associated with the mischievous Little People. Fireflies are usually seen from May through September. If you want to tell a certain story out of season, you must make a small offering, perhaps a pinch of tobacco or cornmeal with a prayer, and use great caution and respect. Otherwise imbalance or harm may result.

Many different Indian tribes tell their own version of this creation story, which comes from the northeastern Algonquians.

Thousands of miles away, the Navajo have long told a tale that is surprisingly similar. People in this tribe believe that some of the laws they should live by are written in the stars, who are friendly beings that assist Navajo healing rituals. Stars and star patterns are often pictured in Navajo sand paintings, which receive healing power from the stars shining through the smoke hole in the roof of the hogan where the healing rituals take place. Navajo artists picture the night sky, called the "dark upper," as the black star-filled body of Father Sky.

Sexuality and Taboos

Like Coyote, adolescents can often be impulsive, and at this stage of life a whole new arena of behavior—sex—opens up. Sexuality has long been regarded as a source of human wealth in American Indian societies. Sex is usually treated positively and considered to be the natural and beautiful way that life continues. But sexuality is also a complex reality stretching far beyond its biological dimensions. It involves cultural and moral beliefs as well as psychological and social behaviors. Parents, clans, and extended families play vital roles in each teenager's development. Their teachings unfold in earnest during adolescence, when fertility becomes an issue and the pace of all learning quickens.

In the past, seasonal rituals, dances, and other special occasions brought young people together for social activities and courting. This continues throughout Indian country today with the socials, powwows, dance competitions, rodeos, and church activities. Typically Indian teenagers at these events drift around together in groups, looking cool, seeing each other, and being seen. Like other American adolescents, many American Indians become sexually active at this point. Some postpone marriage, hoping to fulfill career dreams. But others marry and give birth to their first children. To gain the family's approval, a young person must abide by tribal taboos in choosing a partner.

Every tribe has its own unique spiritual traditions, beliefs, and taboos. Violating these taboos can bring physical or mental harm to an individual. It may affect a person's family and even her unborn future family members. A violation of a taboo must be rectified before harmony can be reestablished and health regained.

Some taboos require that certain rites and rituals be performed in a particular manner, for instance, that you must enter the sweat lodge from the east and proceed clockwise around the central fire; the same would hold true for visiting a traditional tipi or a contemporary home. Others specify that you must not go near lightning-struck objects, and there are many tribal taboos, often specific to a tribe or region, related to animals, plants, and mushrooms.

But there is one universal American Indian taboo: You must not marry within your clan. For most native people the major social organization beyond the immediate family was the clan, and each one had a particular symbol and name. Among many tribes, such as the Iroquois, Creek, and Cherokee, clan membership was determined by the mother's people. This principal goal of the age-old incest taboo is to keep bloodlines fresh; it prevents birth defects and other forms of bloodline weakness. During adolescence, many of these taboos are repeatedly addressed.

Teenagers grow up with these essential points of awareness, and are often reminded of them in stories and rituals, so they will not be tempted to make unacceptable choices.

Today many tribes face the opposite problem: A large number of American Indians marry non-Indian spouses, thanks in part to urbanization. And there are other important issues to grapple with when it comes to marriage and childbirth. The increasing number of out-of-wedlock births, and of Indian babies badly affected by their parents' drug and alcohol abuse problems, as well as the growing awareness of fetal alcohol syndrome, has raised red flags of alarm throughout Indian America. Elders, teachers, and parents are working to educate their young people about these staggering disorders. Adolescent men and women are especially important, since they are the vital connecting link both to ancient ancestors and to generations as yet unborn. This is why many traditionalists say that our actions must be considered in light of how they will affect the next seven generations.

Silver maple
Acer saccharinum

Red maple
Acer rubrum

Dance

When I listen to the beat of the drum,
and I am out in the circle fancy-dancing
with other native youths,
and I know my people are watching with pride,
I am proud to be a Native American.

Wunneanatsu, a Schaghticoke/Winnebago teenager in Meriden, Connecticut, reflects on how the vitality of her ethnicity sustains her. "Being a true Native means being a *native at heart.* You must have it in your blood, but you must also have it in your heart. Being a true Native means believing in and supporting your people."

Wunneanatsu comes from a strong Algonquian matrilineal heritage filled with storytelling, herbalism, healing, and dancing. It takes years of study to learn many of the American Indian dances. Most are connected to healing and awareness of special life phases.

Dance is especially important at every stage of American Indian life, but the athletic balance and endurance of youth is especially beautiful when channeled into dance. Many infants are carried in their parents' arms and "danced around the circle." Indians begin to learn, participate, and even compete as toddlers in the "tiny tots" category at countless national powwows.

Among the powerful native drums are many different drum groups, each with its own repertoire of songs. Drums sing the cadences, directing each dance and its many dancers. Every dancer must listen closely to this music, dance, and be judged—in competition, especially—on her ability to recognize and interpret the right details. The secret is that each dancer must also perform with such smooth grace and balance that she makes her performance look easy despite her dazzling athletics.

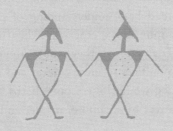

EARTH REMEDIES

Narrow-leaf plantain
Plantago lanceolata

Training for the healing arts begins early in native life and becomes increasingly rigorous in adolescence. Young people are often required to spend special time with a specific medicine person as a trainee, helping with routine chores. If a certain aptitude is demonstrated—by paying close attention, respectfully following orders, and remembering vital points of traditions—the young student may then become an apprentice to the medicine person for a period of years, perhaps her whole life.

We are surrounded by medicine plants, healing fungi, and other valuable earth substances. It takes time to learn their many personalities and benefits. Centuries ago each healer probably knew between fifty and three hundred healing plants and fungi from his particular region. Wherever regions and healers overlapped, the potential healing opportunities increased. Even within one small native village two different medicine people might know the uses of entirely different healing substances. In many areas this continues to be the case.

Often a young person training to be a healer studies with a number of medicine people to gain a broad range of experience. He might apprentice with an herbalist and perhaps then with a healer or a shaman. Often the youth is tested in various ways to determine if he is serious about the work, and to develop his deeper sensitivities to human suffering and how to heal it. A young apprentice may also be required to undergo fasting and feats of endurance to test his resolve.

But even adolescents who are not training for the healing path still have a broad basic understanding of plant use and the applications of some common fungi, especially when it comes to everyday illnesses and injuries. For example, they would know how to use grape and coltsfoot leaves as poultices to lower a fever and relieve a headache. Pressed over a bleeding leg wound, these same herbs will stop the bleeding. The large, cooling leaves of sycamore, maple, and plantain can be used in similar fashion.

Several common shrubs in the Northeast have long been highly esteemed healing plants. Our native witch hazel *(Hamamelis virginiana)*, beaked hazel *(Corylus cornuta)*, and hazelnut *(Corylus americana)* have healing, antiseptic twigs, bark, and leaves. The twigs of these plants are

English plantain
Plantago major

valuable natural dentifrices and chew sticks. Their astringent bitterness is drying and healing for bleeding gums or toothache. Beaked hazel and hazelnut also produce annual crops of delicious edible nuts, whose oil is used medicinally.

Hazelnut oil is a reliable mosquito repellent and a favored insecticide. American Indian teenagers use the light oil for skin and hair care. The large, leathery green leaves of hazelnut make poultices that can be used for everything from headaches to skin sores, tendonitis, and sore muscles. When they are briefly boiled, the leaves and twigs make an astringent, antiseptic liniment rub for skin care and muscle aches as well as a treatment for rheumatism. A mild hazelnut tea relieves headache and reduces fever. Some Canadian tribes pounded and boiled together the bark, leaves, and twigs and applied them as a poultice to treat tumors, abscesses, or ulcers.

The fresh roots of numerous native botanicals can be pounded and poulticed on burns to soothe and reduce swelling, as well as to prevent infections. These include the aromatic roots of wild sarsaparilla, *Aralia nudicaulis;* Canada goldenrod, *Solidago canadensis;* fireweed, *Epilobium angustifolium;* wild hydrangea, *Hydrangea arborescens;* cattail, *Typha latifolia;* and bracken fern, *Pteridium aquilinum.*

The exudations from the leaves of many plants, such as the beautiful leaves of downy rattlesnake plantain, *Goodyera pubescens* (one of our showy native orchids, on the endangered species list), can be applied externally to burned, chapped, or irritated skin to cool and soothe inflammation, treat skin ulcers, and reduce swelling. The fresh leaves of wild quinine, *Parthenium integrifolium;* clintonia, *Clintonia borealis;* the bindweeds *(Convolvulus arvensis; C. sepium);* horse-balm, *Collinsonia canadensis;* horsemint, *Monarda punctata;* rosinweed, *Grindelia squarrosa;* burdock, *Arctium lappa;* and jewelweed, *Impatiens capensis,* are some of the many other choices Indians use individually or in selected combinations to treat inflamed skin. In addition, the clear, colorless, jellylike exudations of cut grapevine, ground sassafras leaves, and fresh-cut cucumbers or aloe stalks also provide therapeutic relief for burns.

You can make antiseptic, soothing teas to dab or spray on burns from the leaves and roots of pearly everlasting, *Anaphalis margaritacea;* Indian strawberry, *Duchesnea indica;* clammy ground-cherry, *Physalis heterophylla;* heart-leaved four o'clock, *Mirabilis nyctaginea;* Labrador tea,

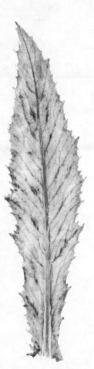

Fireweed or Pilewood
Erechtities hieracifolia

Field bindweed
Convolvulus arvensis

Ledum groenlandicaum; and northern white cedar, *Thuja occidentalis,* as well as red clover, *Trifolium pratense,* and prairie coneflower, *Echinacea angustifolia.* Teas made from the inner bark of certain plants are also used in similar fashion to treat burns. These included the tulip tree, *Liriodendron tulipifera;* white oak, *Quercus alba;* northern red oak, *Q. rubra;* American bittersweet, *Celastrus scandens;* beech, *Fagus grandifolia;* slippery elm, *Ulmus rubra;* and sassafras, *Sassafras albidum.* Various ointments, lotions, and skin conditioners can be readily made from these botanicals.

During adolescence, young people pay more careful attention to their appearance. Many American Indians consider grasses and herbs to be the "hair of Mother Earth," and so they turn to these select botanicals for their own hair care. In the Northeast, the fresh, three foot long, green blades of sweetgrass, *Hiërochloe odorata,* and sweet vernal grass, *Anthoxanthum odoratum,* are frequently braided into young men's and women's hair or worn as hair adornments. People steep the fresh or dried grass blades in light herbal teas and use them to wash and rinse their hair, or comb them through their hair daily for extra sheen and fragrance. Wherever it is found, the dried, strongly aromatic blades of sweet flag (calamus), *Acorus calamus,* which often reach one to four feet in length, are used similarly. In the past, because of their practical and ceremonial functions, these botanicals were valuable items that were traded with tribes who lived beyond their natural range.

Indians also esteemed the green fronds of certain native ferns, especially the maidenhair fern, *Adiantum pedatum,* and the Venus maidenhair fern, *A. capillus-veneris,* for hair treatments. Used to wash hair, the boiled fronds and roots of bracken or eagle fern, *Pteridium aquilinum,* promote lustrous growth. Dried fern fronds are sometimes crumbled over and under a person's sleeping place, especially where she lays her head, for hair care and because they possess some insecticidal properties. Some people insist that they also promote vivid dreams.

The roots of yucca, *Yucca glauca* and spp., contain soapy substances called saponins. Pounded and whipped in water, yucca can be used to treat dandruff and baldness. Yucca-root shampoos are also fine enough to be used for skin and clothing care.

Hedge bindweed
Convolvulus sepium

Red clover
Trifolium pratense

American bittersweet
Celastrus scandens

HAZEL LEAF BODY RUB AND EYEWASH

4 to 6 large leaves
    witch hazel or hazelnut,
    fresh or dried
1¹/2 quarts cool water

You can use this astringent tea, warm or cool, to clean your face, close skin pores, and tighten skin surfaces. It also adds shine and vigor to hair. Add 1 cup to a tub of warm water and soak in it for 20 minutes to relieve fatigue and sore muscles.

This tea also makes a good eyewash. Use it in a sterile eyecup to flush out impurities in your eyes. It also makes an excellent poultice for drawing out redness, calming itching and irritation, relieving eyestrain, and soothing the eyes. Apply it with a cotton ball or gauze compress, placed lightly over the closed eyelids for 10 to 20 minutes at a time. When using this astringent for the eyes, it is best to use fresh tea, and it will feel better if you refrigerate it first.

Crush the leaves and place them in a 2-quart pot. Pour in the water. Place the pot over medium heat and bring to a slow boil, then reduce the heat to a simmer. Stir the leaves and cover the pot. Allow it to simmer for 20 minutes. Remove from the heat and cool. Strain and use this astringent tea immediately, or bottle, label, and date it for future use. Refrigerate to reduce spoilage, but use it up within a week.

Witch hazel
Hamamelis virginiana

Since these plants are deciduous and their leaves are not available for six months of the year, you may want to freeze a supply of this useful herbal remedy. Pour the cool, fresh tea into ice cube trays and freeze overnight. Remove the ice cubes and place them in labeled snap-and-seal freezer bags; then return them to the freezer. You now have little cubes of relief for myriad future uses, especially for treating burns, heat rash, poison ivy, muscle spasms, and cooling off your face and neck on a hot summer day. Try using it on your arms and legs after strenuous activities. Simply take an herbal ice cube from the freezer and lightly rub it over the afflicted areas for a minute or two at a time, until the cube melts away. The intense cold helps to reduce swelling and calm pain. If it is too intense for sensitive skin, use a light touch—alternating a minute on and several minutes off—until you find your own tolerance level.

Hazelnut
Corylus americana

2¹/₂ ounces glycerine

5 ounces emulsifying wax or beeswax

2¹/₂ ounces distilled water

1 ounce dried marigold petals, pulverized

1 ounce dried calendula petals, pulverized

¹/₂ ounce dried mint or bergamot leaves, pulverized

Marigolds and calendula are two flowers long used in skin treatments. Marigolds are ancient natives of the desert Southwest and Mexico; the origins of calendula lie in the Mediterranean, but the flowers escaped to North America long ago. Both have mild pleasing fragrances and soothing mineral healing qualities. This cream is well absorbed into the skin; it is especially pleasant in the heat of summer.

Creams are usually composed and simmered in a double boiler for about three hours in order to create a fine emulsion.

Measure ingredients into the top of a double boiler. Heat at a low simmer, blending everything together.

At the end of the cooking time, pour the cream into a clean bowl. Stir or whip it continuously until it cools and sets. Spoon the cream into sterilized dark glass jars and label.

To counter mold growth or spoilage and extend the shelf life of the cream, you can add 4 drops of tincture of benzoin at the very end of the cooking process.

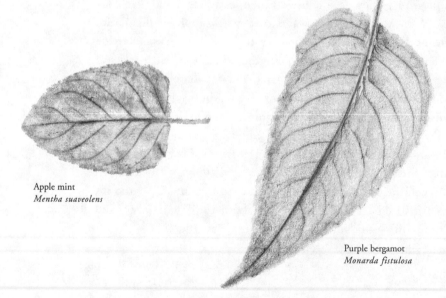

Apple mint
Mentha suaveolens

Purple bergamot
Monarda fistulosa

MARIGOLD-CALENDULA CORNSTARCH BODY TALC

Using the same herbs as in the previous recipe, you can make a remarkably soothing body talc.

Measure these ingredients into a sterile jar or bottle. Cap tightly and shake well; label and date. Keep this in the bath and use it as a choice dusting powder or carry it with you in your gym bag.

2 ounces each dried marigold petals, dried calendula petals, and dried bergamot leaves, pulverized

6 ounces cornstarch

BERGAMOT/MINT BREATH FRESHENER

As a quick and easy digestive aid and breath freshener, try slowly and thoroughly chewing a leaf or two of bergamot or other fresh mint leaves. You can also make one cup of mild mint tea with one cup of water and three leaves of your favorite mint. Use this as a mouth rinse, gargle, and throat spray.

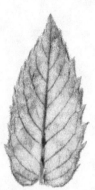

Spearmint
Mentha spicata

WHITE CEDAR SKIN SALVE

A salve sits on the skin surface and provides protective healing benefits. The cooling properties of white cedar are especially rich in minerals that calm burns or irritated skin.

Mix and heat the herbs, cocoa butter, and beeswax together in a small covered pot over low heat for two hours, stirring frequently. If desired, toward the very end add the honey and vitamin E.

Blend the mixture thoroughly and pour it into small containers or onto clean foil in little cookielike pools. Allow it to cool and become firm.

3 ounces powdered dried white cedar leaves

7 ounces cocoa butter or pure vegetable shortening

1 ounce beeswax (use more or less, depending upon the consistency desired)

1 ounce raw honey (optional)

2 or 3 drops vitamin E (optional)

CHAPTER FIVE

Adulthood

"LEAP OVER THE ADVERSARIES OF LIFE"

❖❖❖❖❖❖❖❖❖❖❖❖❖❖❖❖❖❖❖❖❖❖❖❖❖❖❖❖❖

Those who know how to play can easily leap over the adversaries of life. And one who knows how to sing and laugh never brews mischief.

—IGLUILIK (ESKIMO) SAYING

❖❖❖❖❖❖❖❖❖❖❖❖❖❖❖❖❖❖❖❖❖❖❖❖❖❖❖❖❖

Steeplebush, or hardhack
Spiraea tomentosa

Spreading dogbane
Apocynum androsaemifolium

By the time they enter adulthood, most American Indian men and women have a strong sense of their society's traditions and how they fit in. Many choose a life path based on their special talents, such as weaving or pottery. In some cases their roles are determined by their particular culture. For instance, the weavers of ceremonial textiles among the Hopi are men, while according to Navajo custom, this niche belongs to women.

For anyone choosing a path connected to healing, adulthood carries the weight of greater responsibilities. As they come of age, these individuals are considered more trustworthy, able to fully respect and guard many of the secrets of healing, which are only now shared with them. At this point in life, people take on full membership in healing sects or medicine societies and may begin to carry out healing rites.

Commitments to personal relationships also take center stage now. As they move out of adolescence, many individuals begin to think about finding partners and starting families. Not everyone pairs off; some people follow a vision that keeps them single. And others come to terms with their homosexuality, which dictates how their lives will proceed.

Young adults learn the behaviors that are accepted within their own societies, yet some feel pulled to live and express themselves differently. This has always been true. In earlier times gender roles were more sharply defined, especially among hunting and gathering and gardening groups. Commonly the men were the hunters and warriors, while women maintained, and in many societies owned, the gardens and homes. Men's and women's roles were clearly defined and reinforced in general practice and through stories, ceremonies, and certain rituals, such as puberty rites and vision quests.

But not all individuals followed the typical path. In many tribes a woman might choose to follow a warrior's role in order to avenge the killing of a male relative or other family members. Dressing and behaving

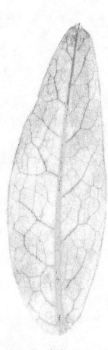

Spreading dogbane
Acocynum androsaemifolium

like a male warrior did not necessarily mean a gender change, but it might. Either way, her decision was generally honored.

A variety of American Indian words acknowledge the subtleties of gender. For example the Sioux term *winkte,* meaning "like a woman," often refers to a man who takes on some feminine roles, such as nurturing children, tanning hides, pottery making, and weaving; he may or may not be homosexual. Among the Mohave Indians in the Southwest, the term *hwame* refers to a lesbian who assumed male roles and married a woman. Perhaps the most familiar native term today is *berdache,* which can mean a male homosexual or a man or woman who dresses and acts like a member of the opposite sex. In contemporary societies, androgynous males and lesbians often refer to themselves as "two-spirited" people.

American Indians were usually tolerant of those who didn't fall into traditional marriage and family roles. Not only were adult homosexuals integrated into their communities, they were considered highly creative, courageous people who were respected for their differences and their determination to express them. Often artists, healers, or both were individuals who exhibited sexual preferences that we might label today as homosexual.

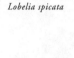

Blue lobelia
Lobelia spicata

Love Medicines

Faithfulness and love are highly valued in every culture. For those who do want to marry, love medicines often hold the key to success. Among many tribes, private rituals employing special plants, herb bundles, amulets, dolls, and personal items evolved to ensure these vital devotions. Some people thought that by using these "love medicines" they could manipulate the magical and spiritual elements of life to enhance the physical and natural. Herbalism mixed with creativity and imagination—as well as a degree of faith—added up to a potent formula for success.

The Iroquois use many plant and animal substances for love medicines and to divine future actions. Some plants are used as "confidence" medicines, or for the power of positive thinking to influence future events. Other herbs are key to "dreaming results" of one's love. To use them, a person places the plants—such as blue lobelia, *Lobelia spicata,* and other species of lobelia, especially Indian tobacco, *Lobelia inflata*—under her pillow before going to sleep.

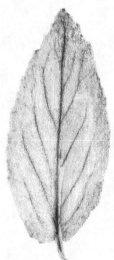

Lobelia
Lobelia inflata

One early-twentieth-century Cayuga method of divination used the roots of two separate plants of boneset, *Eupatorium perfoliatum,* which were held together to see if they would curl around each other. To strengthen this, each freshly dug root was named for the individual intended. If they did intertwine, the two roots were carefully wrapped in a small piece of red calico or red wool and tied securely with a piece of red string or ribbon. Red symbolizes blood, the heart, the sacred fire, and strength. It is often the primary color used to carry prayers to the Creator, and prayer bundles are usually tied in red cloth.

Thanks to its vivid magenta-red color, poke, *Phytolacca americana,* alone or in formula, is a powerful love medicine, as is cardinal flower, *Lobelia cardinalis,* and the halved root of the beautiful orange-red wood lily, *Lilium philadelphicum.* And one of native America's more ephemeral love medicines and good-luck charms is the great scented liverwort, *Marchantia polymorpha.* It may be chewed, sprinkled on articles, or drunk as a tea, in which case the drinker will be able to think only of the secret admirer who "doctored" their tea.

Other Iroquois love medicines, usually used alone, are the dried, powdered roots of knotweed, *Polygonum arenastrum,* and the "pitchers" of the pitcher plant, *Sarracenia purpurea.* Especially popular with men is pepper root, *Cardamine concatenata,* which is considered a "mesmerizing plant" for hunting, fishing, and, in this context, lovemaking success. Such special powers or behaviors are attached to many native plants. Decoctions of white avens, *Geum canadense;* American vetch, *Vicia americana;* partridgeberry, *Mitchella repens;* mountain honeysuckle, *Lonicera dioica;* moosewood, *Viburnum lantanoides;* and the great purple New England aster, *Aster novae-angliae,* are perennial love medicines known and used by many tribes.

Regardless of how they get together, a variety of beautiful wedding ceremonies helps the couple make their commitment to each other. These rituals hail the union of two people in marriage, blessing them with strength, long life, health, and fertility.

Boneset (cross-section)
Eupatorium perfoliatum

Southwestern Marriage Rites

Among the Hopi, Zuni, and other Pueblo tribes, marriage rites continue a tradition that embraces thousands of years of connections to the clouds and spirits, mountains, and other landscape features. These tribes literally wear and inhale their landscape: Its symbols are woven into and embroidered on their clothing and baskets and painted on their pottery and other ceremonial accouterments. The rites, which include families and extended families, focus on all of the key elements—nature, spirit, mind, and body. And in addition to blessing the couple with a good crop, children, and a long life together, wedding rituals also pay attention to the fertility of the village and its surroundings.

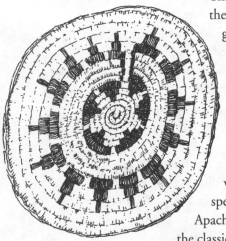

Navajo wedding basket of coiled yucca fiber

Sharing is the cornerstone of Pueblo life. Generations ago, in the days before the wedding feasts, a Hopi bride's family would gather their resources and grind as much as a thousand pounds of corn. Every clan sister and aunt helped as this joyous communal activity became a form of social glue binding them all together. Today the cooking and other preparations for weddings and feast days are still a huge responsibility. In many homes there are so many guests and visitors that they take turns and eat in shifts.

In some tribes people spend time creating ceremonial wedding items for the marriage rites. The wedding basket is a special, sacred item among basket-weaving tribes, especially the Apache, Navajo, and Paiute. There are traditional designs, such as the classic circle patterned with stars and points, as well as original designs that emerge from the weaver's own dreams and imagination.

The Navajo ritual wedding basket is pregnant with symbolism. The large, flat coiled tray is distinguished by dark, pointed, angular designs against its natural rim, encircling the center. The triangular designs are mountains and standing thunderclouds, interspersed with the deep valleys. As you hold it in your hands, its open form signifies the earth; inverted, it becomes the sky dome. A slender opening in the circle design signifies the east, the place of beginnings, sunrise, and power; in Navajo thought, it is the white eastern wind that directs life. This opening invites the power of the east to come into the lives of the newly married couple.

Using the sacred wedding basket during a Navajo wedding draws together real, ideal, and holy influences, confirming the bond of marriage as the couple stands together holding the basket between them. First corn pollen is sprinkled around the basket, blessing it, encircling it and marking the cardinal points with prayers. Then special corn batter is placed in the center. The couple feeds each other, eating from the unique corn preparation in a ritual signifying life, fertility, physical nourishment, strength, and spiritual rebirth. Because corn is life to the Navajo, this ceremony sets the couple on the Pollen Path, or the essential road of life, made holy by the fact that pollen is its symbol.

The joining of a man and woman in this moving wedding ritual reflects the union of the Navajo cosmos, which often appears in symbolic sand paintings that picture Earth Woman and Sky Man side by side. Earth Woman is blue and has the four sacred cultivated plants—corn, squash, beans, and tobacco—radiating out from the center of her abdomen. Sky Man has a black body with the sun, moon, and stars on his abdomen. A fine cord of pollen connects their mouths, indicating their fertility and inseparability. Because speech is so vital, these Holy People are said to speak "pollen words." The paired Holy People represent the unity of complementary energies that are both holy and infinite. This balance comes to people who follow the Pollen Path.

The Sun Dance

Along with marital and familial responsibilities, adults also assume ongoing duties connected to the well-being of their tribe and broader community. In many tribes people reaffirm their commitments each year in a major ritual, such as the Sun Dance of the Plains Indians.

This four-day-long ceremony of fasting, prayers, and dancing is principally a ritual of renewal, community strengthening, and giving to the Creator and to the tribe. Over time, as many tribes were dispersed, and especially today, when only half of American Indians live on their reservations, the Sun Dance has taken on even greater significance. Because it is vital to their own health and that of the community, many people worry that missing it will rob them of strength and wellness.

The vast regions of the Great Plains stretch from the Mississippi River Valley westward to the Rocky Mountains, and from the Canadian provinces of Alberta, Saskatchewan, and Manitoba southward into central Texas. More than twenty bands and tribes ranged across these grasslands, drawn by animal migrations and seasonal food sources. The Assiniboine, Arapaho, Arikara, Blackfeet, Blood, Cheyenne, Comanche, Cree, and Crow Indians dominated much of the central and high plains. The Dakota (Sioux), Hidatsa, Iowa, Oto, Missouri, Osage, Pawnee, Ponca,

At the center of the Earth
Stand looking around you.
Recognizing the tribe
Stand looking around you.

—*Song fragment from the
Lakota Sun Dance*

Mandan, Kiowa, Caddo, Apache, Kansas, Quapaw, and Witchita are also peoples of the Great Plains.

These Plains Indian tribes, with their vast herds of bison, mounted warriors who were superb horsemen with legendary courage, dramatic circles of tipi camps thriving with village life, and women in fringed buckskins with babies snugly fastened in ornate cradleboards, epitomize the "wild west" and the American frontier. Each tribe spoke a different language and had its own unique customs and healing traditions. Most hunted the bison because it provided substantial food, clothing, fuel, shelter materials, and spiritual sustenance.

The Sun Dance evolved out of ancient ceremonies and flourished in the 1800s during the golden age of Plains Indians life. For some tribes it was the only time of the year when all of their people gathered at the same place. Traditionally, the ripening of the Saskatoon berries is the signal to come together for this important ritual. The berries, *Amelanchier alnifolia,* are also called shadblow, juneberry, and serviceberry (and have many other regional common names). These graceful shrubs and small trees can grow up to twenty feet tall. They are one of the earliest native wildflowers to bloom in spring. Profuse, delicate white blooms often yield abundant midsummer crops of dark blue or purple berries that are favored by wildlife.

When the berries were ripe, Indian hunting parties would scout the Saskatoon groves for elk, deer, moose, mountain sheep, and bear, as well as game birds and smaller animals. Frequently there were also communal buffalo hunts to provide the necessary meat for the gatherings, especially the bulls' tongues, which were valued ceremonial offerings.

Although the elaborate ceremonies vary from tribe to tribe across the Great Plains, they all center on sacrifice and self-denial among adult men and women. Some tribal members make a flesh offering at the Sun Dance, and each year, following the original practice, both men and women are pierced or have their chest or back skin slit and tied with a dance cord and prayer bundles. Other participants make different sacrifices, giving up something from their lives to the Creator, especially so that a loved one might be healed.

American Indians have always used sacrifice, accompanied by ritual and prayer, to honor the sacred in their lives. Giving up something, every day or periodically, enhances everything connected to wellness and balance. Sacrificing food and water, fasting for a vision or to honor an ill loved one who is unable to fast or participate in rigorous activities, cutting one's hair in grief—each of these actions is a gift of one's strength. Sacrifice is an ancient aspect of prayer and commitment to the Creator in all traditions. Many Christians and Jews observe this custom when they give up something for Lent or do without bread for Passover.

But in the late 1800s the U.S. government took a dim view of the Sun Dance. Because the ceremony was not understood, it was perceived as a security threat. The authorities pointedly discouraged and ultimately outlawed it, along with the mystical Ghost Dance religion. In its place, Christian missionaries set up churches and schools on the reservations. As a result, many Indians converted to Christianity, which eroded a number of their most important traditions.

Despite its prohibition, many tribes never stopped practicing the Sun Dance. Today, there is a revival of interest in its galvanizing ceremonies, which draw ever larger numbers of Plains Indian people to their reservations every year. The rituals bind their loosely organized tribal bands together and strengthen time-honored traditions. The rites of sacrifice, prayers, and honoring touch both participants and observers in many ways. Wendell Deer With Horns, Cheyenne River Lakota (Sioux), a member of the Two Kettles Band (Oonenunpa), returns to his reservation each summer for the traditional Sun Dance. "As a father and an uncle, I need to remember all the good things of childhood," he reflects. "I have learned that the Creator tests us all in many ways. Perhaps that is how we find out who we are."

Medicine Lodge and Spirit Lodge are also names given to the Sun Dance and to certain aspects of the Sun Dance by some of the Plains Indians. Each tribe celebrates these rites in its own way, but everything is geared toward giving as the people dance around the sacred Sun Dance pole each day and offer their best energies and prayers to the Creator.

American Indian spirituality also attracts many non-native people who find solace and balance in the reverence for earth and respect for all life that is part of native religious traditions. Many of them are drawn to the Sun Dance and its sacred rituals as they examine ways to integrate these beliefs into the fabric of their own personal faith. Although most of these rites are private, some tribes allow the public or invited friends to attend.

The Powwow

Powwow is one of the earliest Algonquian Indian words recorded in the Northeast. Its early meanings were understood to be "medicine man," "conjurer," "ceremonialist," or someone who divines the future, according to seventeenth-century European interpretations. *Powwow* generally referred to a spiritual leader or healer who served to maintain balance and integrity in Algonquian Indian societies in the early 1600s, and probably far earlier.

Powwow could also refer to a special place of healing power, like a giant boulder, a high knoll, or other sacred place where people gathered for ceremonial rites, established strong alliances, or held healing rituals.

Today, the word *powwow* (or *pow wow*) has come through centuries of use to mean big commercial events held by many different tribes throughout the calendar year. They are opportunities for people from many tribes and countries to gather for visiting, trading, swapping gossip, and especially music and dance.

The circle is sacred, and most powwows are set up around a central fire, enclosing the dance circle. Dancing is a major event, and prize money may be given for the best drums and the best dancers.

Powwows have spread far and wide. At any given time, there is probably a powwow taking place somewhere in this country. Many Indians earn a living by dancing, drumming, singing, and selling art work on the "Powwow Highway," planning their year to take them from one powwow to the next.

And many would say that the powwow continues to offer healing, although perhaps in a more subtle way. At powwows, native people reconnect with old friends, mend relationships, and reaffirm their commitment to tribal traditions.

The word *powwow* has also been adapted to modern-day use. When corporate or military people need to plan a special meeting, they often call for a "powwow," where they can discuss their next course of action. But their use of the word is actually quite close to its original Indian definition.

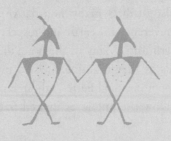

Journey to the Medicine Wheel

The Sun Dance is one of the biggest and most important events during a tribe's ceremonial year. But sometimes individuals need to make special pilgrimages to holy places to renew their spirits, seek divine help in dealing with health problems and life-threatening illness, or to ask for help for another's plight.

For many Plains Indians, respecting the sacred circle of life meant a periodic journey to one of the medicine wheels. These were places of great power and healing energies, where people went to pray, dream, seek visions, and make offerings.

Medicine wheels are made from natural stone. They have a central circle or cairn from which lines of stones radiate outward to a greater enclosing circle, which can be thirty feet in diameter. Medicine wheels made during historic times usually have four main spokes of stones radiating outward, perhaps marking the cardinal directions. Prehistoric examples often have five or more spokes of stones radiating from the central cairn to the outer circle of stones. Most are located in prominent topographic positions.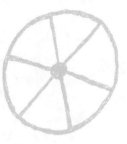

More than sixty-seven different medicine wheels have been found across the northern Plains, including a number in southwestern Canada. They reflect a broad diversity of forms. Limited excavation at some of these sites indicates that they were built over a long period of time, paralleling the prehistoric dates for England's Stonehenge.

Perhaps the most famous is the Bighorn Medicine Wheel, located high in the Bighorns, also called the Shining Mountains, on an alpine plateau known as Medicine Mountain. From here you can look out across hundreds of miles of rolling hills and broad prairies cut by lush valleys and rivers. This immense circle of stones is more than seventy feet in diameter, with twenty-eight spokes radiating from its twelve-foot stone cairn center. Close to the Crow Nation in southeastern Montana, the Bighorn Medicine Wheel is considered a holy site central to Plains Indians' religious needs.

Medicine wheels are strongly associated with many tribes' creation stories. They are respected, like cathedrals, and believed to be the residences of special spirits who can work directly with the higher world. Plains Indians take their sacred medicine bundles and arrows as well as other sensitive ceremonial accouterments to the medicine wheel to be blessed and renewed. As they perform their ceremonial tasks, pray, and make their prayer offerings, people experience healing and renewal themselves.

Many people create beautiful prayer sticks and feathered wands to leave, along with prayers and other offerings, at the medicine wheel. If you visit one of these places, you may see tiny red or flannel tobacco ties and herb bundles tied to fences, shrubs, or tree branches, or fastened to sticks stuck in the ground. To avoid harm, it is important not to touch or remove these items.

People often travel many days and miles to reach one of their holy sites. Some individuals get to a medicine wheel only once in a lifetime. Plants and substances gathered during these trips have enhanced value, especially the various minerals and pigments used in healing formulas and ceremonies. Unfortunately, American Indians have been enmeshed in decades of legal wrangling as they seek to have their sacred sites protected so they can remain free and accessible for private use.

The Green Corn Ceremonies
and Stomp Dances

Creek, Cherokee, and Seminole tribe members reaffirm the commitments that bind their communities together at the Green Corn Ceremonies and Stomp Dances. As with the Sun Dance, growing numbers of people return to their reservations from all over the country for these annual rituals of purification and forgiveness. Although many of them are Christians, they continue to observe their ancient customs as well. And as interest in the sustaining value of these events has grown, so too has respect for traditional foods and medicines.

Descendants of the prehistoric Temple Mound Builders in the southeast, the Creek lived in villages along the rivers throughout their extensive territories. Although there were many different bands and groups, the early traders and explorers gave them the name "Creeks" because of their settlement patterns. Many of these tribal groups organized themselves into the Creek Confederacy in the 1700s.

The Seminole were primarily Creeks who migrated farther south during the settlement pressures and upheavals of the 1800s. Their name means "runaway" or "those who camp away from the regular towns."

The Jingle Dress Dance

The Jingle Dress Dance is an extraordinary expression of beauty that is performed today at many powwows. The story of its origin comes from the Mille Lacs Band of the Ojibway tribe.

Long ago, a man from this tribe journeyed to Canada to seek help from the medicine men for his only child, who was very ill and near death. While he was there, sacred spirits came to him in a vision. They told him to go back to Mille Lacs and have the Ogitchiedahquay women sew a special ceremonial dress for his daughter. The spirits gave him instructions for making the dress, which was originally made from the cast-off lids of tobacco cans. Anemone, a Narragansett woman from Rhode Island and a contemporary Jingle Dress dancer, explains that there were 365 jingles, each representing a day of the year.

The spirits also gave the man several songs to accompany the dress and told him how his daughter should dance while wearing it. When his daughter danced in the sacred Jingle Dress, she was cured of her illness, which is why the Jingle Dress is considered a healing dress.

Their proud history records successive waves of migration, persecution, forced removal, and, most of all, endurance. Along with their close relatives the Miccosukees, they have five reservations today in southern Florida, along with significant settlements in Texas and a nation capital in Oklahoma.

Seminole clan names—Alligator, Bird, Deer, Fish, Sweet Potato, Panther, Turtle, and Wind—originate in their primal environments in the Florida Everglades. Because of the way their tribe is scattered in villages, settlements, and reservations around the country, closeness with the earth and its seasonal rhythms helps to center the Seminole, keeping them aware of who they are and where they came from. Their ceremonies, like those of the Green Corn, are closely tied to natural observations.

The Green Corn Ceremony was one of the most important rituals celebrated by American Indians of the South; for many agricultural tribes, it was the turning point of their year. Near the end of summer, when the last corn crop was ripe, villagers prepared for the four- or eight-day ritual, which was often called the Busk, from the Creek word *boskita*, meaning "to fast." People repaired and cleaned their homes, the ceremonial grounds, and everything possible. Renewal and forgiveness were, and continue to be, the touchstones of the Green Corn rites.

Once everything was ready, people extinguished all hearth fires in their villages. Important leaders and medicine people drank decoctions of purifying herbs, primarily the Black Drink, which they prepared from the leaves of a native holly, *Ilex vomitoria*.

To honor the supernatural forces, fasting and praying followed for several days. Afterward, every family received coals from the sacred fire, usually located in the center of the village, to rekindle their hearth fires. Now, since everything and everyone had been ritually purified, it was possible to eat the ripening corn crop. The entire village gathered for a feast of many corn dishes, venison, and wild green onions. There were ceremonial games of lacrosse, running games, archery contests, and hand games, followed by dancing.

Everyone bathed in the nearby river for purification, then dressed for the Green Corn Dance, which celebrated the new year. Taking part gave people a fresh start where all was forgiven, except for serious crimes. Today contemporary rituals continue to follow these ancient practices.

Treating Disease: The Navajo Night Way

There is a downside to adulthood: As people grow older, they get ill. According to current statistics, nearly half of the U.S. population suffers from some form of chronic illness, such as diabetes, arthritis, heart disease, or alcoholism. Among many American Indian tribes, rates are even higher. Many native people choose to go through healing rites, either alone or in addition to conventional medical treatment. These rituals may be quite complex. Certainly among the most amazing and lengthy—lasting as many as nine days and nights—is the Navajo Night Way.

Transformation and restoring healing balance are central to the Night Way. These great ritual dramas draw together the Holy People and the earth-surface people along with crowds of onlookers by the last night. The nine days and nights of the Night Way become an initiation into the chantway path through life for Navajo and other participants.

The long nights and short days of winter are the time when these complex rituals are performed for patients who suffer from paralysis, epilepsy, arthritis, or from loss of hearing or vision problems. Other sensory disorders and ailments of the nervous system may also be treated in a

The ceremony has a lot to do with purification of the patient. Chanters say, "If you haven't been purified—cleanliness inside and out—the Holy People won't come near you."

—*A Night Way Chanter*

Night Way, after the patient or family seeks the help of a diviner who diagnoses the problem and determines the proper rite(s) for treatment.

Illness and disorders are considered far more than mere organic or physical manifestations. An individual's body, mind, and spirit must be realigned for true healing to occur.

The Night Way is a costly undertaking, and its complicated details require months of careful planning. Hundreds of people come to support these elaborate rites, and they all must be fed and cared for. It is often more than one patient, or the "one-sung-over," can afford, so several patients, along with their families and friends, pool resources and share the massive obligations.

The chanter who will conduct the Night Way directs the sand painters to work out the complex series of vital sand paintings of the *yeis*—the guiding deities, or Holy People—that will be used over the course of the Night Way. The rites are determined by the number of nights prescribed to work the healing transformations.

Besides the sand paintings, there are *yei* impersonators, dancers wearing ornate buckskin masks, whose bodies are painted with white clay and decorated with animal fur and sacred herbs. Other dancers, their bodies also adorned with white clay, wear simple buckskin masks topped with eagle feathers; they represent the four directional Thunderers. Their presence brings in the sky energies: dark cloud, lightning, rain, and wind. The Thunderers sing of the cosmos and the relationships between earth and sky.

The Night Way's prayer of transformation, sung on the first night of the rites, speaks of the glorious details of the one-sung-over's restoration and transformation into beauty. The ceremonies continue with night feasts, prayers, chants and sand paintings, herbal infusions, sweat baths, and offerings. Events culminate on the last night with the great public Yeibichei Dance. Yeibichei is Grandfather of the Gods, Talking God. His appearance signifies the final night of the Night Way, where teams of spectacular masked dancers sing and dance all night until the dawn.

All who attend are encouraged to believe that the real and the ideal will mesh, and that one can achieve a holy state by living the Beauty Way. The Night Way is a major journey to fuller empowerment and restored health. It often brings considerable improvement or even full recovery to the one-sung-over.

In the house made of dawn,
In the house made of
  evening twilight,
In the house made of
  dark cloud,
In the house made of
  he-rain,
In the house made of
  dark mist,
In the house made of
  she-rain,
In the house made of
  pollen,
In the house made of
  grasshoppers,
Where the dark mist
  curtains the doorway,
The path to which is on
  the rainbow,
Where the zigzag lightning
  stands high on top,
Where the he-rain stands
  high on top.
Happily I walk.
Impervious to pain, I walk.
Feeling light within, I walk.
With lively feelings, I walk.

—*Fragment from*
a Night Way prayer

Oto Peyote Ceremony
and the Peyote Spirit

Peyote became popular as a recreational, hallucinogenic drug among the "youth culture" of the 1960s and 1970s. But among certain American Indian tribes, peyote has long been a revered part of healing and religious rituals.

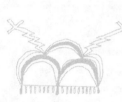

Peyote, *Lophophora williamsii* var. *Lemaire,* is a pale gray-green spineless cactus native to Texas and southern New Mexico and areas southward along the Rio Grande Valley in Mexico. This buttonlike cactus grows barely an inch or so above the ground and has a long carrotlike taproot. The name *peyote* comes from the Aztec word *peyotl,* and it was used by the Aztec and perhaps other earlier peoples in Mexico for many centuries. The surviving Aztec Codices, the earliest books of their religious practices, detail the uses of peyote as it was consumed by the priests and offered to the deities in their temples. At least five centuries of religious and cultural uses have been documented in Mexico and the desert Southwest, and it has spread selectively northward through Indian America.

Peyotism refers to the earliest use of this small native cactus for diverse medicinal, ceremonial, and ritual purposes. People chewed small pieces of peyote, called mescal buttons, to enhance their visions and spiritual experiences. The early use of peyote enhanced tribal rites of dancing and singing because it supported greater endurance.

Of the more than fifty alkaloids in peyote, the most active is mescaline, which is a drug that can alter the mind in both positive and negative ways. Most people who use peyote experience feelings of exaltation and spiritual awareness. Many individuals believe that it deepens their insights into the world around them and gives them a clearer sense of themselves. Many of those who practice peyotism experience color visions and hear special voices and singing. Because of its ability to increase endurance, native midwives have long used peyote during childbirth to ease delivery and relieve the birth mother's anxieties.

During the late 1800s a new movement toward religious use and contemplation evolved; this came to be called peyote religion. Perhaps the earliest tribes to use and adopt the peyote religion, sometime before 1890, were the Lipan Apache, the Kiowa, and the Comanche of the southern prairie.

The late nineteenth century was a cataclysmic period of change for the Plains Indians. Following the suppression of the Ghost Dance religion during this period, the peyote religion became a pathway toward greater peace and understanding among all people. Gradually this developed into the Native American Church, which was incorporated in 1918. Peyote is considered a sacrament in this church. Those members who follow it travel the "peyote road." A "road man," with knowledge of the songs and protocol, is the leader of the peyote rites. The Peyote Spirit Ceremony is said to be very powerful in working for peace and deeper understanding. The Oto Peyote Ceremony and the Peyote Spirit are vital healing and praying occasions; they may be planned and held anytime a pressing need is felt.

Originally people of the Great Lakes regions, the Oto once lived among the Winnebago, Iowa, and Missouri tribes, until they migrated toward the Southwest. Legends say that the tribes split from each other during periods of great change. A final historical rupture occurred, some say, when two chiefs quarreled over the seduction of one's daughter by the other's son. One band splintered away as the Missouri, while the other traveled into distant territory as the Oto. For hundreds of years some of these prairie peoples lived in permanent farming villages, and many adapted to the tipi-living, seasonal hunting lifeways of the Plains tribes. Settlement pressures during the past 160 years forced them away from their lands in Nebraska, Missouri, and Iowa, and today the Oto and Missouri have joined together as the Otoe-Missouria tribe, sharing trust lands together near Pawnee, Oklahoma.

To conduct the Peyote Ceremony, the Oto set up a ceremonial tipi with a central fire and crescent mound, as they have done for more than a hundred years. Perhaps a dozen people sit around the fire and give a tobacco offering while they pray to God. Some may smoke a cigarette, while others offer a pinch of tobacco. The placement and use of the peyote within the ceremony is usually planned by the road man who leads these activities. A particularly large peyote button is placed on the west side of the altar in the very beginning to honor the peyote spirit. Then the peyote is passed around and everyone takes a piece to chew, contemplate, and swallow. The road man begins singing and drumming. Gourd rattles keep a certain rhythm with the music as people sing song cycles and pray. Peyote is passed again, and participants may take as much as they want. Many of these ceremonies begin at sundown and last until dawn, as people pray and sing, intently focused on the visions and healing. Traditional foods and water are served at intervals throughout the latter part of the ceremony. The effects of peyote wear off within twenty-four hours and leave no harmful aftereffects; nor is it habit-forming.

Humor

Despite or perhaps because of their participation in serious and highly respected healing rituals, humor is an important aspect of life for all adults. And some individuals become clowns.

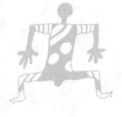

Because many American Indians believe that too much seriousness can lead to imbalance, visible, even slapstick, humor is a thread that runs through most of their cultures. As Sioux holy man Lame Deer explains, "A clown in our language is called a *heyoka*. He is upside-down, backward-forward, yes-and-no man, contrariwise . . . All you have to do is dream about the lightning, the thunderbirds . . . you are a *heyoka*."

Sacred clowns societies and fools societies are found in many tribes. Their members are among the most mystical and sacred of all practitioners because of their essential role in maintaining everyone's equilibrium.

These are the people who sing one or two beats behind. They dance out of step and out of order with the others, mimicking ceremonial procedures and taunting respected protocol. They are chosen characters in a class of their own, and they attract attention with their every motion. They are both wise and innocent, dressed ridiculously or else naked from head to toe, their bodies smeared all over with mud or colored with dark stripes. They paint their faces with freakish features or cover them with a fool's mask. With their clumsiness and outrageous conduct, they remind us of our worst traits and force us to examine our own behaviors.

Clowns use their antics to release the tension among the crowds of onlookers at ceremonial events, but they are also the guardians of rituals in many medicine societies. Black Elk, the Oglala Lakota medicine man and holy man, explained the role of the clown: "The *heyoka* presents the truth of his vision through comic actions, the idea being that the people should be put in a happy, jolly frame of mind before the truth is presented."

Most American Indian cultures have their own fools, who are key characters in sacred ceremonies. The Pueblos have Summer Clowns and Winter Clowns, who are mediators for the life-giving rain of the Southwest, and who are important in the origin story of the people's emergence into this world. Other Pueblo clowns play similar roles: the Acoma and Zia have their Koshare and Kwiraina Clowns; the Hopi have the White Cloud Clowns and the Mudheads; and among the Zuni are the Koyemshi and Newekwe Clowns.

Similar clowning traditions exist in other parts of the country. The Navajo have the Mud Clowns and the Water Sprinkler. The Blue Jay Clowns dash about acting crazy during serious rituals of the Gros Ventres, Spokane, and Sanpoiel tribes of the Plateau region. And on the Northwest Coast, the wild Kwakiutl Noo'nlemala, or Fool Dancers, stir things up during the Cedar Bark Dances of the Winter Ceremonies.

These dynamic individuals affect everything that goes on during the rituals. With their outlandish and sometimes aggravating disruptions, they bring in an element of confusion, making it impossible for people to remain passive. In the midst of highly solemn rites, they strut about, taunting serious beliefs. But at the same time their behavior is oddly reassuring, because the enduring authority of the ceremonies is strong enough to overpower their antics.

Clowns aren't always humorous. The awesome, masked Apache Crown Dancers, or personators of the Mountain Gods, posture and sway around the ceremonial fire, brandishing their lightning swords in each hand. The Apache Mountain Gods govern the winds, weather, and healing when they dance for their people. They perform during the sacred puberty rites of the Apache maidens, bringing good health as they drive away sickness and evil. Each team of black-hooded dancers is followed by one or more white-hooded clowns who represent innocence and purity. It is these little clowns who carry the wisdom of the healing medicines. They dance to the throbbing drums and the old traditional chants as the energies build throughout the night.

In some tribes, being the fool can be onerous. Clowns often bear the difficult task of defusing tensions or problems at a large gathering. And their roles are sometimes physically hazardous. The Cheyenne Contrary Society members were originally noted warriors who lived separate lives of sacrifice. Their backward and contrary actions often place them at great risk of personal harm. They do ridiculous things, like going down a ladder upside down or riding a horse backward. Through their wrong behavior they show people what not to mimic, but they are respected and powerful individuals.

The role of the fool is usually carried out with great pride because the clown helps lighten the people's burdens. And clowns are often far more than jokesters; they are potent healers in many societies. They frequently have special abilities to cure many health and spiritual disorders. Traditional followers who do not want to go to the medicine man or shaman with their problems often seek healing from a clown.

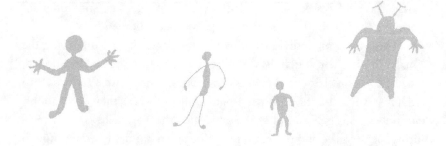

EARTH REMEDIES

Native men and women held great respect for life, and especially for their children, who represented the tribe's continuing survival. To best sustain them, many tribes developed various practices to limit family size. The diversity and sophistication of American Indian contraceptives have long fascinated observers, and we have learned a great deal from their practices. Native contraceptive herbs have been the basis for the development of modern oral contraceptives. Some of these plant extracts terminate the normal estrous cycle, can decrease the weight of the sex organs, and affect other glands' size and function. Scientists studying birth control in the early 1950s actually suggested PPUs, or "Papoose Preventative Units" as a standard measure of effectiveness. (**Caution: Many of the herbal remedies used were and are highly toxic.**)

Many of the key contraceptive herbs were called squaw root or papoose root. These names gave special distinction to their contraceptive energies, since some of these perennial herbs have numerous other properties, applications, and regional names. Both men and women regularly drank small amounts of tea made from the boiled or chewed roots of dogbane, *Apocynum androsaemifolium;* milkweed, *Asclepias syriaca* and other species; wild ginger, *Asarum canadense;* stoneseed, *Lithospermum ruderale;* or antelope sage, *Eriogonum jamesii.* **Note: Both milkweed and dogbane are extremely toxic and not recommended for self-medication.**

The roots and herbal parts of yarrow, *Achillea millefolium,* were brewed into strong contraceptive teas, as were the leaves and roots of false Solomon's seal, *Smilacina racemosa;* and water hemlock, *Cicuta maculata;* the entire plant of poison hemlock, *Conium maculatum;* the leaves and bulbs of trout lily, *Erythronium americanum;* and Indian paintbrush, *Castilleja linariae;* and the seeds and roots of Queen Anne's lace, *Daucus carota.*

Perhaps one of the most valuable herbs in modern medicine is the common twining perennial vine wild yam, *Dioscorea villosa.* Diosgenin from this plant is used to manufacture progesterone and other steroid drugs used to treat asthma and eczema, regulate metabolism, and control fertility. Synthetic products created from this plant's alkaloids effectively

Common milkweed
Asclepias syriaca

Solomon's plume, or
false Solomon's seal
Smilacina racemosa

treat many other diseases and common ailments and provide our modern contraceptives.

Gossypol, an extract from the seeds of cotton, *Gossypium hirsutum,* has been synthesized into a male contraceptive that is used in China today. Many of our southern Indian tribes knew and used cotton seeds and cotton root in similar ways centuries ago.

When all else failed, cases of infanticide and abortion were known to occur among some tribal peoples. These were largely due to the fear of poverty, inability to support a larger family, or the shame or fear of unmarried women. An infant was sometimes killed if it was deformed or suspected to be "not right," or if the father was non-Indian.

Naturally, physical and mental well-being encompass far more than an individual's sexual and reproductive life. One of the many benefits of adulthood is the growing awareness of the many dimensions in our lives. But as we age, we discover that there are more ailments—physical, emotional, and spiritual—that can befall us. Maintaining balance becomes more challenging, and dealing with various health problems can be a commanding focus. Thankfully, American Indian healers were wise in the ways of prevention.

Today interest in native immune-enhancing herbs, some of which have been used for centuries, is creating multibillion-dollar industries. Our most famous are the stunning perennial prairie coneflowers, *Echinacea angustifolia, E. purpurea,* and *E. pallida.* Plains Indians used these rugged plants as vegetables, symbolic and ceremonial foods, and for countless medicinal needs. The roots were chewed for toothache relief and made into poultices for burns, wounds, tumors, and snake and insect bites.

Echinacea products are used to treat a broad range of human needs. Teas, extracts, and tinctures from its taproots are extensively used in many preparations. Echinacea is also made into creams, ointments, salves, sprays, and lozenges, and its seeds are eaten for food and processed for their valuable oils.

Root-bark teas and the oil from the seeds and fruits of black currant, *Ribes americanum,* enhance immune function and treat kidney ailments. Root teas and tinctures of wild quinine, *Parthenium integrifolium,* and of boneset, *Eupatorium perfoliatum,* stimulate the immune system, and their leaves can also be poulticed on tumors and burns. The same is true for an-

Queen Anne's lace, or wild carrot
Daucus carota

other *Eupatorium,* joe-pye weed, *E. maculatum* and *E. purpureum.* Root teas and extracts of wild indigo, *Baptisia tinctoria* and *B. leucophaea,* and of blue false indigo, *B. australis,* also boost the immune system, but they must be used with caution since they can be toxic.

Root teas, extracts, and tinctures of yellow root, *Xanthorhiza simplicissima,* help lower blood pressure, treat some forms of diabetes, and stimulate the immune system. This plant has also been used as a treatment for skin cancers and a liver tonic among some tribes.

People often wish they had more energy in order to better accomplish certain tasks. Basically, a good, well-balanced diet is the best investment you can make for optimum energy. But there are a few additional supplements that may help. Be sure not to push your body beyond its natural capacity to function, or fatigue and burnout will result.

Although it was once considered an aphrodisiac, many people today take American ginseng, *Panax quinquefolius,* as a tonic and stimulant that enables them to maintain a general feeling of well-being. The dried roots are chewed, tinctured, or powdered for capsules, teas, and other health beverages. These products are used as gentle restoratives and preventives to better deal with stress and anxieties. Many athletes and corporate executives take ginseng supplements regularly so that they can maintain peak performance.

Today our native ginseng is rarely found growing in the wild. Instead, it is a valuable shade-grown crop farmed in more than six states, and on various Indian lands and reservations, where it is a profitable business. Much of it is sold in Asia.

An ancient Mayan energy food still sought after today is the blue-green algae spirulina. Species of this single-cell vegetable are grown from the tropics of Mexico and the Caribbean to the alpine lakes in the Northwest Coast regions. Spirulina is marketed in numerous health food preparations. The early Maya peoples in Mesoamerica dried their blue-green algae in the sun, then mixed it with wild raw honey and cornmeal into ceremonial cakes. Spirulina health shakes and energy bars are delicious modern variations of this early native ceremonial food.

The early Maya collected wild honey long before European honeybees were imported. Spanish

Purple coneflower
Echinacea purpurea

Spotted joe-pye weed
Eupatorium maculatum

explorers and priests noted that the Maya had numerous beehives in their fruit groves, from which they brought quantities of fine white honey in large gourds. Through the ages, honey has been used to enhance and sweeten other energy foods as well as to moisturize and soothe the skin.

Many other vitamin and mineral-rich supplements come from our native plants, and many more are formulated today with choice herbs and fungi from India, Africa, Asia, and Europe. Perhaps one of the more unique is the ling chih, or reishi, *Ganoderma lucidum,* an attractive, corky fungus known to the ancient Chinese as the "herb of spiritual potency" or the "mushroom of immortality." This nonedible, fibrous fungus is tinctured and formulated with licorice root, *Glycyrrhiza glabra;* ashwagandha root, *Withania somnifera;* and kava kava, *Piper methysticum,* to make a valuable rejuvenating tonic that you can use when you feel stressed out or depleted.

If the responsibilities of adulthood threatened to become overwhelming, native healers used, either alone or in formulas, mushrooms, cacti, and herbs that had mood-enhancing and relaxing capabilities. Today we have inherited an extensive array of natural remedies that can be used to find greater peace and balance, relieve stress, and reduce anxiety. It is vital to seek trusted professional advice about which of these treatments to use, in what strength, and with what frequency, so that they can best suit your particular needs.

One of the most valuable herbal sedatives and antidepressants extensively used today is St. John's wort, *Hypericum perforatum,* whose fresh flowers are favored in teas and tinctures. Long used by Indians and Europeans to treat myriad internal and external problems, St. John's wort is used, especially in Germany, to elevate mood, relieve anxiety, and promote sleep. And in controlled clinical trials, preparations of St. John's wort have been shown to be more effective than placebos and as effective as conventional antidepressants. St. John's wort flowers in corn, sunflower seed, or olive oil provide a great pain-relieving massage oil that is especially good for treating nerve pain, sciatica, and muscle spasms. One slight drawback is that the plant's compound, hypericin, can cause skin photosensitivity in some people.

Another herb with a long history as a tranquilizer and sleep aid is valerian, *Valeriana officinalis* and *V. sitchensis.* Clinical studies have also demonstrated its effectiveness. Root and blossom teas, extracts, and root

Herbs to Alter Mood

Native people knew and used various herbs to alter moods, much as we do today, from tobacco to ephedra, sage, yarrow, morning glory, and various hallucinogenic mushrooms. Some were natural remedies for anxieties and depression, like St. John's wort. Others were considered the "flesh of the gods," enabling those who ingested them to make spiritual journeys into other realms of knowing and divining information about curing illness.

The unique fungi in the genus Psilocybe are among those considered "flesh of the gods." This group of little gilled mushrooms can often be found on lawns, although very few of them are hallucinogenic. Some, when eaten, may cause transient changes in vision and in one's sense of time and space. It is important not to experiment with anything you are unsure of. And never eat any mushroom you cannot positively identify as safe.

tinctures of this herb are valued sedatives; they also relieve headache and depression for many users.

You can brew the roots and fruits of passionflower, *Passiflora incarnata,* for a relaxing tea. Tinctures of the roots of black cohosh, *Cimicifuga racemosa,* are sedative and anti-inflammatory, as are several mints, especially bugleweed, *Lycopus virginicus,* and catnip, *Nepeta cataria.* The leaves and flowers of rabbit tobacco, or sweet everlasting, *Gnaphalium obtusifolium,* are valued sedatives when chewed or taken as a tea; they also provide asthma and flu relief. You can also drink a mild tea of feverfew, *Chrysanthemum parthenium,* as an analgesic and sedative.

Two of our native orchids, yellow lady's slipper, *Cypripedium calceolus,* and the pink moccasin flower, *C. acaule,* are noted sedatives and antidepressants. These stunning wild flowers are avidly cultivated for their beauty as well as herbal virtues. Their blossoms, seeds, and bulbs are all valued medicinally. Unfortunately, they are on the environmental protection list in most states. At least in the Northeast, this is due in large part to extensive deer predation, which has almost exterminated them from many natural areas. The *Cypripediums* are valuable nervines, with good tonic effects on the nervous system and digestive tract.

People drink the root tea of elecampane, *Inula helenium,* for its sedative effects, and apply it externally as a fungicide. This trusted anti-inflammatory also calms facial neuralgia. The sticky flowers of gumweed, *Grindelia squarrosa*, can be used to make a medicinal tea with sedative value. Each of these herbal teas also helps to relieve rheumatism and asthma. Herbal tea made from wild lettuce, *Lactuca canadensis*, and related species can calm the nerves, relieve pain, and sedate, but these bitter herbs can cause dermatitis in some people.

Wild lettuce
Lactuca biennis

The flower teas and tinctures of red clover, *Trifolium pratense*, are mild, calcium-rich sedatives, which also provide some antidiabetic and anti-AIDS activity. Herbal teas and tinctures of skullcap, *Scutellaria lateriflora*, are valuable sedatives that help relieve anxiety and insomnia. Also the teas and tinctures of the dried fruits (strobiles) of hops, *Humulus lupulus*, are sedative; they provide beneficial relief for rheumatism, cramps, and insomnia.

Leaf teas and root tinctures of New Jersey tea, or red root, *Ceanothus americanus*, are valuable sedative and tonic treatments, as well as trusted lymphatic cleansers. Bark teas and tinctures of catalpa, *Catalpa bignonioides*, provide sedative and antiseptic value. Their large, heart-shaped leaves are also valuable wound dressings and poultices for skin irritations.

DREAM SPIRITS AROMATHERAPY PILLOW

To make an aromatic, sedative, sleep-enhancing pillow, fold equal amounts of the dried leaves of catnip, rabbit tobacco, selected mints, and sage into a small calico or plain cotton pillow case. This pillow will also enhance your dreams, which accounts for its name. The addition of dried rosemary leaves, lavender, and mugwort will make your dreams even more vivid and memorable. Each time you rest your head on this pillow you will experience the additional virtues of aromatherapy, which are much more pronounced in humid weather.

You may want to place a small three-inch-square pillow filled with these blended dried herbs on the back of your favorite easy chair to enhance your meditations and contemplations. Place another in the back-seat of your car for a soothing, calming effect on the children who ride with you. These dried herbs also make fine additions to homemade stuffed animals for babies and children.

Mugwort
Artemisia vulgaris

SUMMER MEADOW RELAXING TEA

Singly or combined, a tea made from the fresh or dried leaves of catnip, sweet everlasting, or yarrow will help you relax after a hard day's work or just before bedtime. The tea can also relieve gas or other digestive problems, and it may help premenstrual syndrome and menstrual cramps. Another bonus is that, cool, it is also good for your pets as a mild sedative, especially before car trips.

Place the fresh ingredients in the bottom of a 1-quart teapot. If you are using dried herbs, use about half as much, since they are more concentrated. Pour the boiling water over the herbs, cover, and steep for 5 minutes, allowing the botanicals to infuse together. Savor their aroma.

Pour a cup or mug of this herb tea and sip it slowly. Try it plain first; you may not need honey. If you have leftover tea, you can drink it cool later on or add it to a relaxing bath, so it is best not to sweeten the pot.

3 fresh leaves catnip or
   other mint
3 small fresh leaves sweet
   everlasting
1 or 2 small fresh leaves
   yarrow (optional)
1 quart freshly boiled water
1 tablespoon raw honey
   (optional)

Yarrow
Achillea millefolium

Aromatherapy

Aromatherapy takes advantage of the fact that fragrances alone can trigger memories and emotional responses, often lifting people's spirits or changing their moods. For example, the fragrances of sage and yarrow can relax and calm you, while the aroma of mesquite might energize you.

Select native plants which lend themselves to aromatherapy are sweetgrass, *Hierochloe odorata;* sweet vernal grass, *Anthoxanthum odoratum;* red cedar, *Juniperus virginiana;* and white cedar, *Thuja occidentalis.* These are primary herbs for incense, smudging, tea, and *kinnikinnik* (special mixtures). Alone or collectively, their fragrances can remind you of ceremonial times, sweat lodge rites, or a particular prayer.

The bark scrapings, pitch, and green leaves of Canadian hemlock, *Tsuga canadensis,* and balsam fir, *Abies balsamae,* bring the scent of Christmas and winter holidays and purification. The leaves and twigs of bayberry, *Myrica pensylvanica;* sweet gale, *Myrica gale;* and sweet fern, *Comptonia peregrina,* are fragrant medicines and aromatic botanicals that have long been steeped in teas and decoctions to banish sadness and celebrate friendships.

The aromatic leaves and twigs of spicebush, *Lindera benzoin,* and sassafras, *Sassafras albidum,* are sweet chew sticks and calming insect repellents. Sagebrush, *Artemisia tridentata* and species; bee balm, *Monarda didyma* and species; pennyroyal, *Hedeoma pulegioides;* and mesquite, *Prosopis glandulosa,* have remarkable scents often exploited in smudges, in incense, and to flavor certain herbal healing formulas. The bee balms and wild bergamots were especially esteemed perfumes of the Delaware, who often packed their ceremonial clothes in these fragrant dried herbs.

And despite the fact that it is strongly discouraged as a recreational drug, tobacco has for countless centuries been a valued American Indian ceremonial herb, used for praying and making offerings. Its fragrance alone triggers respect among traditional people, who do not need to smoke it or burn it in order to find enjoyment.

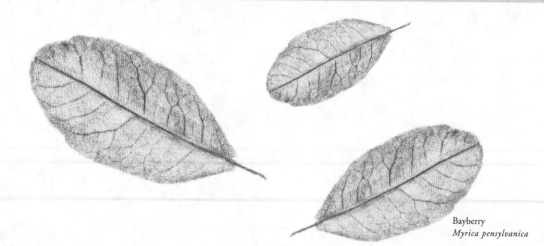

Bayberry
Myrica pensylvanica

SOAPWORT SHAMPOO

You can make this fine shampoo for your hair from the roots and above-ground herbal parts of soapwort, *Saponaria officinalis.*

1 cup fresh soapwort or
¹/₂ cup dried
2 cups warm water

Soak the soapwort in the water for 30 minutes. Process in a blender for about one minute, or until it is pureed. Strain through several layers of gauze or a coffee filter. Bottle and label. Use up within the month, and keep in the refrigerator to retard spoilage.

To use for shampoo, warm about ¹/₂ cup (use more or less, depending upon the length and quantity of your hair). Pour it through your wet hair and work it in thoroughly, then rinse out. This will not lather as much as conventional shampoos.

VARIATION: You may substitute an equal quantity of fresh or dried yucca roots, *Yucca* spp., for the soapwort in this recipe.

Soapwort
Saponaria officinalis

CHAPTER SIX

Fertility, Midwifery, and Childbearing

"FOR IT IS SHE WHO GIVES BIRTH"

Motherwort
Leonurus cardiaca

May all things move and be moved in me

and know and be known in me.

May all creation dance for joy within me.

—A CHINOOK PRAYER

Comfrey
Symphytum officinale

For centuries, everything connected to conceiving a child, pregnancy, and giving birth has been surrounded with particular blessings. Special practices are nearly universal among American Indians, although the specifics vary from tribe to tribe. This vital phase of life is especially important: It strengthens the union of a man and a woman as well as their extended families. And children also ensure the continuation of the tribe.

Many tribes had fertility rites and rituals to help create new life when the time was right. These included distinct ceremonies, symbols, and specific substances designed to enhance this life passage for both men and women. And while many people were fortunate enough to conceive easily, others needed special amulets, medicines, prayers, and guidance to help them.

For most women, pregnancy is a time of radiant good health; many men also thrive as they await the birth of their child. Sometimes it seems as if both parents are glowing with the awareness of creating new life. But these are not always months of perfect tranquility. Health challenges or other worries may confront the birth couple. Many women face pregnancy and birthing alone.

Whatever the circumstances, many women or couples seek a medicine person's help following conception or when a pregnancy becomes obvious in order to create a birthing amulet and, sometimes, a ritual to ensure success. These pregnancy and birth rites may be reassuring songs and prayers of strength and healthy passage, accompanied by some of the life-giving female herbs, like wild yam root, *Dioscorea villosa,* and blue cohosh root, *Caulophyllum thalictrioides* (also called squawroot). These symbolic items strengthen the individuals and the household and provide good luck. Also at this time special new medicine bags are made for the birth mother and for the soon-to-be-born family member.

Special care has always been focused on the body and breasts of the pregnant woman. Women are perceived to be much more powerful dur-

Motherwort
Leonurus cardiaca

Midwives

Long before the advent of formalized medicine, midwives were assisting women in childbirth. Midwifery is one of the oldest continually practiced health care professions in the world. Today it is a tradition that still flourishes; more and more frequently, midwives are requested and respected as alternatives to the care provided by obstetricians.

Midwives are often healers and caregivers not only in their own communities, but also in surrounding settlements. Before they were formally recognized with the term *midwife,* these esteemed individuals accumulated and practiced what was known as "life's lessons" among native peoples. Mothers and grandmothers were midwives for their families and others. Many midwives were knowledgeable health care practitioners who continued to give advice and help well beyond childbirth.

Today there are both lay midwives and certified nurse-midwives practicing in every state. Among them is a healthy network of American Indian midwives, many of whom apprenticed with clan elders, grandmothers, and healers in addition to their academic and scientific study. Some feel drawn to this career because of outstanding experiences they have had with their own home births.

Midwives provide careful prenatal care and supportive coaching during labor and delivery. They are excellent caregivers, whether you choose a hospital birth or join the growing number of women who opt for home birth.

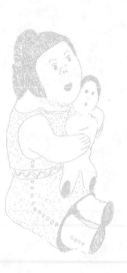

ing pregnancy and yet also more vulnerable. Gentle herbal oils and creams are massaged on the expanding abdomen; applying them guides extra strength and love to the fetus. Light liniments rubbed on the woman's legs relieve the burden of carrying extra weight. When needed, women use herbal poultices, oils, and creams for breast care.

In the past, in many tribes women gave birth alone, removed from the family living areas or in a specially prepared area. If needed, the husband, other women, or both might assist. Native midwives, who helped to bring most of the newborns into the world, were especially coveted.

Today sacred rituals, prayers, chants, and ceremonies of strength and good fortune still bless this vital period in people's lives. And many tribes continue to perform gentle, beautiful blessing rites for the pregnant woman and her unborn child.

The Navajo Blessing Way

Among the Navajo, the Blessing Way (Hoshooji, or Long-life Empowerment Ceremony) restores vitality and well-being during several key life passages. Like other major Navajo healing ceremonies, this is a major event whose throbbing rhythmic chants and prayers envelop everyone attending. Most important, though, is what it does for the "one-sung-over," the person for whom it is done.

A traditional Navajo may experience all or part of this nine-day-long ceremony four times during his life, the first time while he is still in his mother's womb. The Blessing Way is performed again at puberty, and later in life it may be used to help restore a person's balance. When someone marries or is preparing to have a child, the Blessing Way is done to ensure health, fertility, long life, and good fortune.

The essence of this sacred ceremony is to promote spiritual, psychological, physical, and emotional harmony. It reminds people that the goodness that surrounds them is accessible when they live their lives in balance. The beautiful songs from the Blessing Way rites are mesmerizing as they call in the forces of benevolent power for the participants. Often as Navajo people go about their daily work they softly sing these holy songs to remind themselves of the precious balance of life and their closeness with supernatural forces. The Navajo invest their homeland's natural geography with holy power and significance. Blanca Peak, Mount Taylor, the San Francisco Peaks, and Hesperus Peak mark the cardinal points of their spiritual vista. Within their sacred landscape stands Spruce Mountain (Gobernador Knob) in northwestern New Mexico, considered to be the birthplace of Changing Woman and the heart of the earth, according to some Blessing Way chanters. The Navajo revere Encircled Mountain as the lungs of the earth and the place where Changing Woman's children, the holy Warrior Twins, were born. Finally there is Mirage Mountain, believed to be the source of powerful protection and healing. The Navajo use stones from it, called mirage stones, in many sacred rites and healing sand paintings.

This geography is the outer manifestation of Navajo holy traditions. Through sand paintings, songs, chants, visualizations, and the medicine bundle, it is brought into the Blessing Way during an all-night-long ceremony known as a No Sleep, which is performed in the Navajo hogan. Throughout the night, the chanter intones the powerful Earth Woman

When people have a ceremony done for them, it relaxes their body; it relaxes their mind; it—you might say—takes them into another world for a while and, if they give their full attention, they can be healed.

—*Navajo Chanter*

You inhale the dawn four
   times
and give a prayer to
   yourself,
the dawn, and everything
   that exists.
Everything is made holy
   again.

—*Frank Mitchell, Navajo*
   Blessing Way chanter

Prayer while holding a sacred healing bundle known as the Mountain Earth Bundle. The No Sleep ends when the one-sung-over walks out of the hogan's east-facing door and inhales the dawn's light. Taking in four deep breaths, she visualizes the perfect world first seen by the Holy People at the dawn of the Fifth World—the world of beauty, thought, and knowledge. The one-sung-over has become filled with and restored to beauty.

Although they favor specific herbs for the Blessing Way, the Navajo believe that every plant is useful. Contemporary herbalists continue to use many of them today. For example, Mary Begay, a Navajo traditional healer, herbalist, and weaver from Keams Canyon, in the Four Corners area of Arizona, gathered medicinal plants and learned about healing from her father, who was a noted healer, singer, and performer of intricate Navajo chantways. She knows and uses about eighty-eight plants, which is only a small part of the considerable Navajo herbal heritage. It is the Navajo Way that Mary cannot use the herbs for herself, but she earnestly teaches others, hoping to pass on her store of knowledge.

Over the years the Navajo have found both ceremonial and practical applications for many botanicals. For example, rabbitbrush, *Chrysothamnus nauseousus,* is used in rituals as well as for relief of afterbirth cramping and menstrual pains. It can also be used as a hot tea for treating colds, coughs, fevers, and headaches.

Juniper, *Juniperus scopulorum,* is also used during the Blessing Way. One of the most important times to use juniper as a remedy—from the Pueblo to the Navajo—is during birthing, when it is customary to drink juniper sprig tea during labor and immediately after delivery. Infusions made with juniper are also favored for bathing both mother and baby immediately following birth. Juniper tea also soothes upset stomach and diarrhea and helps treat chronic bladder infections. **Note: Do not eat juniper berries during pregnancy.**

Pinyon pine, *Pinus edulis,* also produces a fine tea for treating diarrhea, and it is often added to smudging mixtures for its aromatic fragrance and healing benefit as people inhale the smoke. The pitch is used extensively in soothing skin salves and ointments.

Other native herbs used for pregnancy and postpartum are the attractive blue curls, *Trichostema* spp. These woolly mountain mints resemble rosemary and have a pleasant sweet-sour smell. Their flowering tops make a fine herbal tea, good for settling the stomach. The Chumash Indians of California give it to women to help them expel the afterbirth.

A low perennial milkweed of the juniper/pinyon regions is antelope horns, *Asclepiodora decumbens* and *Asclepias capricornu,* which produces a gigantic root much sought after for its healing powers. Besides being a valuable treatment for asthma, lung infections, and congestive heart disorders, antelope horns has extensive uses during childbirth. Native midwives give women in labor a mild tea made from the roots to shorten uterine contractions and ease birthing. The tea also helps increase the new mother's milk production. **Note: Do not use antelope horns during pregnancy because it can be an abortifacient.**

Pueblo Fertility Rites

The nineteen native pueblos strung along the fertile Rio Grande River valley in New Mexico share many distinctive traditions connected to fertility and childbearing. Among some early Pueblo peoples, a pregnant woman wore a turkey feather in her belt. First domesticated among prehistoric Pueblo peoples, wild turkeys were associated with long, healthy hair. They are also strongly linked to fecundity and Mother Earth, since they nurture large flocks of young nestlings. Feathers continue to be significant in some of the personal practices many individuals observe today. Following an ancient custom, some Zuni families place a feathered prayer stick in a house shrine to bless, protect, and bring special energy to this period of life.

At all key points in the lives of Pueblo peoples, the kachina come into play. Masked kachina dancers sometimes give a pregnant woman or one who desires to conceive a tiny carved *oaka*, or baby, along with a miniature cradleboard. The simple carved wooden image is believed to be a spirit doll that contains the spirit of a new baby wishing to be born.

During women's fertile periods many tribes used special rites, rituals, and herbs to bring about conception. Prairie coneflower or purple coneflower, *Echinacea* spp., and the climbing annual vine wild cucumber, *Echinocystis lobata,* are two native wild herbs whose ripe fruits look like striking ovaries filled with fertile seeds of healing and promise. As in the old European doctrine of signatures—the belief that an herb's appearance indicated its healing properties—native healers took the shape of these fruits as signs from Mother Earth of abundant fertility. Including them in love medicines or fertility medicine bundles is supposed to ensure successful conception within the growing season or year. These two plants also appear in childbirth and healing formulas.

Prairie coneflower, or purple coneflower, is one of the superior native herbs widely in use today, though for other purposes. *Echinacea angustifolia, E. purpurea,* and *E. pallida* are all sought for their perennial taproots, as well as their aboveground plant parts, to make tinctures, teas, and decoctions to strengthen the immune system. Echinacea tea tastes pungent and dry; it is a fine antiseptic, anti-inflammatory, and antiviral treatment.

Wild cucumber
Echinocystis lobata

Iroquois Childbirth Practices

American Indian women prepare for childbirth before and during their pregnancies, according to Katsi Cook, an Akwesasne Mohawk midwife and mother of five. Katsi found a rich heritage of midwifery in her family through listening to her womenfolk's stories. She has devoted herself to carrying on this tradition in her own work.

Among the Akwesasne, pregnant women have long paid close attention to diet. "The old people knew that a woman needed to prepare her body to carry a pregnancy," says Katsi. "They believed that the food eaten by the mother, and to some extent the father, would affect the development of the unborn child's character as well as its body."

Native foods from seasonal sources nurture both the body and the soul of the pregnant mother and her unborn child. This is the child's first introduction to the sacred and ceremonial foods of the family and tribe's diet. The Three Sisters—corn, squash, and beans—are vital, along with strawberries, blueberries, bearberries, maple syrup, venison, and muskrat. The Akwesasne Mohawks, whose homelands were along the fertile St. Lawrence River, relied heavily on fish, and especially the seasonal roe, or fish eggs. Today we realize that these foods are high in vitamin A and essential fatty acids and that they are crucial to blood and cellular development. Unfortunately, since the building of the St. Lawrence Seaway, pollution and industrialization have seriously eroded the availability and safety of traditional food supplies, making it difficult for the Akwesasne to continue some of their customs.

Among the Iroquois, birth confers awe and respect on women. "For the women, the sacredness of fertility and the ceremony of birth itself are aspects of the community and the family which empower us, which are opportunities for transformation. This is a responsibility that truly belongs to the women," says Katsi. And it is a deeply spiritual event: "My grandmother knew that when there's a birthing going on, the spirits come to give the baby gifts," she adds. According to traditional beliefs, a host of spirits attend the birth. Besides the spirits of the people and healing plants who are actually there, the spirits of family members who have passed over as well as those surrounding the birthing place, including the Little People (see Chapter 8) and other supernaturals, may be present.

Of course, the men's role is not ignored. Mohawk men have always participated in the birthing process. As Katsi maintains, this is "because they themselves have all been born of a woman, and they themselves carry the seed of the people's future."

An Inuit Birth in the Canadian North

Part of preparing for childbirth is deciding who should attend the event. Some people believe that these decisions will have a considerable impact on the future of the as yet unborn child.

Before I was born, my mother had to decide who would be involved at my birth. During her pregnancy, many people came to ask for her consent to attend. Customarily, such decisions are based on a number of considerations. People who have asked for consent have to be considered by close relatives and immediate in-laws. Those who are believed to have wisdom in life, who are successful economically and socially, are usually favored. The first person who has to be there is the midwife, man or woman. In my case it was my grandmother. While I was being born, she had to study how I came into the world. According to her, I moved all over, which she took to mean that I would be in strange lands one day. Also present at my birth was the person I was named after, my other grandmother. This automatically meant that I would never call her "grandmother," nor would she call me "grandchild." Instead we called each other *sauni*, namesake, bone-to-bone relation. This brought my parents and me that much closer to her. I was their security against in-law problems.

Then someone had to dress me in my very first clothing. It can be a man or a woman. Since I was a girl, the person who dressed me has to call me *arnaliak*, bringing-you-up-to-be-woman. This person, for the rest of his life and mine, has the heaviest responsibility. Just how I turned out to be as an adult is his job. He guided me in acquiring knowledge of the ways of people and taught me how to know myself. He lectured me on how to approach different kinds of people. He was responsible for shaping my mind. As long as I remained a child, he brought me presents on special occasions such as his hunting successes, or on the first and last trading trips to the Hudson's Bay store in the fall and spring. In return I call him *sanariarruk*, he-forms-me-into.

The most serious part of my birth involved another child. By an arrangement between my parents and his parents, we two called each other *angilissiak*, waiting-for-you-to-grow-up. That is how the Inuit child is born, and with all these people to guide me I began to grow.

—Minnie Aodla Freeman
Quallunaat, 1978

Pueblo Childbirth Practices

Like the Mohawk women's attention to their prenatal diet, other practices we consider modern have been used by American Indians for centuries. For example, among many Pueblo tribes, immediately after a baby is born the birth attendant wraps the newborn in warm blankets before giving her to her mother to nurse. They rest snuggled together for the first hour of the baby's life before they are both cleaned up. This demonstrates an early understanding of bonding, which is now encouraged in hospital delivery rooms.

In most Pueblo tribes, the newborn infant is carefully cleaned, the umbilical cord is tied off and cut, and the cord's end is briefly singed with the embers from a young corn cob. Because corn will always be a vital part of every Pueblo child's life, this act symbolically brings healing blessings from the touch of the earth's staple food. As a gesture of welcome, the newborn is gently soothed and massaged, using a light coating of corn oil or bear grease to protect his skin. Afterward, carefully wrapped in soft cotton cloth and deerskin, he goes into his cradleboard. For protection, he is laced in with a perfect ear of corn tied to one side and a stirring stick or paddle on the other.

Most Pueblo peoples light the hearth fire at birth. The husband—as guardian and protector during this critical time—continually tends it and keeps it going for the first four days of the baby's life. Native traditions like this, handed down for generations, bring a sense of peaceful reassurance and powerful magic to those who believe in and live by them.

Remember, remember
  the circle of the sky
the stars and the brown
  eagle
the supernatural winds
breathing night and day
from the four directions

Remember, remember
  the great life of the sun
breathing on the earth
it lies upon the earth
to bring out life upon
  the earth
life covering the earth

Remember, remember
  the sacredness of things
running streams and
  dwellings
the young within the nest
a hearth for sacred fire
the holy flame of fire

—*Pawnee/Osage/Omaha*
Indian song

The Paiute Childbirth Ritual

Men play a significant part in childbirth in many tribes. The San Juan Paiute are among the most traditional of the ten modern Paiute groups in Arizona and Utah. Despite the fact that today many babies are born in hospitals, the first childbirth is still an important rite of passage for young men and women in the San Juan community. It is the symbolic counterpart of the woman's menarche ritual (see Chapter 3). Each of these time-honored practices marks a major turning point in the life cycle.

In this tribe, a pregnant woman observes certain taboos during her

Prenatal and Pregnancy Beliefs

Diverse beliefs, often dictated by religious or traditional taboos, governed prenatal behavior from tribe to tribe and region to region. Some traditions prevented a pregnant woman from doing certain chores, eating particular foods, or touching lightning-struck wood for fear of bringing harm to her unborn child. Among the Navajo, Seminole, and many other tribes, similar restrictions also applied to the expectant father. At the center of most of these traditions was the desire to keep a natural respect and balance within the family, tribe, and ecosystem.

Many tribal groups believed it was important to abstain from eating salt, sugar, or grease (rendered meat fat) during pregnancy. Some also avoided meat, either altogether or, in some regions, specific game meats such as alligator, rabbit, possum, eels, turtles, or frogs.

preparations for childbirth, and for a period following the birth of her first child. Her husband must also abide by these prohibitions. Neither can take any meat, salt, or cold water for thirty days following the birth, and they may only touch their hair and faces with a scratching stick; they cannot use their hands. The task of training the new father falls to the kinship networks. His wife's family instructs him by giving him specific tasks, which begin with running east each morning toward the sunrise and running west each evening toward the sunset.

When the thirty days have passed, the young couple bathe in cold water, trim the ends of their hair, and paint their faces with red ochre. Now that the baby has completed his first month of life, these practices will strengthen them for the challenges of parenthood.

During the childbirth rites, people tell traditional stories in order to introduce them to the newborn and to review them for the parents. Many Southern Paiute rituals and traditional beliefs are framed by these sacred stories, especially the cycle of Winter Stories or Coyote Tales, which continue to be vital community threads. These treasured tales, set in earliest mythic time when animals and people could speak together and influence supernatural events, provide explanations for the origins of life, cosmology, and many rites. Many see the stories as the special glue that holds the family fabric together and keeps everyone well.

EARTH REMEDIES

The medical specialties we call gynecology, obstetrics, and pediatrics have always been areas of primary concern to Indian women. Although their herbal medicine chests varied considerably depending on where they lived, native women used many valuable herbs to enhance pregnancy and ensure a shorter, gentler labor than what many women experience today. Many early explorers observed the apparent ease with which American Indian women gave birth. Dr. Virgil Vogel, a noted American Indian historian, has said: "The Indian practices associated with childbirth have been called more rational than those of Europeans of an earlier period. Christians long held that it was contrary to the will of God to ease the pain and discomfort of labor, for it was the intended penalty of the Almighty for original sin." American Indians had a much more forgiving attitude.

The cleansing astringency of uterine herbs such as blue cohosh roots and red raspberry leaves has long been valued for use throughout pregnancy and childbirth (see also Chapter 1). While they are pregnant, American Indian women use the leaves of various species of raspberry, *Rubus idaeus* and others, in infusions and tinctures for several purposes. Raspberry leaf tea taken daily eases morning sickness for many women. This superior and safe native herb helps prepare the womb for birthing, is an effective uterine relaxant, relieves cramping, and can reduce hemorrhaging. Today many physicians and midwives, especially in England and Europe, use raspberry to treat morning sickness and avoid a threatened miscarriage. Later on it also stimulates the mother's breast milk.

Red raspberry
Rubus idaeus

Another fine tonic for female reproductive systems is squaw vine or partridgeberry, *Mitchella repens.* The aboveground parts of squaw vine are used to make tinctures and infusions. Women appreciate its cool, slightly bitter taste, and drink it during the last two months of pregnancy to prepare the uterus for childbirth. This herb often strengthens contractions and shortens labor. Later on, women use squaw vine teas and salves to treat sore nipples during breastfeeding.

Dwarf mallow, *Malva neglecta,* and cheese plant, *Malva rotundifolia,* are ubiquitous, dense, matting herbs noted for their many soothing applications during pregnancy and childbirth. A warming tea made from their leaves and blossoms is a mild diuretic and expectorant, traditionally given to facilitate labor. Used as a gentle wash for mothers and babies, the tea can also calm skin irritations.

Many southern tribes, from the Maya and Aztec to the Alabama, Koasati, and Pueblo, used a tea of cotton root, *Gossypium hirsutum,* to ease childbirth labor. The same was true for corn smut fungus, *Ustilago maydis.* Also known as maize mushroom, corn smut fungus is considered a virulent and undesirable windborne parasite by most farmers. But Indian farmers in the Great Lakes regions and the Southwest have long cultivated it in certain corn patches. It is a highly esteemed vegetable food when underripe, and a powerful medicine when fully ripe. In the past, when a pregnant woman reached full term and wanted to induce labor, she used ripe maize mushroom, with extreme caution. Today knowledgeable American Indian midwives still use it during labor to speed and ease contractions and control hemorrhage.

Certain mushrooms and plants are considered to be beneficial, especially during the later stages of pregnancy, to enhance the mother's production of milk. The milkweeds, lettuces *(Lactuca),* and milk mushrooms *(Lactaria)* can be carefully used in light teas, as washes, or as amulets. These plants must be selected with caution: Know your species.

The ongoing but selective use of peyote by American Indian midwives recognizes the many therapeutic virtues of this sacred native botanical. Although it has been controversial, peyote continues to be highly esteemed within the Native American Church (see Chapter 5). This herb relaxes uterine pain while strengthening contractions, and it is a legendary herb of endurance.

Nursing mothers must be careful what they eat and drink because so much passes through their milk to their babies. Mild herbal infusions of certain plants have long been used by Indian women to increase their milk flow. Doubtless this also adds minerals and vitamins, too. Increased fluid intake is the best stimulant to milk supply, but a cup or two of tea made from the blossoms and leafy tops of calendula, *Calendula officinalis,* or skeleton weed, *Lygodesmia juncea,* will provide additional benefits.

Along with calendula and skeleton weed, the blossoms and leafy tops of the following herbs can be steeped in water and made into a skin wash. Worked into simple ointments, they will relieve swollen or inflamed breasts or sore nipples:

Herb Robert
Geranium robertianum

Comfrey, *Symphytum officinale* (not for internal use)
Black raspberry, *Rubus occidentalis*
Red raspberry, *Rubus idaeus*
Field sow thistle, *Sonchus arvensis*
Fox grape, *Vitis labrusca* (leaf poultice)
Prickly lettuce, *Lactuca scariola* (not for internal use)
Turtlehead, *Chelone glabra*
Herb Robert, *Geranium robertianum* (leaf poultice)
Wild geranium, *Geranium maculatum* (leaf poultice)

The roots of these herbs can be made into herbal poultices for breast problems:

Canada lily, *Lilium canadense*
Lady fern, *Athyrium filix-femina*
Lizard's tail, *Saururus cernuus* (breastweed)
St. Andrew's cross, *Hypericum hypericoides*
  (not for internal use)
Evening primrose, *Oenothera biennis*
Daylily, *Hemerocallis fulva*

Wild geranium
Geranium maculatum

Wild Foods Eaten During Pregnancy

There has long been a belief that eating bright, wholesome foods and fungi will benefit an expectant mother and her unborn child. Berries and fruits are especially symbolic of the female, life-giving forces in nature. During this time, women also favor the sacred Three Sisters—corn, squash, and beans—eating them in soups, stews, breads, cakes, spreads, or on their own, lightly steamed.

Lamb's-quarters
Chenopodium album

There are a host of delicious wild foods high in fiber, vitamins, and beneficial minerals and oils. Many are great chopped and served with other favorite vegetables, especially corn, squash, or potatoes. Wild greens that are great steamed or stewed are:

Purslane, *Portulaca oleracea*
Lamb's quarters, *Chenopodium album*
Wild garlic, *Allium sativum*

Wild onion, *Allium cernuum*
Wild strawberry, *Fragaria vesca*
Wild woodland violet, *Viola canadensis*
Stinging nettle, *Urtica dioica*
English plantain, *Plantago major*
Narrow-leaf plantain, *Plantago lanceolata*
Garlic mustard, *Alaria officinalis*
Dandelion, *Taraxacum officinale*
Evening primrose, *Oenothera biennis*
Prairie coneflower, *Echinacea angustifolia*
Chickweed, *Stellaria media*

Stinging nettle
Urtica dioica

Steamed, boiled, or roasted roots of wild seasonal resources are also vital in a healthy pregnancy diet. Some of the choicest are:

Arrowhead, *Sagittaria latifolia*
Burdock, *Arctium lappa*
Catbrier, *Smilax rotundifolia*
Cattail, *Typha latifolia*
Chicory, *Cichorium intybus*
Cucumber root, *Medeola virginiana*
Groundnut, *Apios americana*
Hog peanut, *Amphicarpaea bracteata*
Jerusalem artichoke, *Helianthus tuberosa*
Oyster plant, *Tragopogon porrifolius*

Wild woodland violet
Viola canadensis

Never pick anything edible or medicinal from roadside margins—go at least fifty feet or more away from the road—because of the real dangers of toxic pollutants and systemic poisoning. Roadside margins serve as filters to absorb gasoline emissions, road runoff, oily dust, and other windborne pollutants.

Many women have also long esteemed certain wild mushrooms, which some thought to be special gifts from Mother Earth. As we now know, naturally grown mushrooms (as opposed to commercial mushrooms grown in the dark) contain folic acid, which helps to prevent birth defects. These delicious and abundant choices, which do not have any poisonous look-alikes, can be eaten when they are underripe:

Angel's wings, *Pleurocybella porrigens*
Oyster mushroom, *Pleurotus ostreatus*
Fairy ring mushroom, *Marasmius oreades*
Horse mushroom, *Agaricus arvensis*
Meadow mushroom, *Agaricus campestris*
Blewit, *Clitocybe nuda*
Black morel, *Morchella elata*
Yellow morel, *Morchella esculenta*
Purple-gilled laccaria, *Laccaria ochropurpurea*
Grayling, *Cantharellula umbonata*

Some of the large, meaty mushrooms are best when they first emerge. If they are picked young, they are still fragrant, "milky" or "juicy." Once they get old they may still be edible, but they're no longer a memorable treat, and a few may become toxic. **It is always best to avoid old mushrooms, raw or cooked.** These delicious woodland treats are:

Honey mushroom, *Armillariella mellea*
White matsutake, *Armillaria ponderosa*
Fragrant armillaria, *Armillaria caligata*
Shellfish-scented russula, *Russula xerampelina*
Hygrophorus milky, *Lactarius hygrophoroides*
Salmon waxy cap, *Hygrophorus pratensis*
Shaggy mane, *Coprinus comatus*
Chicken-fat suillus, *Suillus americanus*
Chestnut bolete, *Gyroporus castaneus*
King bolete, *Boletus edulis*
Hen of the woods, *Grifola frondosa*
Chicken mushroom, *Laetiporus sulphureus*

Note: It is most important to positively identify any wild foods, especially mushrooms, before eating them. Mistakes can be fatal.

Modern research shows that certain mushrooms lower blood cholesterol levels, reduce the risk of strokes, and enhance the immune system. In addition, mushrooms also act as antiviral and antibacterial agents, and can stop the growth of some cancerous tumors. Some of these mushrooms are available in supermarkets, and in Chinese, Korean, and Japanese markets in most major cities. Others are available in tablets, capsules, teas,

May the longtime sun shine upon you, all love surround you, and the sweet light within you guide your way on.

—*Old song from the Brush Dance, a Yurok Indian healing ritual* and tinctures. Production of some of our native mushrooms, such as the hen of the woods, *Grifola frondosa,* also known as the Japanese maitake or the "dancing mushroom," has become a multibillion-dollar business in order to meet growing popular and scientific needs.

Squaw Balms and Papoose Roots

Squaw and *papoose* are among the earliest (Algonquian) Narragansett Indian words recorded in the Northeast. The Oxford English Dictionary notes them as early as 1634. *Papoose* means "American Indian baby." *Squaw* or *squa* means "woman" or "wife." Many eastern Algonquian Indian women were and still are *squaw sachems,* supreme rulers of their villages and tribes. These were early words of distinction, but in some regions the words were corrupted by derogatory insinuations and became terms of derision.

Numerous herbs were marked colloquially with the words *squaw* and *papoose,* signifying their specific usefulness by and for Indian women and their infants. Their names reflect vital early human needs. Many are parturients, or substances that induce uterine contractions during labor. Most are also uterine tonics, strengthening and toning the muscles and nurturing the general well-being of the uterus. The papoose roots serve to relieve colic and other infant discomforts. A multitude of these time-honored botanicals survive today as the various squaw balms, squaw vines, squaw roots, and papoose roots:

Papoose root, *Trillium erectum* (birthroot)
Papoose root or squaw root, *Caulophyllum thalictrioides* (blue cohosh)
Squaw mint, *Hedeoma pulegioides* (American pennyroyal)
Squaw root, *Rubus occidentalis* (blackberry)
Squaw root, *Cimicifuga racemosa* (black cohosh)
Squaw root, *Senecio aureus* (golden ragwort)
Squaw tea, *Ephedra nevadensis* (desert tea)
Squaw vine, *Mitchella repens* (partridgeberry)

Canada lily
Lilium canadense

Infanticide and Infant Mortality

Infanticide and infant mortality were age-old concerns among all early tribal cultures, where the natural rigors of life winnowed out all but the strongest and healthiest individuals. There is some documented evidence of mercy killings of deformed or weak infants, as well as babies who lost their mothers in childbirth. During the settlement periods there are also records of Indians killing babies fathered by non-Indians, since they would have been shunned in normal village life.

Infant mortality is an ongoing concern among American Indians. They have long suffered high rates of infant death, especially on reservations where sanitation and health care are major problems. In 1911 Indian infant mortality was considered to be a national health tragedy. Diligent work on the reservations, particularly by the Indian Health Service, has done much to reduce these risks. Between 1955 and 1992 infant mortality among American Indians and Alaska Natives dropped by 82 percent; it is now lower than the national rate.

Cherokee health writer J. T. Garrett has said, "There must continue to be a coming together into the circle in a sacred way to begin to solve the problems and concerns." Tribal involvement at every level in their own health services will make essential improvements possible.

Another serious health crisis to reckon with is fetal alcohol syndrome (FAS) and fetal alcohol effect (FAE), which have devastating results on American Indian populations. Alcohol use and abuse robs the users as well as their offspring of certain aspects of physical, mental, and intellectual clarity. The probing personal study done by native writer Michael Dorris in his book *The Broken Cord: A Family's On-Going Struggle with Fetal Alcohol Syndrome* (1989) reveals much about this growing problem that is not unique to Indian America. Many Indian elders lament that the increasingly high rates of alcohol abuse and teen pregnancy among native populations will severely undermine the culture.

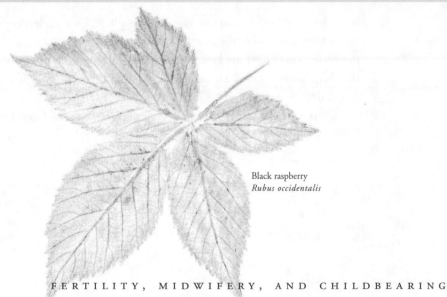

Black raspberry
Rubus occidentalis

2 cups fresh goldenrod
blossom tops, or 1 cup
dried

1$^{1}/_{2}$ pints or 24 ounces
sunflower seed oil or
corn oil

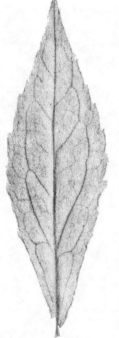

Canada goldenrod
Solidago canadensis

Essential oils (those distilled from the plants themselves) are highly potent and should not be used directly on the skin or taken internally. For example, an essential oil of wintergreen would be poisonous if consumed. Many essential oils are principally for medicinal use; sometimes you can use a few drops to add fragrance to an herbal product.

During pregnancy, and especially during the first three months, it is best to avoid essential oils altogether. A wiser choice is to infuse your favorite herbs and blossoms in a neutral cooking oil.

Place the blossoms in a large glass bowl or pot and gently crush them with a clean teacup or mug. Pour the oil over the herbs and stir well.

Place this pot inside another, larger pot of water (or you can use a double boiler), cover the herb and oil mixture, and simmer over low heat for two to three hours.

Remove from heat, uncover, and allow to cool. When cool, pour the oil mixture through a sieve or colander lined with gauze, positioned over a large sterile pot or jug. When it is finished dripping, gather the gauze and press the remaining oil out of the herbs. Discard the herbs and pour the infused oil into clean dark glass bottles. It will have a pale green-gold color and a naturally pleasing aroma. Seal and label the bottles. This infused goldenrod oil will last for many months, but it is most potent when used fresh.

VARIATIONS: You can vary this simple recipe by selecting other favorite blossoms and herbs, but if you are pregnant, be sure to confirm that the herbs you choose are safe. If you have sensitive skin, use only the gentlest ingredients. Good choices are calendula flowers, pink or red clover, or evening primrose blooms and leaves.

Pour a teaspoonful of oil into your cupped hand and gently massage

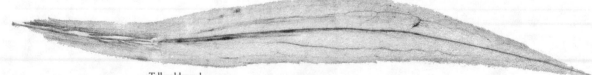

Tall goldenrod
Solidago altissima

your legs and arms, first stroking down toward the feet and fingertips, and then back up toward the heart. As you do your massage, clear your mind of all concerns and problems. Focus all your thoughts on glowing good health and new life. Give very special attention to your face and feet, especially the soles of your feet, as you massage away all tension and pain. Finish with a gentle circular massage of your shoulders, breasts, abdomen, and hips. If you can, get someone else to do your back, or you can use a long-handled bath brush or sponge to apply the oil. To minimize stretch marks as your body expands, gently massage your abdomen with oil, and add some aloe vera gel to help your skin maintain its elasticity and promote good circulation.

Uterine Tonics

Pregnancy is a time of bodily changes and heightened sensitivities. It is best not to take anything you do not need and to choose your herbs and foods very carefully. You should strictly avoid the more powerful herbs, such as blue cohosh, yarrow, goldenseal, sage, and pennyroyal. Here are two mild infusions you may want to try.

Early goldenrod
Solidago juncea

Corn Silk Tea

Corn silk is the long, silky, threadlike styles on an ear of corn, each one leading to a ripe kernel. It symbolizes the female fecundity of the corn plant. Like its counterpart corn pollen, which represents male fertility, it is used extensively throughout American Indian healing. When used in medicines, both the silk and the pollen add the mineral qualities from the earth in which the corn was grown.

Many women use corn silk tea as a mild diuretic during pregnancy. It is one of the finest, lightest herbal teas. This herb also strengthens the bladder and uterus and acts as a kidney and liver tonic.

2 teaspoons fresh corn silk or
1 teaspoon dried
1 cup boiling water

Put the corn silk in a cup. Pour in the boiling water and cover. Infuse for 5 to 8 minutes. Uncover and sip. This is fine as it is, or you may sweeten it with honey or maple syrup. You may have three or four cups daily.

RASPBERRY LEAF TEA

1 fresh raspberry leaf
(3–5 leaflets) or
1 teaspoon dried
1 cup boiling water

During the final weeks of pregnancy you may want to drink this mild tea daily to strengthen uterine muscles for delivery.

Crush the herbs in a cup and pour in the water. Cover and infuse for 5 minutes. Do not make a strong infusion. You may drink one or two cups daily.

GREEN GODDESS SKIN WASH

2 or 3 large sunflower or
Jerusalem artichoke leaves
2 large plantain leaves
1 quart cold water
1 tablespoon apple cider
vinegar

If you are fortunate enough to live in a place where you can readily pick your herbs, try this lightly antiseptic skin wash.

Wash the leaves, crush them to release their healing energies, and place them in a small pot. Pour the water over them, cover, and place the pot over medium-low heat to simmer for 10 minutes.

Remove from the heat and cool, with the cover still on, for 30 minutes. Pour this decoction into a clean bottle or jar, straining it through clean gauze or a coffee filter. Add the apple cider vinegar to produce a slightly acid pH and a more perfect balance for your skin, face, and hair. The vinegar will immediately "bleed" much of the color from the decoction, producing a lovely green liquid.

Store this soothing skin wash, labeled and dated, in the refrigerator, and use it within a week. During the cold winter months, keep some on the back of the stove to warm for daily use. During the heat of summer, use it right from the refrigerator. You can keep this in a small spray bottle to refresh your face, neck, and hair. When the week is up, use what remains in the bath, a footbath, or to rinse your hair.

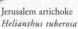

Jerusalem artichoke
Helianthus tuberosa

VARIATIONS: Try substituting witch hazel or hazelnut leaves, or the leaves of bergamot, bee balm, spicebush, Carolina spicebush, goldenrod, heal-all, slippery elm, basswood, sassafras, echinacea, or black-eyed Susan. Toward the end of pregnancy or afterward, you might try the leaves of bayberry, smooth sumac, jewelweed, sensitive fern, boneset, or joe-pye weed.

Sunflower
Helianthus annua

HERBAL HAIR CONDITIONER

You can use the skin wash recipe above to rinse and cut any soapy film on your hair after shampooing. To further enhance your hair's health and shine, you can use it as a base to make a conditioner.

4 ounces green goddess skin wash
4 ounces flat beer

Measure liquids into a plastic measuring cup; stir well and apply to your clean, almost-dry hair. Do not rinse out. Set or style your hair as you normally would, or pat your hair dry.

CHAPTER SEVEN

Middle Age

FACES IN THE LANDSCAPE

❖❖❖❖❖❖❖❖❖❖❖❖❖❖❖❖❖❖❖❖❖❖❖❖❖❖❖❖❖❖❖❖❖❖❖

Hops
Humulus lupulus

Lame Deer, commenting on the love of the land, suggested

that as the Sioux get older their faces begin to reflect

the landscape on which they live, the wrinkles of their faces

resembling the rolling plains and Badlands of the Dakotas.

He might equally well have described the people as

aging buffalo or as reflecting the granite of the Black Hills

which contain some of the oldest rocks on earth. It is

important to note that many of the traditional Sioux regard

these ancient relationships as being so powerful as to be

capable of dominating and largely determining the course of

individual human lives and fortunes.

—VINE DELORIA JR., LAKOTA SIOUX SCHOLAR AND WRITER

❖❖❖❖❖❖❖❖❖❖❖❖❖❖❖❖❖❖❖❖❖❖❖❖❖❖❖❖❖❖❖❖❖❖❖

Hops
Humulus lupulus

Although the midlife crisis has become a cliché, it is true that many people, especially during middle age, need to renew themselves and sometimes to reevaluate their lives. Some individuals decide to stop drinking, change harmful eating habits, give up other dissolute behaviors, or even take up a new life path. People do this in a variety of ways; many American Indians undertake a journey to a sacred part of their landscape.

Every culture has its sacred places, from Stonehenge in England to the Wailing Wall in Jerusalem. And throughout North America countless sites are imbued with special meaning, heightened energy, and far more than just physical beauty. The fact that these spots are often associated with a tribe's origin stories invests them with even more significance and power. A Taos Pueblo man said it best when he reflected on the return and protection of the sacred Blue Lake in 1968: "We have lived upon this land from days beyond history's records, far past any living memory, deep into the time of legend. The story of my people and the story of this place are one single story. No man can think of us without thinking of this place. We are always joined together."

Oral traditions of storytelling, prayer, and ceremonial song and dance keep these ancient sites vivid in the tribe's collective memory. Native people return to these holy places, as they have for hundreds of years, much the way other people go to church, synagogue, or mosque at prescribed times. Visiting and holding seasonal ceremonies at these sacred sites renews people. Many experience profound physical, mental, and spiritual healing, especially during periods of personal change. Healing minerals, fungi, animals, or plants collected on these journeys are especially esteemed.

Baboquivari Peak in southern Arizona is the home of I'itoi, the Elder Brother of the Papago Indians, O'odham, who gave this arid land to the people. This desert area has been the Papago homeland for millennia. The

Wild geranium
Geranium maculatum

sacred mountain is their center; it is a common thread throughout their ancient songs and stories.

The Hopi, westernmost of the Pueblo peoples, continue to look toward their sacred San Francisco Peaks, directing prayers and their time-honored kachina rites to the sacred place where the kachina spirits reside. Distant ancestors of the Hopi, the Anasazi, or "ancient ones," lived for over 1,200 years in a 160,000-square-mile area we now call the Four Corners region, where the states of Colorado, New Mexico, Arizona, and Utah meet. In this awesome region of striking canyons, mesas, cliffs, and valleys, primal cliff dwellers built huge planned towns with multistoried dwellings at Pueblo Bonito, Chapin Mesa, and Mesa Verde. And in another part of the desert Southwest, Yavapai elders, also descendants of the ancient cliff dwellers, still rise before dawn to pray to the spirits in the four peaks of the sacred Mazatzal Mountains near the Mogollon Rim.

In the heart of Pueblo Indian territory, near Albuquerque, is Petroglyph National Monument, where more than seventeen thousand prehistoric petroglyphs, or Indian rock drawings, can be seen. Today, nineteen pueblos still flourish along the broad Rio Grande Valley and beyond, each maintaining its own religious and healing practices, language, and government.

Where the geography is different, so too are the holy sites. The Mesquakie Indians have long believed that groves of trees in their Iowa homelands are the dwelling places of their ancestors' spirits and that the sounds of wind in the trees are the voices of their grandparents. As a result, they consider wood and objects made from certain wood, like tree burls, sacred. The Mesquakie make fine feast bowls, clan spoons, and masks from burl wood to be used as ceremonial items.

The Delaware Indians (Lenape), whose homelands were in the Eastern woodlands, believe there is a powerful race of "little people," known as Wood Dwarfs, *wemahtekenis,* who inhabit the trees. The Delaware had to perform special rites and rituals to pass safely through the forests and take the trees they required for medicines, tools, weapons, and ceremonial items. The bark, roots, and seeds or fruits of many hardwoods are still vital in healing preparations, and the fungi and lichens growing on certain trees continue to be valuable foods and medicines.

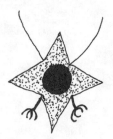

Four-point star beings from West Mesa, Petroglyph National Monument

Plains Indians Journey
to the Black Hills for Renewal

Sometimes the ancient geology of a landscape appears to take a human shape or to resemble someone we have known. Some say these areas are inhabited by ancestors' spirits watching over us. Whatever the explanation, in certain regions the earth seems to have much to tell.

The ancient rock formations in and around the Black Hills of South Dakota have been sanctuaries for native people over a long stretch of time. Like great spirit cathedrals, they stand as reassuring sentinels jutting out of the flat prairie lands. For this reason, during critical life passages people from more than twenty Plains Indian tribes travel from all over North America to sacred sites in the Black Hills. They fast and pray at Bear Butte, called the "Gathering Mountain," Harney Peak, known to the Sioux as "Mountain at the Center Where One Comes to Speak," or the Devil's Tower, known as the "Bear's Lodge." They also hold healing and vision rites. Visions are great guiding gifts from the Creator, born of prayer; they often bring a return to clarity and wellness.

People make these trips at special times during their ceremonial and personal year. Many return throughout their lives, as often as they can, because of the powerful sense of renewal they receive in these holy places. To them, the land is strength. Mother Earth has unlimited healing and nurturing capacities, especially when people honor her. The minerals, medicinal fungi and plants, and animals that continue to materialize across the earth reassure people of her amazing fecundity.

Prayers, fasting, and sweat lodge rituals are vital parts of these renewing pilgrimages. Many people make offerings of sacred tobacco, sage, cedar, and sweetgrass, which they bind into small prayer bundles of red or calico cloth and tie up into shrub and tree branches. Sometimes they place the bundles on rock outcroppings along the trails in the Black Hills or in other holy places. If you visit these sites, you may see some of these prayer ties fastened onto vegetation or sticks. These are sacred and should never be touched by visitors.

Grandfather Great Spirit,
All over the world the faces
   of living ones are alike.
With tenderness they
   have come up out of
   the ground.
Look upon your
   children that they may
   face the winds
And walk the good road to
   the Day of Quiet.
Grandfather Great Spirit,
Fill us with the light.
Give us the strength to
   understand,
And the eyes to see.
Teach us to walk the
   soft earth
As relatives to all that live.

—Sioux prayer

Hopi Prayer Offering Ceremony
at Winter Solstice

Mirroring these individual ceremonies, many tribes practice rituals to cleanse and ensure the healthy continuation of the entire community. These tribal cycles of renewal are especially vital in the desert Southwest, where ceremonial concerns often center on rain. Because barely ten inches of precipitation fall each year on their 1.5-million-acre reservation in northeastern Arizona, the Hopi annually petition the heavens to get the life-giving rain they need for their melons, squash, beans, gourds, peaches, and corn.

While many Hopi men and women have trained since childhood for their kachina societies and rites, it is during middle age that they assume responsibility for these vital healing ceremonies. The men weave the sacred kilts and blankets and make the other prayer and ritual accouterments. The women determine when the rituals will take place. As the acknowledged leaders, it is up to both to teach the younger generations and perpetuate their ancient traditions.

For the ten thousand members of the Hopi tribe, winter is a deeply spiritual time when they conduct special communications with the Spirit World through rituals, prayers, healing herbs, special foods, and other offerings. Some of the most important Hopi rites occur during the winter cycle, while the people endure the long, cold nights and shorter days. A major turning point in Hopi ceremonial life is the winter solstice ritual called the Soyal.

The winter solstice is the day with the fewest hours of daylight, the beginning of winter in the Northern Hemisphere. It occurs on December 21 or 22, when the sun is farthest south of the equator and almost appears to be standing still. Earlier people observed this natural phenomenon with concern and used prayers, rituals, and ceremonies to encourage the sun to return and warm their lands. In the desert Southwest, where the sun shines brightly during most of the year, Pueblo farmers keep track of where the sun rises and sets each day in order to plan the year's activities.

The Soyal consists of private rites held in the *kiva,* a large circular subterranean ceremonial chamber. Hopi priests pray and prepare the *kiva* for days before the ritual. During the rites, the men purify themselves and abstain from eating salt, grease, or meat. In or near all pueblo plazas, two tall, thin ladder poles stand above the *kiva* opening, serving as sacred hallmarks and reminding the people of their original emergence place from the last world through, the *sipapu*.

The *kiva* is the hub of ceremonial activities designed to spiritually prepare the arid land for the new planting season. The clean-swept earthen floor of the *kiva* is sprinkled with sacred cornmeal and healing herbs. Flowers are placed around the floor in patterns symbolizing the universe, along with perfect ears of corn, eagle feathers, and other holy objects. The entire *kiva* becomes an altar.

The men make exquisite prayer sticks, incorporating feathers and other symbols of renewal. They smudge them in the smoke of burning herbs and tobacco. They also prepare small sacred bundles of snakeweed and other healing herbs wrapped around wood or an ear of corn, and take them to selected homes as healing gifts. Messengers visit every Hopi home with corn-husk boats filled with cornmeal and surrounded by prayer feathers dusted with corn pollen. Corn kernels and other vegetable seeds are blessed and sprinkled with earth from the *kiva* to ensure good crops for the coming growing season. People pray to the Creator for the fertility that will allow the cycle of life to continue.

At the solstice, the entire village enters the *kiva* for the final Soyal rites, guided by the Soyal kachina. Dressed magnificently and painted with heavenly symbols, his head crowned with a stunning corn-husk star, he carries a shield representing the sun. As he dances around the villagers gathered in the *kiva,* they combine their prayers and energies to draw the sun back toward summer from its distant journey to the south. These rituals strengthen and renew the people's bonds with both their supernatural and natural worlds.

Hopi Basket Dance

After the kachinas have returned to the San Francisco Peaks, the women's dances begin. These ceremonies are largely controlled by women in their middle years, who are also the primary dancers.

Slow, thoughtful, and methodical, the Basket Dance proceeds throughout a hot August day. It is devoted to generating respect for the

Hopi Kachinas

Kachina cults are possibly the oldest continuing healing and horticultural societies in the Northern Hemisphere. More than three hundred kachina spirits inhabit the sacred San Francisco Peaks, north of Flagstaff in northwestern Arizona. With prayers and ceremonies, the Hopi beseech these supernatural beings to live with them in their villages from winter solstice until summer solstice and to enhance their crops, work, and health.

The kachinas work with the Hopi people to secure their vital life needs. And the people strive to achieve personal balance, harmony between themselves and their family, clan, friends, and villages as well as with the natural and supernatural worlds. This is the Hopi Way.

The great pantheon of Hopi kachinas takes many awesome forms, from the sacred Corn Mother and Soyal kachina to various vegetables, birds, animals, demons, and ogres. Each spirit being plays a vital role. They are often joined by raucous clowns and mudheads who defuse tension and tease the crowds during rituals, teaching through their misbehavior.

Inspired by these spirits, men and women in the kachina societies carry out the rituals and ceremonies as masked, costumed human forms of the kachinas. Before the ceremonies, they prepare the *kiva,* carve and paint the fantastic kachina masks and *tablitas* (headdresses), dance sticks, and other items, and weave their dance kilts and sashes.

The Hopi also represent their sacred guardian spirits in carved wooden dolls, infused with the supernaturals' energies and blessings. They carve pieces of cottonwood root into these unique kachina beings, adding arms, legs, beaks, ears, horns, rattles, and even bits of turquoise, shell, coral, and feathers. During some of the rituals, the kachina dancers wear small kachina dolls dangling from their wrists and fingers, and they present the dolls to Hopi children as gifts and reminders of the future roles they will undertake. Many kachina dolls are remarkable pieces of art, displayed in some of the finest museums and private collections in the world.

As dancers, dolls, spirit messengers, and sources of supernatural blessings, the kachinas come to life in Hopi ceremonies during the first half of the year, returning to their spiritual homes in the mountains in late July. Kachinas are the intermediaries between the Hopi and the Rain People and other vital spirits. Although they are more than a hundred miles away, people in most Hopi villages can see the volcanic peaks of the mountains. They know that the kachinas are doing their work when storm clouds build over the peaks and drift eastward filled with showers for their parched fields and orchards.

Hopi Way and abundance for the seasons' crops. Wearing their *mantas,* traditional black dresses embroidered with bright red and green threads, fastened over one shoulder, the women dancers enter the plaza carrying traditional yucca basketry plaques, which are traylike baskets. Forming a circle, the women seem to be kneading the earth with their moccasined feet and slow, shuffling dance steps. Their nasal songs pray for the land's fecundity.

Creating a cornmeal trail as they walk, a Hopi priest leads three other women carrying gifts, but no baskets, into the center of the circle. As the circle closes around them and the singing continues, the three women hurl various gifts—bread, corn, and other objects—out to the crowd of onlookers, who leap and shout as they try to catch something. The enthusiastic exchange goes on as the circle of women continues to dance, chanting and moving their plaques in rhythm with their prayers, eyes cast down to the ground.

As the day proceeds, the men enter the plaza, returning from their footraces. Hopi runners are legendary for their endurance, and footraces are a significant part of many Hopi ceremonies. The men begin before dawn in the east, the direction of sunrise, many miles away. They seem to run with the sun back to their village. Young boys often run with their fathers, uncles, and grandfathers, demonstrating their physical abilities for the women.

Puffing from their exertions, the men run around the circle of singing women and back out of the plaza. Later, the first ten runners get coiled baskets made of yucca. Every runner receives a gift of appreciation, which he holds over his head. Amidst applause they run out of the plaza again, while the circle of Basket Dancers continues to chant their prayers for the harvests.

Prayers, strength, and endurance are necessary during the hot summer days of gardening and harvesting, when the Hopi collect and process their healing plants and nurturing foods. This tribe grows various colors and varieties of corn, and each has symbolic and nutritional significance. They are most identified with blue corn, which is part of their origin story. Ages ago, when their ancestors arrived in this world, the Hopi were allowed to choose one color of corn that would determine their destiny. They selected the short blue ear of corn. Rugged enough to survive in their arid region, blue corn signifies an arduous life for the Hopi, but one filled with enduring strength, enabling them to survive and outlast all other peoples.

Corn sustains Hopi society and blesses their tables, ceremonies, and prayers. And just as the Hopi inveigle annual corn crops from the desert, Hopi wisdom coaxes healing from the numerous native plants and minerals in their environment. Some of their healers say that people are literally surrounded by the healing relief that their bodies need, and they are drawn to it as they dream and pray.

The same plants used by Hopi basket makers and weavers are also noted for other uses. Two of the native yuccas, the narrow-leaf yucca, *Yucca glauca,* and the banana yucca or Spanish bayonet, *Y. baccata,* provide prodigious amounts of fiber from their swordlike leaves and food from the young fleshy fruits. They are highly esteemed for the saponins in their roots, which yield soap for washing clothes and hair. Yucca root shampoos add shine and strength to hair, and may even prevent baldness. Because it is a reliable anti-inflammatory, yucca tinctures and infusions also provide relief for arthritis.

Throughout this region grow numerous native species of sagebrush, especially the sand sagebrush, *Artemisia filifolia,* a willowy shrub that can reach two feet tall, and the matlike fringed sagebrush, *Artemisia frigida,* which ranges from Mexico to Alaska. The Hopi smudge the dried twigs, branches, and leaves of sage to ceremonially purify a gathering of people. The same aromatic oils that make sagebrush a good smudging herb also contribute to its insecticidal and antifungal properties. Made into a hot tea, sage can be inhaled as a decongestant or used to relieve a headache or sore throat.

Another valued herb is broom snakeweed, *Gutierrezia sarothrae,* common throughout much of the desert Southwest. Its crushed foliage emits a turpentinelike odor. Snakeweed teas are cleansing emetics, useful for treating snake and insect bites and eye problems. Snakeweed is also used in sweat baths to relieve sore throats, colds, aching muscles, and rheumatism.

Native people favor the beautiful wild shrubby masses of four o'clocks, *Mirabilis multiflora,* for their showy magenta-purple flowers, and seek them for their large medicinal roots. Used in various ways at the different pueblos to treat eye infections, relieve stomach distress, and soothe sore muscles, they are also esteemed for their sedative properties. Indian tea, *Thelesperma megapotamicum,* the slender perennial of pinyon and juniper regions, serves many of these same therapeutic needs. It makes a delicious wild tea that has mild diuretic benefits.

Flowering saltbush, *Atriplex canescens,* is one of the most valuable shrubs in this arid region. It is eaten raw, cooked, or rendered to ash, which the Hopi favor for their blue cornmeal *piki* bread, a sacred ceremonial food. The crushed roots and flowers of this herb can be applied directly to skin sores and irritations for relief, or worked into healing salves and ointments.

Plants vary in their chemistry and forms as well as their uses in different parts of the country. Like many of the fragrant grasses, viburnums, and oaks across North America, junipers are significant to tribes in many regions. In the southwest, the junipers range from shrubs to small trees. One-seed juniper, *Juniperus monosperma;* Rocky Mountain juniper, *Juniperus scopulorum;* and the alligator juniper, *Juniperus deppeana,* are all of great economic value. The fragrant wood and bark have endless uses for fuel, construction, digging sticks, prayer sticks, bows, and basketry. In the past, the shredded outer bark provided disposable baby diapers, sanitary napkin material, cradleboard padding, and winter insulation materials.

Juniper is still used for aromatic smudges and incense. Many people burn it in their home fires to purify their dwellings and relieve colds and respiratory problems. Depending on the strength of the brew, medicinal teas made from juniper berries and green sprigs are mild diuretics, or produce relief for stomach problems, colds, constipation, and even rheumatism. Some native peoples, including certain Navajo artists who call them "ghost beads," use juniper berries in necklaces to avoid seeing ghosts or having bad dreams.

Juniper mistletoe, *Phoradendron juniperinum,* the unique yellow-orange parasite often found clustered on some juniper branches, also has medicinal value. When eaten, the translucent berries provide a cure for diarrhea and stomach problems. Some Pueblo men and women use them in teas and other concoctions to prevent baldness. Like the more northerly American mistletoe, *Phoradendron flavescens,* an evergreen parasitic shrub with white berries, Juniper mistletoe can be toxic. Despite this, effective treatments for epilepsy, palsy, stroke, and tuberculosis come from native mistletoes, which also serve as sedatives and can help reduce high blood pressure.

Middle Age and the Medicine Path

Middle age is a time when many healers find that they can devote themselves more fully to the Medicine Path. Some admit that they've spent years exploring other life paths, ignoring the original call to healing that came to them in their youth. Whether it's because such a calling cannot be denied forever or because healers must have a wide range of life experiences before they can take possession of their powers, it is often during midlife that these individuals go through the requisite training to use their gifts to help others.

Other native healers first come into their powers at this time. Some individuals become more open to psychic and multisensory awareness after recovering from a serious illness or shock, such as surviving a lightning strike or suffering a major loss or upheaval in their personal lives. Sometimes native people experience personal growth and change through an illness and the special medicines and rituals used to cure it.

This may also be a time when healers and seers gain added strength and intuitive capacity. They may more frequently experience dreams that are filled with healing knowledge of certain plants, mushrooms, and minerals or that foretell future events.

And as they age, some people experience a sharpening of certain faculties even as others diminish or fail. Those who have lost sight or hearing may gain deeper ability with touch. Much like Western practitioners of therapeutic touch or massage, these healers can discern where someone's energies are blocked and massage away the problems.

Navajo Mountain Way

Mountains define boundaries and are spiritual guideposts as well as terrestrial markers. They govern weather conditions and can overwhelm with their power and mass. They seem to possess strong energy vortexes for those who live in and near them.

Mountains frame the Navajo homelands, and their sacred strength enters many chants and sand paintings, especially the Mother Earth sand painting. Navajo history relates how First Man and First Woman fastened the Sacred Mountain, Choli'i'i, to the earth with a streak of rain and decorated it with pollens, dark mists, the female rain, and mixed chips of precious stones.

Dealing with the darker side of human nature is essential to healing. The Mountain Way (Dzix K'ihji Ba' aadi) addresses violence, sexual excesses, depression, or quarreling, and is connected to the Male Beauty Way, a multiple-day healing rite used to treat specific ailments, life-threatening diseases, and disorders of men of advancing age.

Navajo sacred practitioners include herbalists, hand tremblers and other diagnosticians, sand painters, and *hataalii,* or singers. *Hataalii* study all their lives to learn the histories of their healing ceremonies as well as the prayers, chants, herbs, masks, and medicine bundle contents necessary for performing them. They are keepers of traditional knowledge who share their myriad practices in many ways, especially when they perform the ritual chantways, or sings.

Hosteen Klah, the noted Navajo medicine man, recalled that it took him years to learn the male Mountain Way. The singer must know the names and habits of the animals who live in the sacred mountains and speak their languages, especially that of the bear.

The Bear Chant (Zilthkayji-bakaji) and its sacred symbols require many long hours of memorization. The ceremonies, which last nine days and nights, include hundreds of chants, many long prayers, and several elaborate sand paintings. One pictures an arching rainbow guarding and enclosing three sides of a complex design, the eastern opening of which is guarded by two bears. The bear is one of the most protective spirits for the Navajo, and its power is used to diagnose illness. This Navajo rite invokes the bear's energy in cases where ill will or even witchcraft is suspected. But out of respect for bears' awesome power, this expensive ceremony can be held only in the late fall and winter, after they have entered hibernation.

The Bear Chant once called for a live bear cub to be led through as part of the rituals. Today healers bring the bear's presence into the rites symbolically. There are four types of bears protecting the Navajo rites, symbolized by their colors: black for the east, white for the south, blue for the west, and red for the north.

Hosteen Klah used many wild plants to brew his tonics, emetics, and other medicinal formulas, especially desert goldenrod, *Solidago spectabilis* and other species; water grass, *Heteranthera dubia;* grass daisy, *Chrysanthe-*

The plan was made in the home of the First Man.
The planning took place on the top of the Beautiful Goods.
They planned how the strong earth's heart should be formed;
How the Mixed Chips should be used, and
How the Sacred Mountains should be made.
How she should be made like the Most-High-Power-Whose-Ways-Are-Beautiful.

—*From the Mountain Way*

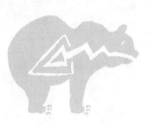

Navajo Sand Paintings

In all the ceremonies that have sand paintings, not one has the same sand painting. The figures, the lines, colors, sizes, they all differ.

—Tom Ration, Navajo hataalii

It takes countless hours of human labor and a lifetime of training to get from hard rock to a painstakingly detailed, finished sand painting. Navajo sand painters who work in natural earth colors usually know where to locate the specific rock they need. They require a truck as well as family and friends who are willing to spend their summer days collecting rocks. Some stones need to be roasted, because the hot fire alters and deepens their minerals' colors. All must be separately pulverized and finely ground, then carefully stored until they are needed.

Many Navajo sand painters earn additional income by creating, showing, and selling designs they create on pressed particleboard, brushed with glue and sanded. These commercial paintings are beautiful renderings, but they can never exactly copy the sacred patterns. Whole families work together, sharing their artwork and healing legends with a growing field of collectors.

Five generations of the Ernest Hunt family, Navajos from Sheep Springs, New Mexico, are involved in their expanding family business. The children learn by doing: "I go halfway with the children, even down to the little ones. I will help them with anything they want, but they must be taught to care for themselves in life," says the soft-spoken Mr. Hunt. Many of their sand paintings show the four holy plants—corn, squash, beans, and tobacco—that sustain the Navajo people.

mum leucanthemum; and dwarf sage, *Salvia eremostachya.* These plants are valuable astringents with antimicrobial properties.

Many other Navajo herbs continue to enrich healing practices, especially when applied to the needs of middle age. Like the Hopi, the Navajo use sagebrush. Navajo sage or big sagebrush, *Artemisia tridendata,* is the tallest and most prolific native sage growing west of the Mississippi River. It is especially plentiful through much of Navajo country. Thanks to the aromatic oils, including camphor, in its small threadlike leaves, it is one of the sacred herbs used in purification rites and numerous native ceremonies throughout America, probably for thousands of years. Medicinal teas from this rugged perennial are valuable in treating Rocky Mountain spotted fever and have long been dependable treatments for colds, sore throats, aching muscles, and stomach disorders. **Note: Like most powerful native herbs, this should not be used during pregnancy.**

Several native North American ephedras are known as Navajo tea, desert tea, or Mormon tea. These American species do not contain the drug ephedrine, like the related and more controversial Chinese ma-huang, *Ephedra sinica,* which is a stimulant of the central nervous system. *Ephedra nevadensis, E. torreyana,* and *E. trifurca* are profusely branched, broomlike shrubs growing throughout the deserts and dry mountainsides of the Southwest and Mexico. They have been used by various tribes—as far back as the early Aztecs—for burn poultices and in ointments to treat sores and stop bleeding. Ephedras are frequently made into a medicinal tea and used as a headache remedy, as well as a mild diuretic and cold and fever cure. Both the tea and a poultice made of the plant's twigs are analgesic, providing relief for rheumatism and arthritis pains. Today we continue to get decongestant and asthma relief from these plants.

Many tribes consider diseases and disorders to be special pathways of learning. For some patients, an illness and its cure serve as an entry into secret medicine societies. This is especially true among the Iroquois of upper New York State and Canada.

Iroquois Longhouse Curing Ceremony

The bark-covered ceremonial longhouse was a magnified symbol of the Iroquois' everyday, working homes and it embraced the geographic symmetry of their homelands. Doors were positioned at either end: One opened to the east, the rising sun, and the Hudson River, while the other opened to the west, the setting sun, and Lake Erie. The north side faced the St. Lawrence River, and the south wall faced the Susquehanna River. The central walkway through the middle of this structure signified the Mohawk River.

In most cases only traditional families—those who followed native customs—could enter their community's ceremonial longhouse, which was a sacred place of worship and periodic rituals. This is still true today. Tribal members belonging to other religions and nontribal visitors are usually excluded from longhouse rites. Keeping the congregation focused and devoted to the rites and rituals deepens their healing power.

Black flint together with
lightning,
stands as a shield for me;
Black flint, with your five-
fingered shield moving
around,
With this keep fear away
from me,
keep the fearful thing away
from me;
Hold it and stop it!
Black flint, the power you
possess in your medicine
pouch,
at the point where the black
snakes meet and cross,
put up a shield of
protection in front of me;
I'll be safe behind it, then
I'll be safe.
Behind this the fearful thing
will not reach me,
will not get me.
The fearful thing did not
reach me.
The Fear missed me.

*—From the Song of
the Black Bear*

The Mask Societies of the Iroquois

Ancient legends and dreams determined the designs of the masks these societies use. The False Faces have very large eyes, usually accentuated with tin or brass plates, which stare out over a prominent nose and a large-lipped mouth. Animal fur or long clumps of horsehair frame the spirit face, creating a formidable demeanor. The False Face can be carved only from a living basswood tree. It must be done by a chosen carver who knows the correct prayers and offerings to be given to the tree so that its spirit will live in the mask.

Buffalo Mask, Hunchback, Long Nose, Whirlwind, Scalp Mask, Harvest Mask, and Laughing Beggar Mask are some of the masks representing spirits. Perhaps the most awesome is Old Broken-Nose Mask. He represents a powerful spirit being who argued with a mountain—and lost. His long nose and large mouth were permanently squashed sideways by the mountain.

Most masks have open mouths so that the wearer can blow hot ashes over ill patients during the curing rituals. These masks are blessed and adorned with small ceremonial ties of tobacco. They are usually painted ghostly white, red, or black. Some are painted half red and half black, signifying the duality in life.

The charming Husk Faces, called "Big Heads" or "Bushy Heads," are cousins and helpers of the False Faces. They are more closely associated with farming and gardening, but they have the same curing powers. Hollow or protruding eyes stare out over big noses, puffy cheeks, and smiling or circle mouths, usually surrounded by a thick corn-husk mane or wreath. Husk Faces are braided and sewn, or tightly woven of natural corn husks. Some are adorned with puffs of white cotton, to symbolize Old Man Winter, or with satin ribbons, to indicate a fine lady or young woman.

Special amulets or personal talismans, which are tiny versions of both Husk Faces and False Faces, may be used in the Dream Guessing Rites at the Midwinter Ceremonies (see Chapter 4). These tiny three-inch masks may also be given to new members when they are inducted into one of these healing societies. These are usually people who have been healed by the society's rituals. The tiny maskette is given to them after the healing ritual as a charm to protect them against the ailment's return.

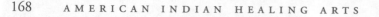

Traditional Iroquois believe that illness is a disorder of the natural world caused by unhappy supernatural spirits or by people's failure to do the right things in life. Beneficent spirits work to restore health and order among the Iroquois.

The sacred Hadooes (Hedowe), potent supernatural beings from the ancient pantheon of Iroquois cosmology, are one of the oldest healing cults in the Northeast. These beings—represented by medicine society members wearing stunning carved wooden False Faces—enter longhouse ceremonies during curing rites. People wearing the unique Husk Faces assist them. The Faces share their healing powers with the people, who feed them cornmeal, sacred tobacco, healing herbs, and cornmeal mush. Strawberries, huckleberries, and sweetgrass also play a part in longhouse rites.

Because they symbolize the spirits that bring order and balance and restore health, the masks are alive with power and require proper handling, feeding, and resting. According to Iroquois tradition, they cannot be displayed publicly or reproduced artistically, except in miniature, and minus their sacred symbolism.

Many False Face Society rituals pertain to purification and making new. The Traveling Rite, performed in the spring and fall each year, cleanses and renews the village. After a sequence of longhouse rites, the False Faces go out publicly to visit each traditionalist house, shaking their large snapping-turtle-shell rattles, and symbolically sweeping away all negativity and disease.

Amazing acts of healing take place at these times. Frequently the masked beings will reach into a woodstove and cup glowing coals in their bare hands, blowing charcoal dust over troubled or sick people in order to cleanse and cure them. Afterward the Faces and the traditionalists return to the longhouse for concluding rituals and prayers, ending with an honoring feast for the Masked Spirits.

The Iroquois legacy of healing herbs is enormous, beginning with the white pine, *Pinus strobus*. When the Six Iroquois Nations (Tuscarora, Mohawk, Seneca, Onondaga, Oneida, and Cayuga) formed the confederacy known as the Iroquois League to resolve conflicts and combine their collective strengths, they symbolically buried all weapons of war beneath a magnificent white pine tree, considered the "White Roots of Peace," one of the Iroquois' sacred trees. Not surprisingly, white pine is a powerful healing plant of the Iroquois and all other tribes within its wide range.

Then Dekanawida taught the people the Hymn of Peace and the other songs. He stood before the door of the longhouse and walked before it singing the new songs. Many came and learned them so that many were strong by the magic of them when it was time to carry the Great Peace to Onondaga.

—*From* The Iroquois Book of the Great Law, *by Arthur C. Parker, a Seneca*

White pine
Pinus strobus

Like other conifers, the needles of white pine are bitter but tasty chewing herbs and dentifrices. They are a good source of vitamin C. The long green needles, which grow in bundles of five, can be used year round. They are especially good during long, cold northern winters, when you can pick them fresh and chew them daily for a refreshing herbal mouthwash and throat treatment, or use them to prevent colds. Dr. Ella Wilcox Sekatau, a Narragansett medicine woman, remembers that her father, a noted chief and medicine man, instructed her to chew some needles while walking to school every day. Children in her tribe knew that when chewed like gum, the needles would refresh their mouths and strengthen their teeth.

Brewed in hot water, a small handful of white pine needles makes a bracing, refreshing tea, especially if you add a touch of maple syrup. A stronger brew makes a fine face, hair, and body wash, and it's great added to your bathwater.

Along with the short-needled Canadian hemlock, *Tsuga canadensis;* white spruce, *Picea glauca;* balsam fir, *Abies balsamae;* and tamarack, *Larix laricana,* the white pine is considered a year-round medicine factory for those who need and know the many therapeutic virtues of its other parts. In fact, the green twigs and needles of most native conifers are rich sources of vitamins and minerals. When chewed until soft or boiled with other botanicals or bits of charcoal, the gummy, resinous sap can be applied as a poultice for blisters and other wounds.

In this same evergreen family of trees are the Southern or Atlantic white cedar, *Chamaecyparis thyoides,* and red cedar, *Juniperus virginiana;* the latter is also known as juniper. The Iroquois boil or steam cedar needles in water to relieve head colds, headaches, sinus infections, congestion, and other forms of respiratory distress. They also dry and smudge the needles for ceremonial use or dry the peeled outer bark and add it to fragrant *kinnikinniks* (herbal smoking/smudging mixtures). People used the cedar berries (the blue-green, conelike fruits) to treat bladder and kidney complaints, and today you can try tinctures made from the green needles and berries to treat these same needs.

Contemporary healers from the Chinese, Ayurvedic, European, and African traditions use a profusion of Iroquois herbs in their healing formulas; many can be found in naturopathic medicines as well. For example, lobelia, *Lobelia* spp., which mimics nicotine, helps patients quit

Canadian hemlock
Tsuga canadensis

Curly dock
Rumex crispus

smoking by inducing a slight nausea. It is also a vital cardiotonic herb and a valuable treatment for asthma, bronchial spasms, and tightness in the diaphragm. Usnea lichen, *Usnea* spp., acts much like penicillin and is used to treat bacterial infections. Because it has antifungal properties, it can also relieve yeast infections. The ubiquitous jewelweed, *Impatiens biflora,* which has long been cherished as an antidote to poison ivy and stinging nettle, is also a treatment for yeast infections.

Curly or yellow dock, *Rumex crispus,* is a powerful perennial herb that is especially valuable during middle age. It is a vital kidney tonic and blood purifier, as well as a treatment for skin conditions such as eczema, psoriasis, ringworm, and acne. It assists fat metabolism and increases iron absorption, helping to reverse anemia. Burdock, *Arctium lappa,* is useful for most of these same needs and is effective in treating gout and high cholesterol.

The Adirondack mountains take their name from the Iroquois word meaning "bark eaters," reminding us that the inner bark of many trees and shrubs can be used medicinally. Infusions of wild cherry bark, *Prunus* spp., relax and soothe coughs, sore throats, and other bronchial conditions. Lozenges made from bark infusions have long enjoyed considerable commercial healing use. Infusions of willow bark, *Salix* spp., and meadow rue, *Thalictrium polygamum,* which are natural aspirins, provide headache and pain relief, and are trusted anti-inflammatories that reduce the discomforts of arthritis. The twigs of both shrubs provide highly esteemed chew sticks or dentifrices.

Jewelweed
Impatiens capensis

Delaware Big-House Curing Ceremony

Called the Delaware Indians by early Europeans, the Lenape's origins lie in the northeast regions that became New Jersey, lower New York, eastern Pennsylvania, and northern Delaware. Archaeological evidence indicates that ancestors of the Lenape lived on the northeast coast as long as twelve thousand years ago. This tribe was considered the "Grandfather People" by many Eastern woodland Indians. They were respected peacemakers, and their medicine tradition and healing rituals influenced many tribes throughout the East. There are unique parallels between Iroquois and Delaware healing and curing ceremonies.

The centerpiece for the Lenape ceremonial year was their

Gamwing, or annual Big-House Ceremony, performed to maintain harmony within their universe. For centuries this twelve-night ceremony of thanksgiving and renewal drew the people together. Every family that could get there came to the Big House. This homecoming provided spiritual enlightenment and strengthened time-honored traditions for everyone attending.

The Big House structure was filled with symbolism representing the Lenape universe. Its four walls were the four quadrants of the universe, and the roof represented the Sky World, abode of the Great Spirit. The floor was the earth, beneath which rested the realm of the underworld. A carved centerpost suggested the staff of the Creator, with its base in the earth and its top reaching toward the Creator's hand. Two carved human faces adorned the top of this post on its east and west sides, watching the two Big House doors. The eastern door signified the sunrise, day's beginning, and the origins of things; the western door represented sunset, conclusion of the day, and the end of all events. North and south Big House walls symbolized the respective horizons. Twelve great Masked Beings, or Mesingw, faces symbolizing the guardian spirit of game animals, adorned vital positions within the Big House. The masks were carved of hard burr oak and painted half red and half black. This symbolized the duality in life: day and night, female and male, east and west, good and bad.

The Big House rituals contained healing powers capable of curing any disorders, especially the growing needs of people in their middle years. And as people of middle age came more fully into their healing powers, they were often called upon to lead the curing ceremonies.

Ceremonial rites often began with purifying cedar smudging and a deer hunt before the sacred feast. Healers collected herbs and minerals for a variety of individual needs and harvested mushrooms and lichens for medicinal tonics and astringents. Delaware herbalists had well-developed medicine bundles, songs, and charms, which they carefully guarded as aspects of their personal power; this continues today.

Gathering sacred medicinal plants requires respectful rituals. A Lenape herbalist first prays for spiritual help and guidance, often mentioning the patient and his or her problems, as well as the plant(s) needed for the cures. Along with the prayer, he sprinkles a pinch of tobacco or cornmeal in each of the cardinal directions, including heaven and earth, drawing in the spirits of the four winds. When he finds the first specimen, the herbalist offers another prayer and more tobacco directly to it, and then passes it by, hoping it will intercede with its relatives. As he finds additional plants, he takes them, offering a final prayer and more tobacco to the plant spirits and the earth in exchange for allowing the plants to continue to flourish.

Sacred, thoughtful practices also accompany the preparation of herbal remedies and formulas among the Delaware. Following strict protocols has long been a part of their curing process; it also ensures that remedies attain their maximum healing potency and spiritual qualities.

Sadly, the Delaware no longer practice the Big-House Ceremony. "The Delaware people have lost so much," says ninety-year-old Lucy Parks Blalock, also called Oxeapanexkwe, or Early Dawn Woman, of Quapaw, Oklahoma. During the nineteenth century, growing settlement pressures, conflicts, and epidemics forced some, but not all, Lenape to leave their homelands. Many traditional Delaware went west and north, eventually settling in Oklahoma, Wisconsin, and Canada, where they actively continued their religion. But fragmentation of their customs was an inevitable result of their migration. Keepers of the Big House built their last log frame structure in a remote location near the Caney River, west of Copan, Oklahoma. The last Big-House Ceremony ended in 1924, but today there is interest in bringing it back.

Despite their losses, descendants of the Delaware living in the United States and Canada today continue to honor their herbal traditions. And other contemporary healers use a myriad of Delaware plants, fungi, and lichens, especially throughout the middle years.

American angelica, *Angelica atropurpurea;* sweet flag, *Acorus calamus;* black walnut, *Juglans nigra;* gentian, *Gentiana* spp.; Virginia snakeroot, *Aristolochia serpentaria;* and hops, *Humulus lupulus,* are excellent digestive tonics and metabolic aids. Black walnut is especially effective for controlling yeast infections, while hops exert a sedative influence on nervous stomachs and spastic colons. We continue to use goldenseal, *Hydrastis canadensis,* and elecampane, *Inula helenium,* for respiratory infections, and American wild ginger, *Asarum canadense,* to treat motion sickness, nausea, and as a warming circulatory stimulant. American ginseng, *Panax quinquefolius,* and sarsaparilla, *Smilax* spp., help detoxify and boost sluggish, stressed systems, and provide excellent tonics for both men and women. Hawthorn, *Crataegus* spp., is a fine heart tonic, assists tissue repair, and gently reduces hypertension.

Sarsaparilla
Smilax officinalis

Because the bear was believed to have supernatural power, American bearberry, *Arctostaphylos uva-ursi*, known internationally as uva ursi (the term is Latin for "bear's grape") has long been one of the Delaware people's sacred herbs. Both animals and people consume its edible berries, and tinctures and teas made from bearberry's evergreen leaves relieve chronic urinary tract infections and dissolve kidney stones. Bearberry is also one of the best herbs for diabetics, helping to regulate excessive sugar and assist the body's natural production of insulin. *Kinnikinnik* (see Chapter 9), an herbal smoking mixture often made from dried bearberry leaves, has a mild sedative effect on respiratory problems and relieves headaches.

Bayberry, *Myrica cerifera*, has proven to be a strong astringent for the gums, as well as a fine treatment for inflamed mucus membranes. Extracts of bayberry can reduce swelling and painful arthritic inflammations. Horsetail, *Equisetum* spp., another common herb, has a high silica content and is good for skin and hair and as an internal styptic to control bleeding from the kidneys or urinary tract. A mild diuretic, horsetail aids the body's absorption of calcium, reducing the risk of osteoporosis, which can begin during middle age. External treatments using horsetail help keep skin, nails, and hair smooth and shiny as well as strong and healthy.

EARTH REMEDIES

May all I say and all I think
be in harmony with thee,
God within me, God beyond me,
maker of the trees.

In me be the windswept truth of shore pine,
fragrance of balsam and spruce, the grace of
  hemlock.
In me the truth of Douglas fir, straight, tall,
strong-trunked land hero of fireproof bark.
Sheltering tree of life, decar's truth be mine,
cypress truth, juniper aroma, strength of yew.

May all I say and all I think
be in harmony with thee,
God within me, God beyond me,
maker of the trees.

In me be the truth of stream-lover willow, soil-
  giving alder,
hazel of sweet nuts, wisdom-branching oak.
In me the joy of crab apple, great maple, vine
  maple,
cleansing cascara, and lovely dogwood.
And the gracious truth of the copper-branched
  arbutus,
bright with color and fragrance, be with me on
the earth.

May all I say and all I think
be in harmony with thee,
God within me, God beyond me,
maker of the trees.
                    —*Chinook prayer*

Native healers were not perfect, and not everything they tried worked. But they did have centuries of accumulated empirical knowledge. Researchers today continue to study native treatments for age-old disorders and illnesses such as cancer, kidney and bladder ailments, diabetes, and diseases of the heart, liver, circulatory, and respiratory systems.

For example, contemporary European studies of saw palmetto berries, *Serenoa serrulata,* which have long been used by the Seminole and other southern Indian tribes, have found them to be a successful treatment for an enlarged prostate. It produces increased urinary flow, decreased frequency of urination, and other beneficial effects. In Germany, men use a saw palmetto tincture to relieve their symptoms.

Many health challenges occur during our middle years. Men and women may experience problems with libido or sexual enjoyment, as well as cyclical periods of depression, fatigue, memory loss, stress, and anxiety. Gentle restoratives such as American ginseng, *Panax quinquefolius;* American wild ginger, *Asarum canadense;* St. John's wort, *Hypericum perforatum;* and wild yam, *Dioscorea villosa,* are useful native resources, individually or in formula. Various wild fungi such as wood ear, *Auricularia auricula,* and the hen of the woods, *Grifola frondosa,* have noted uses for strengthening the immune system and heart and helping to maintain normal vigor.

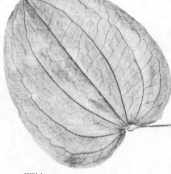
Wild yam
Dioscorea villosa

Menopause, or the "change of life," is the cessation of a woman's menstrual flow. Although all women experience menopause differently, this can be a sensitive time. Driven by decreasing estrogen levels, this journey through physical, emotional, and spiritual changes can last for a while. Some women experience mood swings, hot flashes, night sweats, and vaginal dryness both before menstruation stops and for several years after. For some women, it can also be a period of self-discovery, when they feel great freedom and experience renewed sexual interest.

Black cohosh, *Cimicifuga racemosa,* which is a fine antispasmodic used for menstrual cramps and to stimulate labor, also decreases hot flashes in menopause. This is one of several highly therapeutic squaw balms and squaw roots (see Chapter 6) found in American Indian women's medicine chests. Many women also use the roots of blue cohosh, *Caulophyllum thalictroides,* especially in herbal tea and tincture formulas, to curb hot flashes and balance mood swings.

Today many people mix our native herbs with botanicals introduced from other healing traditions, just as our native American plants are often incorporated into European, African, Chinese, and Ayurvedic formulas. In some complex mixtures, the roots of black cohosh and blue cohosh are formulated with equal amounts of wild yam, sarsaparilla roots, crampbark *(Viburnum opulus),* red raspberry leaf *(Rubus idaeus),* and dandelion roots *(Taraxacum officinale),* along with the root of dong quai *(Angelica sinensis),* to help support estrogen and progesterone levels and minimize hot flashes.

To treat dry skin, eczema, and other skin ailments that may show up during menopause, you can try evening primrose oil. Made from the seeds of evening primrose, *Oenothera biennis,* it is available in capsules that can be taken internally or applied externally. **Caution: Do not take evening primrose oil if you have epilepsy.**

Evening primrose is a rugged, self-sowing biennial or perennial. It has a long, white, carrotlike taproot that is a delicious vegetable. Indians ate this for obesity and digestive disorders. Numerous lance-shaped leaves crowd around the sturdy, fibrous stalk, which grows from one to eight feet tall, often branching out in shrubby fashion. Tubular yellow flowers with four broad petals open after sundown to entice evening pollinators. Long, ridged seed capsules ripen throughout summer and into autumn.

Evening primrose oil is a good source of gamma-linolenic acid (GLA) and other essential fatty acids (EFAs), which are vital to cell structure. Deficiencies of EFAs may be responsible for cardiovascular ailments, arthritic inflammations, and rheumatic disorders. Recent studies show that evening primrose oil can be useful in treating these serious medical problems as well as premenstrual syndrome, migraines, diabetes, alcoholism, and asthma.

Whether "male menopause" actually exists at all is controversial. Men don't usually experience sharp hormonal changes or significant symptoms like those of female menopause. In fact, there is great variability among men, with some retaining full reproductive capacity into extreme old age. For those with problems, however, American ginseng, *Panax quinquefolius,* is practically legendary as a dependable restorative and an antistress herb. It has long been considered a valuable aphrodisiac to stimulate the male sex drive—a testosterone tonic for men over forty. Both men and women use ginseng products today during periods of change, stress, and anxiety.

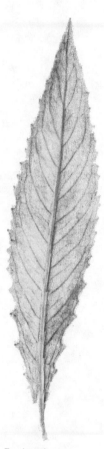

Evening primrose
Oenothera biennis

Nutraceuticals for Modern Needs

Nutritious healing foods or nutraceuticals abound in many natural environments, including home gardens. Many of them may be the "weeds" you are pulling out and throwing away, unaware of their value. Evening primrose, chickweed, purslane, plantain, nettles, burdock, and yellow dock are a few common examples. You can also make tonics and digestive aids with Jerusalem artichoke, lamb's-quarters, epazote, pigweed, garlic mustard, cinquefoil, dandelion, and chicory, all of which have high vitamin and mineral content.

Small amounts of one wild edible daily, along with your conventional foods, may be just what you need for robust good health. Dine on particular ones to target a personal need, or selectively enjoy the ones in your area. Choctaw/Apache Claude Medford Jr. used to say: "The elders believe that when we see increases in some of the wild medicine plants, this is the Creator's way of showing us that we will have an increasing need for these plants."

Wild chicory
Cichorium intybus

Lamb's-quarters
Chenopodium album

Epazote
Chenopodium ambrosioides

Dandelion
Taraxacum officinale

HERBAL CHEER MOOD AID MIXTURE

A formulation including both native and introduced herbs gives the best results. This mixture will help elevate your mood and moderate depression.

One part each:
dried St. John's wort
flowers passionflower
blossoms devil's club bark

Put the herbs into a glass jar; mix, and seal it tightly.

To make tea, measure 1 tablespoonful of the herb mixture into a mug, pour boiling water over it, and steep, covered, for 10 minutes. Strain and drink, up to two cups a day.

HERBAL CHEER TINCTURE

Use about 1 ounce of each herb listed in the recipe above; if herbs are available fresh, use 2 ounces each. Put the herbs into an 8-ounce glass jar. Fill the jar three quarters full with vodka and top with water. Seal tightly and shake gently. Store the jar in a cool place and shake it gently once a day, allowing the mixture to steep and infuse for at least two weeks.

Filter off the liquid. Label and store it in a clean glass bottle, away from the sun or heat. Use about $^1/_2$ teaspoon in tea or water, three times each day.

CALENDULA SKIN OIL

3 ounces fresh ground
calendula petals, or
1$^1/_2$ ounces dried petals
10 ounces sunflower seed or
corn oil

Calendula, *Calendula officinalis* and *C. arvense,* are cheerful, orange-gold "pot marigolds" noted for their antiseptic and healing properties, especially for the skin. These flowers are bright garden favorites and wild roadside escapees long sought for their therapeutic qualities.

Use this calendula skin oil to gently rub on irritated skin, minor burns, acne, or fungal conditions.

In a medium heat-proof glass bowl, pour the oil over the herbs. Stir well. Place in a 150-degree oven for about 4 hours. Check and stir the mixture once an hour.

Calendula
Calendula officinalis

Remove from the oven and pour through a gauze or muslin strainer. Allow the oil to drip clear and squeeze the remaining oil from the herbs. Measure, bottle, and label half of this oil. With the remaining half of the oil, you can make calendula salve, a topical skin dressing for sensitive areas, especially chapped lips.

Calendula Salve

Calendula oil reserved from previous recipe

Grated beeswax, 1 ounce for each ounce of oil

1 tablespoon aloe vera gel

4 drops tincture of benzoin

Measure the oil into a small pot. For each ounce of oil, add 1 ounce of grated beeswax. Place the pot over low heat and warm it, stirring gently, until all of the wax is melted. Remove from the heat and quickly add the aloe vera gel and tincture of benzoin. Blend well. Pour the salve into a small jar, cool, label, and cap tightly.

Calendula Tea and Eyewash

3 teaspoons fresh calendula petals or 1 teaspoon dried

2 cups boiling water

A tea made from calendula is especially good for the liver and gallbladder, where its detoxifying effects help prevent skin problems. You can also use this tea to settle digestive disorders. Use freshly made tea for best results.

Put the herbs in a small teapot. Add the water, cover, and infuse for 7 to 8 minutes. Pour a cup of this soothing blossom tea and savor the steaming fragrance as you sip it slowly.

To use this tea as a soothing eyewash for swollen, irritated eyes, carefully strain 1/4 cup through fine muslin and cool. Put it in a small, sterile eyecup. If it smarts when you try it, dilute it further with distilled water. Be sure to sterilize the eyecup with boiling water after each use. In the heat of summer, refrigerate the tea briefly and use it to calm allergy-reddened, itchy eyes.

10 green nettle tops and leaves

20 green evening primrose leaves

6 young green evening primrose seed capsules

STEAMED EVENING PRIMROSE AND NETTLE GREENS

Morning is a good time to pick wild greens, before the day's heat has robbed them of some of their vitality. Wear gloves to pick nettles. Once they are cooked, they lose their sting.

Place the plants in a small saucepan and pour 1 cup of cool water over them. Cover and place over medium heat.

As soon as the liquid comes to a bubbling boil, remove it from the heat. Allow the pot to sit, covered, for 10 minutes. Strain the amber-green tea into a mug and drink while it is still hot. Try it first unseasoned and unsweetened. If you prefer, season to taste.

Dab this warm herb tea on troublesome skin rashes, poison ivy, insect bites, or eczema, or put it in a mister to spray on your face and hair in hot weather. It is a great facial rejuvenator and toner.

If you don't want all of the tea, puree the greens with some of their juice to make a warm or chilled soup. Or spoon the steamed vegetables onto a small plate and enjoy them warm, perhaps with several drops of apple cider vinegar over them. Alternatively, you can chop and stir-fry them with eggs.

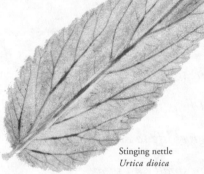

Stinging nettle
Urtica dioica

VARIATIONS: If you have a circulatory problem, headaches, digestive troubles, or arthritic or rheumatic conditions, add 1/2 teaspoon of cayenne pepper, *Capsicum frutescens,* to your vegetables before you steam and eat them.

> May the earth continue to live
> May the heavens above continue to live
> May the rains continue to dampen the land
> May the wet forests continue to grow
> Then the flowers shall bloom
> And we people shall live again.
>
> —*Hawaiian prayer*

CHAPTER EIGHT

Old Age

THE OLD WOMAN
WHO NEVER DIES

Sensitive fern
Onoclea sensibilis

O Great Spirit

Whose voice I hear in the winds,

and whose breath gives life to all the world,

hear me! I am small and weak,

I need your strength and wisdom.

Let me walk in beauty, and make my eyes ever

behold the red and purple sunset.

Make my hands respect the things you have made

and my ears sharp to hear your voice.

Make me wise so that I may understand things

you have taught my people.

Let me learn the lessons you have hidden in

Sensitive fern
Onoclea sensibilis

every leaf and rock.

I seek strength, not to be greater than my brother,

but to fight my greatest enemy—myself.

Make me always ready to come to you with

clean hands and straight eyes.

So when life fades, as the fading sunset,

my spirit may come to you without shame.

—TRADITIONAL NATIVE AMERICAN PRAYER

Sensitive fern
Onoclea sensibilis

In many American Indian societies, elevated status accompanies old age. Elderly people and elders—people of distinction, who are not necessarily old—are considered precious, unique reservoirs of accumulated knowledge. People treat them with respect, giving them the choicest foods and other special privileges. In some tribes, individuals of advancing age are given the honor of naming babies, and, because of their life experiences, younger people seek their sage counsel.

One of the tribal customs of the Yakima people, for example, is to designate an elder guardian or guide who prepares each young boy and girl for their vision or spirit quest. The Yakima, whose name means "runaway," continue to live in camps and settlements along the Yakima River, a tributary of the mighty Columbia in southern Washington.

Even when they are not the focus, rituals frequently recognize and honor elderly people. This is especially true in many key ceremonies when the generations all come together, such as spring renewal rites, planting

The Storyteller Doll

The classic Pueblo storyteller clay doll, which has become a collector's item, was originally created by Cochiti artist Helen Cordero. These dolls portray a traditional grandparent telling the old stories to grandchildren and friends. Ms. Cordero fashioned her grandfather sitting with his head tilted back, eyes closed and mouth open, as if singing or telling a story. Small Pueblo children sit in his lap, on his legs, and along his arms and shoulders.

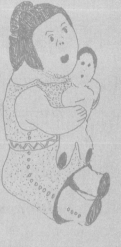

Her classic depiction has quickly become quite famous, and countless Pueblo and other American Indian potters and artists now fashion their own interpretive versions for contemporary markets. Many people keep one or more on their private altars, desks, or computers to remind them of the importance of traditions and the charms of remembering. Each time one of these dolls is painted, drawn, or fashioned in clay, it is a celebration of Pueblo traditions and an honoring of the elders and old ones.

and harvesting celebrations, solstice and equinox observances, and the midwinter or new year rituals. An honor guard of American Indian veterans and elders leads the formal procession that officially opens and sometimes closes traditional American Indian powwows and fairs, and sometimes respected elderly individuals ride in a decorated parade car or truck as a mark of distinction.

At this advanced stage of life, people sometimes struggle to maintain their best physical and mental capabilities while dealing with limitations or disabilities. Many have an urgent desire to pass on their knowledge to those who will continue to use it, especially for healing and spiritual practices. While some people enter old age with anger, resistance, or a sourness about life, the aging process can bring a quiet serenity; some people seem to be filled with a special light or aura.

In some cultures visions and dreams prepare the way for each stage of life, and getting ready for the final passage is no exception. Many elderly people relate eerie, strangely beautiful stories of seeing the Little People, traveling to the Spirit World, or speaking with the spirits of dead loved ones who "are coming back for them."

Many tribes associate certain colors with death. In some, black symbolizes death and the Spirit World; in others it is white; for some Cherokee people, purple carries the same significance. Particular animals are also associated with dying. Some of the eastern Cherokee and Creek Indians and the Northwest Coast peoples consider the owl a harbinger of death or even a sign of witchcraft, since it foretells a person's passing by calling his name in the night. Likewise, among some northeastern Algonquian people the mournful cry of the loon signals someone's demise. And some of the Plains Indians, Cherokee, and Delaware peoples connect the nighthawk with impending death and night-roaming ghosts.

While these animals are symbols of death, others are protective. Among many peoples, turtles are a sign of enduring long life and old age. Turtle-shell rattles are honored ceremonial instruments and a part of the apparel of tribes in many regions, including the Pueblo peoples of the Southwest, the Iroquois and Algonquian in the Northeast, and the Creek, Cherokee, and Seminole in the Southeast.

Because bad omens can reveal themselves at any time, it helps to carry special amulets, fetishes, milagros, and medicine bags to ward off harm and guard against dark energies. People make these spiritual gifts for friends, family members, or even themselves during troubled times. They meditate as they work, investing the item with prayers for special protection and well-being and incorporating personal love and healing energies.

Journey to the Spirit World

When their lives end, people eventually journey to the Spirit World. But holy people and other special shamans can go there at other times in their dreams and trances. Often native people prevail upon them to make the journey to retrieve valuable healing guides, plants, and curing ceremonies. Sometimes a person travels to the Spirit World to find and communicate with the ancestor spirits or a loved one who has recently passed over. Holy people are seers whose travels let them see the future. They can foretell critical events and occasionally save people from accidents or other un-

Crazy Horse dreamed and went into the world where there is nothing but the spirits of all things. That is the real world beyond this one, and everything we see here is something like a shadow from that world.

—*Black Elk,*
Oglala Lakota holy man

The Little People

Around the world, different peoples have their own unique races of Little People. Among the many forms these magical, seldom-seen, tiny beings may take are elves, gnomes, fairies, leprechauns, pixies, banshees, brownies, and dwarfs. A variety of Little People inhabited the diverse environments of Native America. Almost every tribe has distinctive tales about their own Little People, and some tribes have more than one group. They may be mystical hunters, artists, traders, stonemasons, or plant guardians, but they are always storytellers and teachers.

Some native traditions say that the Little People were the First People, and they remain the guardians of the bigger, clumsy people, we who live today. Most tribes felt that only children and elders who had a good heart and a deep spiritual connection with the earth could see the Little People; others thought that these beings were themselves the spirits of earlier children. In some tribes' stories, there are giants who share similar realms. They may still be seen in rock outcroppings and powerful stone formations across the land.

The Little People can be found throughout American Indian folklore. They are mysterious changelings who can appear as salmon, fireflies, mosquitoes, or medicine plants. They are shape-shifters, emerging as wood dwarfs peering out of a living tree, a face in stone, or a presence in the water or soil.

happy fates. And if they can't do that, they can at least prepare people for mishaps before they actually occur.

Throughout time, people have wondered what, if anything, follows death, and many native stories sought to explain the afterworld. A host of customs governed everyday behavior, especially where animals were concerned; people hoped that these observances would guarantee that their final journey would lead to peace. Most hunters have long respected the custom of making an offering of tobacco or pollen and saying a silent prayer before killing an animal whose flesh and hide were needed for food and clothing. Herbalists and gardeners follow these same protocols. Everything is a careful dance of reciprocity. Something is always given in gratitude for something taken.

Long ago, the Eastern Delaware (Lenape) believed that it was vital

The native Hawaiians have the Menehunes, who are magical stonemasons, always creating special things in their Pacific island archipelago and then suddenly disappearing. They lead healers to special medicine plants and reveal secrets of healing.

Some say that Kokopelli, the prehistoric humpbacked flute player pictured in stone throughout the desert Southwest, was a little dancing storyteller. S/he charmed the animals and plants for the First People to help them survive in earliest times. Certainly Kokopelli, pictured everywhere now, is the ultimate survivor.

The Makiawisug of the Mohegan were tiny woodland guardians. They used their special powers to guide healers to medicine plants and mushrooms and to the tastiest berries. People left them respectful offerings of corn bread and meat in tiny baskets placed near berry bushes. These Little People still look after the sacred landscapes of southern New England.

And Cherokee children hear about the Thunderers, Yunwi Tsunsdi, who have been dancing and drumming in the Great Smoky Mountains for thousands of years. They control the mushrooms and medicine plants, and manage the game animals—and some say they manage the people, too. The Thunderers bring knowledge of healing to chosen people in their dreams.

not to abuse dogs or other animals because you might be confronted by their spirits as you made your own final journey and passed over into the Spirit World. According to their beliefs, after the body died and the spirit departed, there was a long pathway to reach the Creator, Kishelamakang. First the spirit must pass over a huge bridge to the Sky World, leading into the Milky Way, which was guarded by the souls of all the departed dogs. Lenape who had lived their lives well could walk over the bridge and the road beyond without trouble. But people who had not lived a good life were prevented from crossing the bridge. They were forced to take a different road, on which they could never stop. This, the Lenape said, was a well-worn trail that never ends.

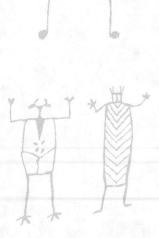

We Hidatsa believe that our tribe once lived under the waters of Devil's Lake. Some hunters discovered the root of a vine growing downward; and climbing up it, they found themselves on the surface of the earth. Others followed them, until half the tribe had escaped; but the vine broke under the weight of a pregnant woman, leaving the rest prisoners. A part of our tribe are therefore still beneath the lake.

—Buffalo Bird woman (Maxidiwiac), Hidatsa Elder, born about1839 in North Dakota, reflecting upon her tribe's origins

Hidatsa Old Woman Who Never Dies and Corn Dance Ceremony

Origin stories are carefully handed down to each new generation. Many tribes have a living sense of hallowed geography, a reverence for the land of their beginnings. Sacred medicines and foods from a people's homeland have enhanced value and often work in deep and amazing ways.

Corn has long been central to the survival of many tribes. Among these are the Mandan and Hidatsa Indians, village-dwelling farmers who lived in large earth lodges on high bluffs along the upper Missouri River. They shared similar customs and rituals, especially the ancient Corn Dance Ceremony, which, unfortunately, is no longer performed. This spiritual rite, keyed to the urgencies of spring, was vital to a successful planting season. It sustained and motivated everyone, but especially the elder women, who were its most important performers. To be old enough to participate in this dance was an honor.

Each spring, the eldest women of the Hidatsa performed these special rites along with a dance celebrating the Old Woman Who Never Dies, who long ago gave their tribes the seeds for their gardens. The women gathered in the village and attached dried meat offerings to the tops of tall poles to feed the Old Woman's spirit. These were left in place throughout the growing season until after harvest time. During the dance, younger women fed the older women dancers a special meat preparation, and they received corn to eat in return. And at planting time, they mixed some of these ceremonial corn kernels into the tribe's garden seeds for a special blessing.

Going further back in time, Hidatsa legend relates how the very first seeds were acquired for their earliest gardens. Wild geese brought the first corn kernels to plant, wild ducks brought the first beans, and swans brought the earliest gourd seeds. This is symbolized each year by the migrating waterfowl. Annual Hidatsa rituals honor these cycles, which weave together nature and the tribes.

The name *Hidatsa* is said to mean "willows." The god Itsikama'hidic first gave it to an early Hidatsa village, promising that the people would become as numerous as the willows along the Missouri River. Despite this, the Hidatsas and Mandans were nearly exterminated by a smallpox epidemic in 1837–38. The few hundred survivors in each tribe united and moved farther up the Missouri River in 1845, settling near the trading post of Fort Berthold, where they were joined by the Arikaras in 1862. To this day, we rely heavily upon their medicines and healing practices.

Willows, like people, are adaptable and easily hybridized. Although some will grow almost anywhere, they favor cooler, wet northern regions; there are about three hundred species found across the Northern Hemisphere. *Salix* is the genus name for the willow family (Salicaceae). The bitter, astringent bark contains a natural aspirinlike substance called salicin, which acts as an anti-inflammatory and reduces pain. The human body metabolizes salicin much as it does acetylsalicylic acid, which is aspirin.

Salicin is especially useful for easing headache and arthritis. Using a willow twig as a toothbrush or chew stick calms a toothache, inflamed gums, and mouth sores. Willow bark teas can relieve diarrhea and treat some cancers of the esophagus and stomach. And placing a poultice made with willow bark tea on skin tumors, abcesses, and even poison ivy rash will provide relief while it dries and heals the skin.

The Arctic willow, *Salix arctica,* and bearberry willow, *S. uva-ursi,* are two of our more northerly species. Their leaves, bark, twigs, catkins, and roots have long been prominent in countless native healing preparations. The various red willows (osiers) are highly esteemed in many tribes for use in ceremonial medicines, *kinnikinniks* (the incenselike smoking mixtures made, since prehistoric times, from fragrant healing botanicals), and artistic constructions. Sandbar willow, *S. interior;* the tall red willows, *S. laevigata* and *S. lasiandra;* the arroyo willow, *S. lasiolepis;* and the shining willow, *S. lucida,* whose canes and branchlets are more golden to brown in color, all carry special healing energies. And the tall black willow trees, *S. nigra,* which can reach heights of thirty-five feet, are also highly valued pharmaceutical factories and craft resources.

In our way of life it is the elders, the grandparents, who are seen as the bridge to the past, just as the young are the bridge to the future. And both are necessary to complete the circle of life.

—Trudie Lamb Richmond,
Schaghticoke Algonquian Elder,
historian, teacher, and
storyteller

Iroquois Midwinter Rites

The influence of the Iroquois tribes once extended from the Atlantic seaboard to the Mississippi River region, and from southern Canada to the Carolinas. Today, most Iroquois live on reservations and trust lands in New York, Wisconsin, and Canada. Traditional Iroquois people celebrate the longest, most important event in their ceremonial year at midwinter.

No outsiders are permitted to visit the longhouse during this time, and no one may sketch, photograph, tape-record, or take notes.

Midwinter Ceremonies involve everyone in the tribe, but they are governed by the elders. Many of the events can take place only with certain elders playing the key roles. The ceremonies begin each day with a prayer of thanksgiving and the ritual offering of tobacco. Over the course of a week to ten days, the people perform eighteen ceremonies entirely in the native language of the tribe that is hosting the rituals. There are six Iroquois nations: Onondaga, Oneida, Cayuga, Seneca, Mohawk, and Tuscarora. Each nation has its own unique variations that come into play when the rites occur on its reserve in Canada or its reservation in the United States.

Midwinter marks the new year of the Iroquois. It is the end of the old ritual year and the beginning of the new one. It starts on the fifth day after the new moon following the winter solstice, usually in January. This is the time when the seven Star Dancers—which we know as the Pleiades—are directly overhead in the crisp, dark night sky. More than forty distinct constellations are visible from the Northern Hemisphere; the Pleiades and other constellations are vital in countless American Indian legends (see Chapter 4). Their appearance in a certain part of the sky often signals the time for key tribal events and ceremonies.

Today, the dates for Midwinter Ceremonies must also take into account people's schedules, especially those of the chiefs. Iroquois people are spread around the country, and it is hard for many of them to get back home for these traditional rites.

Because Midwinter Ceremonies are a time of renewal, many take them as their birthday time. Naming ceremonies for newborn children are also common at this period. David Richmond (Snipe Clan), an Akwesasne Mohawk historian and teacher, recalls that 166 Mohawk babies received their names during the Midwinter Ceremonies in 1997. Once a walker of high steel (see Chapter 4) and a Vietnam veteran who fought as a Green Beret, Dave speaks with quiet dignity about his tribe's religious practices. He is proud to see that more of his people are observing their traditions.

According to Mr. Richmond, the intent of Midwinter Ceremonies "is to give thanks to all natural and supernatural beings in this world." This is the time for confessions, for curing ceremonies, and for giving thanks to the False Faces, the Hadooes (Hedowe) (see Chapter 7). The Feast for the Dead is held in order to offer favorite foods and native tobacco to the spir-

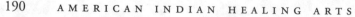

Iroquois Little Water Society

The Seneca prophet Handsome Lake was born in 1735 into the Turtle Clan, in the village of Conawagas on the Genesee River. He was a victim of displacement due to land loss and relocation, poor health, and the ravages of alcoholism. When he was near death he received prophetic visions describing a new social and religious order. This became known as the Code of Handsome Lake. It sought change by, at least in part, banishing or destroying the societies and orders that had preserved the older religious rites of the Iroquois.

The Code of Handsome Lake divided the Iroquois and forced many of the secret medicine societies and their rites underground for preservation. But secrecy seems only to have strengthened them, since they have continued to prosper through the last few centuries.

The Little Water Society remains an important part of the Iroquois' religious system, and their medicine lodge is one of the highest religious mysteries. Although its origins are lost in time, the energies of its members, both men and women, keep it going.

This society, which has no public ceremonies or dances, meets four times each year. At these social gatherings of renewal everyone smokes their native home-grown tobacco. The ceremony begins before midnight and concludes at daybreak; the sun must never see these rites. Instead, the ritual singing goes on in total darkness to conserve the power of the secret medicine, known as the "little water-power," for use by the medicine people in their healing ceremonies. Most of the rituals are chanted in unison by the entire company of members, each shaking a gourd rattle.

its so that their souls will be at rest. The medicine societies are also at their busiest during this action-filled period.

Dreams are treated seriously at every age, but the contents of elders' dreams are given especially serious attention. Each elder is a library of cultural knowledge and tribal traditions, and their dreams have special potency. They can often foretell illness and prescribe minerals, herbs, fungi, or other curing practices. During certain rites, the tribe reviews and discusses old dreams. These are essential threads throughout the ceremonies, culminating in the Dream Guessing Rites (see Chapter 4).

Iroquois medicine societies long ago discovered countless native herbs, fungi, minerals, and animal constituents to treat a wide range of human needs. Among their unique healing botanicals are the bog and wetland plants. The cold winter months brought colds, respiratory congestion, arthritis, rheumatism, and other concerns for the elderly. The bog plants, especially the flags, provided helpful treatments and relief. Today traditional Iroquois healers return to these environments to selectively harvest the resources they need to continue their traditions.

Both sweet flag, *Acorus calamus,* the aromatic calamus root, and its close relative blue flag, *Iris versicolor,* are valued root medicines. Though both have toxic properties, they can be used in small amounts to aid digestion, stimulate appetite, and soothe sore throats and colds. People carry small pieces of the dried roots as amulets to ward off illness and ensure good health. Winter muskrat is a favorite traditional food of the Iroquois because of the animal's tendency to feed heavily on sweet flag, which is also known as muskrat root. Some say the rich, dark meat is so highly perfumed that eating it is like ingesting a valuable medicine. Because many tribes believe that sweet flag has spiritual powers, they use it ceremonially as well.

Among the more fascinating medicine plants of the Iroquois are the Sarraceniaceae, carnivorous pitcher plants. These bog plants have long been vital to tribes throughout the East, who often traveled some distances to get these peculiar native plants in their specialized environments. Today most are on endangered species lists because their fragile habitats are shrinking, and their attractiveness has made them vulnerable to collectors.

The northern pitcher plant, *Sarracenia purpurea,* is a strikingly beautiful plant found in sphagnum bogs. The Iroquois call this "turtle socks" or "turtle shoes." They steep the whole plant in a pot of water to make cold and flu remedies. The resulting liquid yields an effective decongestant as well as a liver tonic. In the past, some tribes used the pitcher plant to prevent smallpox.

The Creek, Cherokee, and Seminole used three other species of healing herbs. These were the trumpets, *Sarracenia flava;* crimson pitcher, *S. leucophylla;* and hooded pitcher, *S. minor.*

Sioux Blessing of the Sacred Pipe

The noted Sioux *heyoka* (sacred fool) Lame Deer once described the Thunder Beings, or *wakinyan*—the Sacred Flying Ones, or thunderbirds—and the power of their lightning. These supernaturals are known as *wakanoyate,* the Spirit Nation, and they lived on the earth when it was new. When they died, their spirits went up into the clouds and their bodies turned into the black stones scattered across the Badlands. Some of their lightning bolts turned into black stone spear points after they brought the first light into the world.

The ceremonial sacred pipe contained some of this potent energy from the heavens because the carver brought an awareness of the tribe's cosmology and creation stories into the making of the body and stem of the pipe. The two pieces of the pipe were wrapped and kept separately. They could be joined only by certain elders during specific holy ceremonies.

The Blessing of the Sacred Pipe was an important annual renewal for various societies among the Sioux and other Plains tribes, who also created magnificent pipes to accompany their prayers. Tobacco societies often held substantial power in setting the time and nature of these events, which might coincide with the tribe's Sun Dance or with a journey to a medicine wheel (see Chapter 5). These ceremonies were often private, attended only by a group of elder men and healers. Occasionally elder women were delegated to assume responsibility for these special rites. Being chosen was a privilege and a burden, because it required days of detailed prayers and travel with some of the tribe's most sacred accouterments to Bear Butte or another point in their sacred landscape.

Contemporary pipe carriers from many Plains tribes continue these sacred rites and traditions. They are often called upon at public and private gatherings to lead blessings and sanctify the events. They too renew their pipes and sacred accouterments, each in their own special ways.

In my dream, one of these small round stones appeared to me and told me that the maker of all was Wakan'tanka, and that in order to honor him I must honor his works in nature. The stone said that by my search I had shown myself worthy of supernatural help. It said that if I were curing a sick person I might ask its assistance, and that all the forces of nature would help me work a cure.

—*Brave Buffalo, a standing Rock Sioux medicine man, describing a boyhood dream that helped him understand he was on a special healing path*

Cheyenne Blessing of the Sacred Arrows

In contrast to the Blessing of the Sacred Pipe, the whole tribe was invited to attend the Cheyenne Blessing of the Sacred Arrows. Various bands of Cheyenne people came together from all over the country for their annual renewal, which took place at the Sun Dance. This was a cherished time of shared feelings, prayers, foods, and goods. A strong communal spirit flourished, and people achieved renewal on many levels.

The sacred arrows were kept wrapped; they stored the energy of the people. They were bestowed on the Cheyenne along with an idea for a special society for their protection and instructions for renewing them every year.

As sacred clowns, the elders set the tone of the event, lightened its seriousness, and wove everyone together. In early times, the Cheyenne Contrary Society of respected warriors would perform daring and often hilarious acts of bravery during these rituals. Their feats often exposed them to danger, but their special responsibilities gave them sacred powers. Society members were required to abstain from sex and many other life pleasures in order to devote themselves to their society and their visions.

Yurok, Karok, and Hoopa (Hupa) World Renewal Ceremonies

The Yurok, whose tribal name means "downstream people" in the Karok language, and the Karok, whose name means "upstream people," originally lived along the Klamath River in northern California. They fished for salmon, hunted, and gathered other resources. They lived in villages of large cedar plank houses in the winter, and in summer they moved around the region to exploit the lush seasonal harvests of acorns and other wild nuts, seeds, and fruits. These tribes were noted for their beautiful, tightly woven baskets.

The Hoopa have retained their original homelands in the Hoopa Valley along the Trinity River near its confluence with the Klamath River in California's highlands. Salmon and acorns were also their traditional staple foods. The Hoopa were famous for their finely twined baskets and hats, cedar-planked houses, and dugout canoes.

All three tribes held annual World Renewal Ceremonies to "firm the earth." This was their way of reaffirming their respect, devotion, and connection to the earth. It was vital to seek this balance, since the people went out into their environs for food, medicine, and even for visions.

Most of the rites could only be led by elders, who retained the knowledge of how to perform them. Elders taught other tribe members about living the good life, reconnecting them with their place and clearing their villages of harm or degradation to ensure the continuation of dependable natural resources. Shamans underwent purification rituals before performing these secret renewal rites in scattered natural locations.

Everyone in the village was engaged in the sacred rites. To accompany them, dancers publicly performed three principal dances. The White Deerskin Dance brought together many performers wearing animal-skin aprons beneath shell-and-tooth necklaces and elaborate feather head-dresses. They carried poles draped with white deerskins and decorated with choice red-feathered woodpecker scalps.

The impressive Boat Dance crowded the participants in long dugouts as they navigated the turbulent rivers, vital sources of salmon and other fish and game foods. The third dance was a ritual Jumping Dance, for which the performers wore woodpecker scalps fashioned into dazzling headbands, and carried wands of sacred plant materials. The heady com-bination of so many people coming together, in conjunction with the rit-ual prayers and dances, was believed to create great powers of renewal for the earth.

A key plant remedy among these three California tribes was the devil's club, *Oplopanax horridum*. This sweetly aromatic ginseng relative is found along the Cascades and throughout the red cedar forests just north of their homelands. The roots and bark of this formidable, bristly shrub have long been used to treat adult-onset, insulin-resistant diabetes. When taken as a tea, this herb seems to lessen food binges and the craving for sugar. Devil's club may also relieve some body/mind stress and increase one's feelings of well-being.

Creek and Seminole Old People's Dance

In the old days, in late autumn, when the purple pokeberries were ripe, Seminole men performed this traditional nighttime masked dance. The vivid magenta dye from the fresh berries provided the colorful stain for their gourd, melon, or bark masks. The men cut holes for the eyes and one for the mouth, which was decorated with teeth made of corn kernels.

The rest of their costumes were no less elaborate. The men created wild, fragrant headgear by fastening sumac leaf stalks together in clumps, attached long earrings on their masks, and wore old, mismatched clothes with a shawl or blanket drawn around them. They wore turtle-shell leg rattles above their ankles. Some dancers carried a bow and arrows—often improvised especially for this dance—as they stalked and postured around the dance ground and pretended to see various game animals and spirits.

Sometimes the older men would tell fortunes. They would clear a patch of ground of all weeds, grass, and trash, and make it smooth. One man would sit at each of the four directions. The man at the west would draw a circle in the earth with his cane and the four would study the surface of the earth inside the circle to predict the future. Maybe a bug would walk across part of the circle. It all had a meaning.

—*Willie Lena*

Their amusing antics were calculated to make people laugh as they performed tricks and struck funny poses. Young children were awed and frightened by these apparitions, but most of the older tribal audiences loved their hilarious presentations.

The Creek and Seminole Old People's Dance served many purposes besides harvest and renewal rites and the honoring of certain perennial plants. The dances sought to recognize the well-loved elders in each tribe, and since the origins of these old-time dances dated back to the earliest rituals, performing them renewed the people's spirits, songs, and medicines.

Unfortunately, Seminole and Creek peoples no longer perform these specific ancient ceremonial dances. But parts of them can still be seen. During the dark periods of the 1800s and early 1900s, when the United States and Canadian governments outlawed some of the most sacred religious ceremonies, American Indians responded by repatterning their dances. Distinctive traces of old Ghost Dance, Sun Dance, and War Dance rites, along with older ceremonial animal, gourd, harvest, and healing dances, live on today, woven into contemporary powwow dances.

Pokeweed, *Phytolacca americana,* is a tall, rugged, large-leaved plant with reddish-magenta stems. It is widespread along roadsides and open woods from Ontario and southern Quebec south to Florida, and west to Texas and Mexico. This ubiquitous herb grows with robust energy into a small shrub, but it dies back to the ground after a killing frost. Its deep, thick taproot is highly esteemed for native medicines, as are the clusters of tiny white summer blossoms and drooping clusters of dark purple berries in autumn.

The whole plant is considered toxic, but all of its parts can be carefully used in various seasons. In spring you can collect the newly emerging green shoots, steam them in several changes of water to eliminate their bitterness, and eat them like asparagus. This *poke salat* is often enjoyed as one of the first spring greens after the wild onions and wild leeks.

Known in the Creek Indian language as *osa',* poke is a powerful medicinal plant that has vital contemporary applications. **Note: Because of its toxic properties, poke, like many healing plants, must be used carefully, in small amounts, and with full knowledge of its beneficial and harmful effects.** Herbalists carefully clean, cut, and tincture the fresh roots in alcohol to extract their healing constituents. The long, sturdy taproot is used in very small amounts to relieve lymph congestion and swollen nodes and to cleanse the blood.

Earlier peoples took natural signs as useful indicators. In addition to its use in the Old People's Dance, Oklahoma Seminole chief and medicine man Willie Lena recalled how pokeweed was consulted as a harbinger of spring. Seminole men cleared the ground around four poke plants and watched them closely to see if they showed any tiny leaves by New Year's Day. A showing of new growth indicated a good growing season ahead for gardens, farms, and wild medicines.

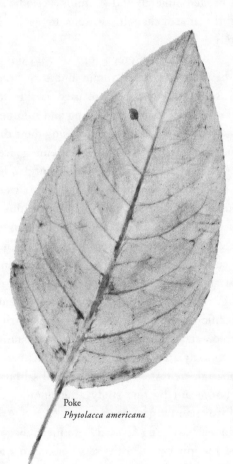

Poke
Phytolacca americana

Centuries ago our ancestors ate seasonal, regional wild foods. They drank tonics and blood thinners like the root-and-bark teas of black birch, sassafras, spicebush, and sarsaparilla in late winter and spring. The twigs of these and numerous other shrubs and trees were valued chew sticks, containing much-needed minerals and vitamins. Periodic light water fasts were important at the time of changing seasons, to rest the internal organs and purify the body.

In the spring, the emerging green tops of wild onions, wild leeks, wild garlic, and the roots of water plantain and arrowhead were coveted vegetables and seasonings, and they were used as skin tonics that also worked as systemic insecticides in early spring and summer. Wild onions were so highly esteemed in native spring cleansing diets that special local festivals and suppers were planned around their emergence in late winter and early spring. Vitamin-rich greens and blooms of dandelion and plantain, wild sorrel (toxic in large amounts), and mints were also used as trusted liver tonics, cleansing herbs, and vegetables at this time of year.

You can eat native wild garlic, leeks, and the ubiquitous wild onion grass fresh in season, or dry or tincture them for future needs. These members of the allium family continue to be vital foods, restoratives, and medicines.

Many American Indians devised special diets to maintain good health. As they age, people's immune and skeletal systems require substances rich in specific vitamins and minerals, so many tribes emphasized fruits and vegetables, such as the potassium-rich amaranths and watercress. They also regularly ate wild onions and garlic; papaya, pineapple, and avocado; chaparral, creosote bush, peyote, and saltbush. Their experience has been borne out by one study after another confirming the health benefits of fruits and vegetables.

Florida Seminoles have long favored "swamp cabbage," which is actually the heart or the inner part of the sabal palmetto and other palms. This was eaten raw and also enjoyed steamed or cooked. Today the vegetable known as heart of palm is an expensive delicacy in many restaurants. This distinctly Seminole vegetable comes from their saw palmetto, *Serenoa repens* or *serrulata,* whose delicious fruits are also highly esteemed treatments for an enlarged, inflamed prostate. Balanced with

Sheep sorrel
Rumex acetosella

Wood sorrel
Oxalis corniculata

other select native herbs, saw palmetto has long been valued as a male tonic. It is also the source for the palmetto fiber extensively used by Seminole artists for everything from their colorful dolls to their Bible and album covers.

Another superior edible resource long familiar to American Indians is the wild mushroom. With their amazing shapes, colors, and presentations, the vast array of these fungi can dazzle an observer. Getting to know these fascinating organisms from the earth is a lifelong devotion for a growing number of people. And they are powerful: They can kill or cure you. Besides tasting good, some of the most choice edible wild mushrooms offer great health benefits.

You may know where to find these earthy treasures growing on trees, but if you run out of wild supplies, they are also available at some supermarkets. In spring and fall you can often find wavy clusters of tree ears or wood ears, *Auricularia auricula,* growing from fallen hickory or hemlock logs after heavy rains. These large, smooth, tan to brown jellylike fungi are smooth; they look like ears, both in shape and in how they grow from their wood host. If you find some, collect them with joy and take them home for a special meal. If you dry them first, their flavor and fragrance become more robust.

Our native wood ears are closely related to the Chinese *mo-ehr, Auricularia polytricha,* which is highly favored in Asian cuisines. Studies show that these fungi have beneficial effects on blood coagulation and may contribute to a lower incidence of coronary artery disease. Many people like eating this mushroom once a week for its therapeutic benefits; its crunchy texture is also appealing.

Mushrooms are entirely different organisms from higher plants and from each other. Puffballs, morels, jellies, chanterelles, and fairy rings are choice edibles, and some have positive effects on health. But one huge polypore stands out especially well in both categories. Hen of the woods, *Grifola frondosa,* is a clustered mass of fleshy, fluted grayish-tan "spoons" with whitish pores beneath. These branching, overlapping fans grow out from the bases of oaks, hickories, and other deciduous trees, looking almost like exploding cauliflowers in the autumn woods. Some clusters can grow to be four to five feet wide and weigh up to a hundred pounds. This choice, meaty mushroom, which often occurs year after year in the same place, is a hunter's delight. (As with the prized morels of spring, mushroom hunters are reluctant to reveal the locations where they find their treasures.)

Black birch
Betula lenta

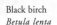

The hen of the woods is known as *grifoni* in Italy, where it is esteemed as a meat substitute. In Japan and the United States it is also called maitake, which means the "dancing mushroom," because people in Japan would often dance with joy upon finding it. Huge specimens—sizable enough to feed a small family for an entire season—come out of our New England woods.

Not only is this mushroom a delicious edible, but research has shown that it helps fight diabetes, cancer, and the HIV virus. Called the "king of mushrooms" by people who know and eat it, the amazing *Grifola frondosa* also lowers blood pressure, reduces obesity, substantially reduces fibroids, and decreases prostate problems. It may also prove to be one of nature's finest immune stimulants.

During old age, medications, illnesses, and other conditions can affect the senses of smell and taste. Appetite stimulants can help people keep or regain the desire to eat. American Indians long used restoratives such as American ginseng, American ginger, sarsaparilla, sassafras, black birch, sweet fern, and other related root plants, either individually or combined in balanced formulas, to raise body heat, stimulate appetite and metabolism, and aid digestion. They also ferment these botanicals to make time-honored elixirs, such as the original root beers, and tonics to cleanse the kidneys and dissolve and expel kidney stones.

Many tribes also use the leaf teas of numerous wildflowers to stimulate the appetite, especially for children and the elderly. You can lightly steep several fresh leaves (or other indicated parts) of one of the following plants for five to six minutes. Sip the tea, preferably without maple syrup or honey, since sweeteners tend to satisfy a desire for food.

American mountain ash, *Sorbus americana* (ripe berries)
Turtlehead, *Chelone glabra*
Downy rattlesnake plantain, *Goodyera pubescens*
Purple gentian, *Gentiana quinquefolia*
Columbo root, *Swertia caroliniensis* (roots)
Wild tarragon, *Artemisia dracunculus*
American barberry, *Berberis canadensis* (leaves and roots)
Hop tree, *Ptelea trifoliata*
Quaking aspen, *Populus tremuloides* (inner bark)

American mountain ash
Sorbus americana

While leaf teas are the best way to use these botanicals, many of them can be easily tinctured (see Chapter 10). Adding between several drops to a half teaspoon of tincture to hot water will produce a great digestive tea. If you wait ten minutes after you've added the tincture, most of the alcohol will evaporate.

Traditional treatments for eczema, emphysema, asthma, Alzheimer's disease, and other ailments of aging have evolved over time. Native herbalists selectively incorporate the best plants from the Ayurvedic, Chinese, European, and African healing traditions, which in many cases are as valuable as our indigenous plants. Many of these "introduced" herbs have now been in use in North America for several hundred years.

Healers blend native herbs that assist memory, such as clematis, chaparral, devil's club, and cayenne, with introduced botanicals such as ginkgo, gotu kola, feverfew, and rosemary. Each of these plants has potential side effects, so herbalists use caution when making their formulas until they achieve the right balance for a particular patient, based upon age, body size and weight, and severity of symptoms.

Dry skin and dry hair conditions call for the use of special oils such as those made from sunflower seed, corn, and jojoba. Mixed with certain herbs, pollen, and minerals and mineral oils, these can be used to treat internal as well as external physical needs. Native people supplement these treatments with skin lubricants made seasonally of various fish oils and animal fats, often mixing the oils with botanicals that have strong insecticidal value, such as the mints, sweet fern, wintergreen, bayberry, and pennyroyal.

Bayberry
Myrica pensylvanica

HERBS TO RAISE BODY HEAT

To raise body heat and stimulate poor circulation you can add small amounts of grated or chopped ginger root to cooked vegetables and soups. You might also try powdered dried cayenne, paprika, or other sweet, mild, or hot varieties of pepper, depending on your palate.

You can also apply dried, powdered cayenne pepper directly on the skin to relieve arthritis or other joint and muscular pains, but do not try it if you have any open sores or cuts. To stimulate circulation in your feet and ankles, try lightly dusting cayenne into cotton socks just before you pull them on your feet.

1 cup fresh wood ears, or
  1 ounce dried,
  reconstituted

3 cups hot vegetable or
  chicken broth, or hot water

2 cups warm water

$^1/_2$ cup chopped dandelion
  roots or carrots

$^1/_2$ cup natural wild rice

2 tablespoons chopped
  onions

1 tablespoon sea dulse,
  chopped

1 teaspoon crushed red
  pepper, or to taste

salt and pepper to taste

2 tablespoons cornstarch

1 egg, well beaten

2 tablespoons cider vinegar

$^1/_2$ cup chopped green onions
  for garnish

This stimulating and warming soup, filled with healthy ingredients, can be a meal in itself. Enjoy this with friends, or savor it yourself.

If reconstituting dried mushrooms first, place them in a glass bowl, cover them with 3 cups of hot broth, and allow to soak for 30 to 40 minutes.

Reserving $^1/_4$ cup of the mushroom broth, pour the rest, along with the mushrooms, into a medium soup pot. Add the additional water and bring this to a boil over medium heat.

Add the vegetables and wild rice, stir well, and lower the heat to simmer. Stir in the sea dulse and crushed pepper, season to taste, cover, and simmer for 35 minutes.

In a small cup, mix the reserved mushroom broth with the cornstarch until smooth; carefully stir this into the soup, and raise the heat slightly, to medium. Stir until the soup just thickens.

Slowly pour the beaten egg into the soup while stirring well. Remove from the heat and add the vinegar. Spoon the soup into serving bowls and garnish with fresh chopped green onions.

Yield: 6 generous cups.

Dandelion
Taraxacum officinale

ARNICA MASSAGE OIL

Every morning and evening, make it a regular practice to gently massage your feet. While you are gently rubbing your soles, concentrate on easing all of their burdens and stimulating healthy blood flow. Use four or five drops of a mild arnica oil in the palm of each hand, and work this well into the skin, going around each toe and massaging the whole foot. Always work from the toes back toward the ankles and up the leg.

You can also use this fragrant oil to massage sore, aching muscles or for total body massage.

Chop or bruise the arnica as you place it in a sterile 8-ounce jar. Pour in enough oil to cover all the plant material. Put the lid on tightly and agitate the jar briefly to mix and thoroughly coat all materials. Place this on a sunny windowsill for three weeks, shaking the jar daily.

Pour this cold-infused oil into a muslin or gauze filter over a clean jar and strain out all plant material. Squeeze the oil through the cloth, then pour the oil into clean storage bottles and label. This should last up to a year if kept in a cool place, but your intent should be to use it daily.

Arnica *(Arnica cordifolia),* enough to fill an 8-ounce jar
Sunflower seed or corn oil

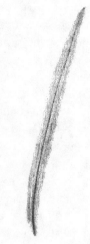

Virginia (grass leaf) mountain mint
Pycnanthemum virginianum

STIMULATING FOOT BATH

Try this just before cutting your toenails.

Crush the herbs as you drop them into a big pan. Pour a kettle of boiling water over them and steep for a few minutes. Add the cider vinegar and fill the pan half full of warm or cool water, depending upon the season and your preference. If you like, add some cayenne pepper.

Sit comfortably with your bare feet immersed for 15 to 20 minutes, if possible. Wiggle your toes, flex your feet, and do simple foot exercises for a minute or two at a time, then relax. Repeat every 3 minutes.

$^1/_2$ cup fresh bergamot or mountain mint, blossoms and leaves
Boiling water
$^1/_4$ cup apple cider vinegar
Water
Cayenne pepper (optional)

Purple bergamot
Mondarda fistulosa

Penobscot Root Clubs
and Root Medicines

For more than three centuries the Penobscot Indians of Maine have carved unusual clubs and walking sticks from young gray birch, *Betula lenta,* and poplar, *Populus balsamifera,* as well as their relatives. These traditional carvers are said to incorporate the spirits of the wood into their distinctive art.

The men journey along the Penobscot River in their canoes to small islands where they select and dig up a few choice, small trees. Cleaning and working with the trees brings them closer to the tree spirits, who tell or teach them what to carve. As they slip off the aromatic bark and scrape the inner bark, they see "spirit faces."

When the carver is done, a small spirit face may appear to stare out from an eagle's wing, flanked by a turtle, bear, or eel surrounding the head of the club, made from the rootball. Multiple personalities emerge from these haunting sculptures, unique to the riverine woods of Maine.

Once all Penobscot men knew the ways of the woods and made these carvings. They created fierce-looking war clubs or ethereal spirit clubs. Although quite a few of them became ornate collectors' items, many people believe there was an ancient connection to healing.

Stanley Neptune, who is Eel Clan, began studying with Penobscot master carver Senabeh Francis in his early twenties. Today Stan and his son Hugga both carve, combining modern skills with the traditions handed down through many generations. Stan's sister Nina knows the spirituality of the old clubs and feels that they still retain the spirits of their makers, just as old baskets, canes, and walking sticks do. Actually, "the tree calls to the carver," says Nina.

The trees used by these carvers also provide vital medicines. Poplar roots and bark contain salicin, which has aspirinlike qualities and can reduce fever, relieve headache, and soothe colds, flu, and muscle problems. Gray birch roots, bark, and twigs yield aromatic oil of wintergreen (even more than the wintergreen plant itself), which is esteemed for treating headache and muscle pain, rheumatism, gout, and bladder infections.

And these and other enduring trees give Penobscot and Passamaquoddy peoples much more than medicines, art, and spiritual foundations. Early legends describe the Creator making these native peoples from tall, deeply rooted ash trees. The Creator had first tried making people out of rock. When this did not work, he broke the rocks, which became Manogemassak, Little Spirits.

MARIGOLD BLOSSOM AND MINT MASSAGE OIL

This is a fine oil for your face, arms, and hands. Simply fill an 8-ounce jar two thirds full of fresh or dried marigold petals. Top with fresh or dried mint leaves and follow the recipe at the top of 203.

➤ ➤ ➤

By the fires that night
we feasted.
The Old Ones clucked,
sucking and smacking,
sopping the juices with sourdough bread.
The grease would warm us
when hungry winter howled.

—*Mary TallMountain, Athabaskan/Russian poet,*
  self-taught writer born in the Yukon in 1918

CHAPTER NINE

Death, the Afterlife, and the Spirit World

FOOTPRINTS THAT FADE ON THE PATH

Smooth sumac
Rhus glabra

When people die they are carried by the moon up to the

land of heaven and live in the eternal hunting grounds.

We can see their windows from on earth, as the stars, but

beyond this, we know very little of the ways of the dead.

—IKINILIK, ESKIMO ELDER

Smooth sumac
Rhus glabra

Very few beliefs were shared among all of the tribes inhabiting the diverse regions of this country, but there was a universal thread of reverence for life and respect for death. Just as there was a path of life, so too there was a road of death. Ceremonies, prayers, and sacred songs blessed the Road of Life and Death with power, grace, and protection.

Although it remained mysterious and difficult to understand, death was accepted as unavoidable. Most native peoples were not afraid of dying, and in many tribes this remains the case. In some areas the elderly held the right to determine when, where, and even how they would die. European colonizers frequently misunderstood this, finding it controversial and alien to their religious beliefs.

Death terminates a person's earthly existence and begins the soul's next journey. Many tribes and individuals believe that immediately after the body dies, the soul starts along the well-worn path to the Spirit World. This can be a complicated trip: A hierarchy of ascent and descent through these realms is a part of many tribal beliefs. Elaborate rituals ease this final passage and ensure that the spirits will not roam about, causing problems for the living.

Native concepts about the afterlife are distinctive. The Navajo people believe that the spirits of their departed go into the Sky World and travel the Milky Way to the Dance Hall of the Dead, where they make a successful transition into the hereafter. They hold elaborate ceremonies to help the soul on its journey. The Hopi House of the Dead and the Eskimo Soul Journey After Death entail similar rituals.

The Menomini are the "Wild Rice People" of the western Great Lakes regions in Michigan and Wisconsin. Early Menomini believed that every human being possesses two souls. One, *agawetatciuk,* or "a shade across," lives in the head and is considered to be the intellect. After death, this soul may linger, wandering about restlessly. Some say that it gives

Fragrant tansy
Tanacetum vulgare

sharp whistling cries after dark. People leave offerings of food and tobacco for this spirit.

The other soul, *tcebai,* lives in the heart. After death, the *tcebai* travels to the hereafter. After departing from the body, it travels westward on a four-day journey along the Milky Way toward the home of Menomini creation deities Manabus and his brother Napatao. These brothers first gave the Medicine Lodge, called the *Midéwiwin,* to the people for worship and as a means of destroying disease. The Ojibway of Wisconsin, Michigan, and southern Ontario shared similar spiritual beliefs.

Ideally, the path of life is long, healthy, and rewarding, but people are shaped by the obstacles they encounter along the way. Physical afflictions or other problems often define who an individual is and how she views life. Death begins the separation of soul and spirit from the body. Each must be looked after according to the person's beliefs.

Some believe the soul and spirit are one and travel together; others see them as separate entities. While the soul passes over immediately following death, the spirit may linger, seeking to finish work left undone. Some say that ghosts, unwilling or unable to leave, roam many parts of our land. In many native traditions special rites, feasts, ceremonies, and ritual feedings are necessary to enable these spirits to find peace and go to rest.

Ceremonies surrounding death are tremendously important because it is so vital that transitions into the afterworld occur properly. This was a particular problem in the past, when warriors were lost in battle or people suffered mysterious deaths—like those in recurring epidemics of introduced diseases—without the suitable attending rituals. Wanting proper care for its safe passage, the restless spirit may be unable to leave and find its resting place in the afterlife. Instead, it may come back to haunt the relatives, bringing them a lingering, wasting sadness akin to what we call grief.

Grief and sorrow over the loss of a loved one has always been a part of human life, and this has shaped many native rites surrounding death. Grieving is natural and cleansing. Regardless of one's strength or stature in life, crying for departed loved ones conveys respect. Many tribes held rites of condolence for their leaders and most tribal members. The Iroquois carved distinctive condolence canes embellished with detailed mnemonics and symbolic pictographs that record the ritual "crys" and other protocol for these ceremonies.

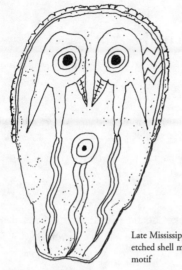

Late Mississippian Mound Builder's etched shell mask with weeping eye motif

In many tribes, the grieving family holds a giveaway, where they bestow most of the deceased's personal belongings on special friends and family members. This generous way of remembering the loved one ensures that something of the person's spirit lives on with everyone. And dispersing all of these material possessions lessens the likelihood that the loved one's ghost or shade will linger.

Some American Indian customs for dealing with grieving reflect familiar traditions from other cultures. Some rituals help people gain closure. For example, the Lutupahko, the Yaqui death anniversary ritual and fiesta that is held one year after a loved one's death, closes the formal period of mourning. This is not unlike the Jewish ceremony, often held one year after a loved one dies, when a gravestone is unveiled.

The Hurons in southern Canada, northern neighbors of the Iroquois, periodically held a Feast of the Dead. They performed this elaborate ceremony for all those who had died since the last Feast of the Dead was held. These major occasions drew together the families of the deceased. The remains of their loved ones were ritually buried in a large common grave and honored once again.

Death and funeral rites are major obligations for the family, clan, band, and tribe. Careful handling of the dead and assembling the necessary grave goods to accompany the deceased's spirit into the afterworld are

The Anishinabe Path

Native beliefs concerning death were diverse, but many tribes held that the soul would encounter numerous obstacles along the passageway or death path.

The sins that you've committed here against animals or your own people will be waiting for you when you go to the happy hunting ground and that would stop your entrance . . . 'cause there will be a big dog waiting for you when you reach the fork in the path to where you are going.

—Harold Goodsky, Anishinabe

The Anishinabe Path was the soul's journey after death. People of this Great Lakes Algonquian tribe believed that the passage to the final resting place took five to seven days.

significant responsibilities, often surrounded by tribal taboos and protocols. For instance, many Plains Indians wrapped their dead and placed them on elevated platforms or in substantial trees to enable the souls to journey upward into the Spirit World. On a more mundane level, this practice also kept the dead body safely away from most predators and, given the wind and weather conditions of the Great Plains, served to embalm it. And because death affects more than the person who has died, the ceremonies must address other areas of health and wellness as well as spiritual and religious needs.

Today some American Indian rituals most familiar to tourists have death at their core. The Yaqui Easter Ceremonies, which take place during the Christian Holy Week in April, blend native interpretations of Christ's death and resurrection with those of their Spanish Catholic conquerors as well as their own pre-Columbian mortuary customs. These Yaqui celebrations reenact centuries of political and religious history with spectacular pageantry. They also deal with good and evil, life and death, wellness and illness. So much transpires during these events that they are the center of the tribe's ceremonial year. Perhaps the most familiar native rituals of death are the colorful Días de los Muertos, the Mexican Days of the Dead, which today are prominently celebrated across the Americas.

The Seneca Ghost Feast

The Seneca, one of the Elder Brothers of the Iroquois Confederacy, are known as the Keepers of the Western Door. Today they are centered in community groups in upper New York state, southern Canada, and with the Cayuga tribe in Oklahoma. More than six thousand Seneca live on their Allegheny and Cattaragus reservations near Buffalo, New York.

If left unexpressed, sorrow and loss can cause problems. The Seneca hold the Ghost Feast to dispel sickness or ill fortune caused by evil ghosts. It can also calm unsettling dreams and nightmares about restless phantoms and spirit intruders. The chief woman of the O'gi'we Oa'no', or Chanters for the Dead, can call for the O'gi'we when a member of the society experiences such a troubling dream. Or a ceremony may be offered to the deceased's clan to treat the spirit needs of all grieving clan members.

As preliminaries to the feast, members of the society sing a set of ritual songs around a large water drum and perform other rites. Someone with special powers divines the identity and problems of the troubling spirit(s) so they can be propitiated and driven away by the use of tobacco and the appropriate songs and chants.

As is the custom with most Seneca and Iroquois ceremonies, the concluding feast nurtures all participants. Among the traditional foods the Seneca prepare and serve following the Ghost Feast are roasted corn soup, *wah-da-sgion-dah,* and boiled cornbread, *ga-gai-te-ta-kwa.* After everyone eats, the leftovers stay on the feast table overnight to, according to custom, satisfy the hungry ghosts that for some reason are earthbound.

Everyone's passing is mourned, but when a Seneca chief dies, in addition to other mourning rites, a special Condolence Ceremony is held at the wood's edge. Here the surviving leaders grieve and speak about the tribe's loss.

The Seneca and other Iroquois tribes had numerous ghost medicines and death medicines. They used these to guard their other healing remedies, guide ghosts away from earthly attachments, protect people and animals from "ghost sickness," and honor good spirits, asking for their help and guidance. In the early 1900s Cayuga herbalist Robert Smoke, of Six Nations Reserve, noted the special uses of boneset, *Eupatorium perfoliatum,* especially if it was found growing near graves. Known as "ghost medicine," young boneset branches are burned in a pot in the house to drive

Yu ni ne-un-ai; ji-bai oke ni ki-pi-ai; ni mus se-chu?
(Here I am; Spirit Land, I am coming; must I pass away?)

—*An old Mohegan Death Chant, usually sung along with a tobacco offering to the Spirit of the Deceased*

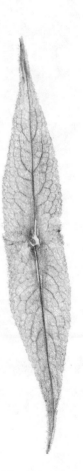

Boneset (cross-section)
Eupatorium perfoliatum

Now we become reconciled
as you start away. . . .
Persevere onward to the
place where the Creator
dwells in peace.
Let not the things of earth
hinder you.

—*From an early Seneca
funeral address*

away ghosts. One may also hang a fresh branch of boneset along with white pine, *Pinus strobus,* over the doorway to keep ghosts away. Iroquois traditionalists sprinkle the dried root of American angelica, *Angelica atropurpurea,* or a strong, fragrant decoction made from the plant, inside and just outside the house for a similar purpose.

In life as well as death, the Seneca were blessed with sacred plants, especially two evergreen trees of the northern woodlands. Canadian hemlock, *Tsuga canadensis,* and balsam fir, *Abies balsamae,* each contain prodigious amounts of healing constituents in their needles, pitch, roots, branches, and inner bark. Their fragrant branches were used inside dwellings for bedding, as well as in sweat lodges for their aromatic purifying qualities. The whitish, aromatic gumlike sap was chewed, or boiled and rendered, for medicinal purposes. The bark was extensively used for poulticing on sores and wounds, and people used the astringent tannins from the bark to tan leathers, produce dye, and strengthen early salves and ointments. Teas and oils made from the needles and bark were used to treat colds, coughs, and rheumatism and as body lotions.

These trees are also associated with death and burials because of their aroma and healing qualities. They have special meaning because they never die. Indeed, our name for these plants—evergreen—signifies their persevering nature. Their oils were used to wash and prepare the body of the deceased, who was often dressed and laid out on their fragrant boughs for burial rites and ceremonies.

Contemporary herbalists continue many of these practices, either following traditions or amending them based on empirical experience. Today many people also fasten a braid of sweetgrass, *Hiërochloe odorata,* over each doorway inside the house. Traditional Cherokee also respect this traditional practice.

Seminole Mortuary Practices

Josie Billie, a famous Miccosukee/Seminole medicine man, knew the traditional uses of many different plants at Big Cypress Reservation in Florida. When he treated people, he made a long bubbling tube or medicine pipe of wild bamboo through which he would blow additional healing energies into the prepared medicine, to "fix it."

He had numerous applications for the fragrant sweet bay or bayberry,

Southern Paiute Cry Ceremony, Cry Songs, and Giveaway

Some say that the Cry Ceremony and Cry Songs first came from the Mohave long before 1870. Others recall that these traditions came from neighboring tribes, the Pahrump and Moapa, and from the Chemehuevi as a memorial ceremony. But no one knows quite how old these ceremonies really are.

Today, when someone dies, the Southern Paiutes hold a memorial Cry Ceremony for one or two nights before a church funeral. On the last night, groups of singers sing two cycles, the Salt Songs and the Bird Songs, from sunset to sunrise. During brief pauses between songs, the family and friends make emotional speeches. The participants share traditional stories, especially those that reveal the origins of rituals usually performed during life crises. And they reflect upon the life of the individual whose spirit they have gathered to sing over into the Spirit World. Afterward, at a giveaway, the family distributes the deceased's valuables among the guests.

Myrica cerifera, which he called *to-li* or *cho-wam a-no-chop-pi.* "I use the leaf of *to-li* when I make medicine for sick people," he said. He administered a fragrant bayberry tea infusion at a family ceremony that he called Miccosukee Purification. And when someone died, family and friends were supposed to drink bayberry tea for three days and wash their faces, hands, and arms with it. In some cases they sprinkled the tea inside the house, or *chickee,* and around the outside perimeter for protection from ghosts.

When a traditional Seminole or Miccosukee dies, his body is carefully washed with *to-li,* then lovingly dressed in his finest garments and buried. If he was a smoker, tobacco or cigarettes are placed beside him. Traditionally, a woman is buried in new clothes adorned with her special beads. Her favorite old clothing is neatly folded and placed in the casket along with her.

Sofki is a traditional vegetable drink of many southern Indians. Considered both a food and a beverage, it is usually made of roasted or parched corn that is mashed or pounded and boiled in water until it becomes fairly thick. There are many variations. It may be seasoned with pounded hickory nuts or pecans. Or it might contain tomatoes, mashed pumpkin, pumpkin seeds, or other regional seasonal roots, seeds, or vegetables. The most common form is made with corn alone and is enjoyed hot or cold. *Sofki* is a favorite of the Seminole, Cherokee, and Creek, who usually prefer it to milk, water, and other beverages.

When made and blessed in a special way, *sofki* is considered sacred, and a jar of it often goes into the casket to nourish the soul as it journeys to the afterworld. Other special foods also accompany the corpse at burial time.

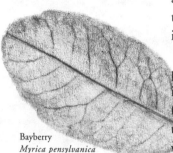

Bayberry
Myrica pensylvanica

Traditional Seminole burials, especially in Oklahoma, take place in private family cemeteries, with small wooden grave houses built over each individual grave. At a Seminole burial each member of the funeral party files by the open grave and throws a handful of soil on the casket. This is their way of "shaking hands for the last time" with their departed. Afterward they sprinkle a decoction of bayberry tea over the grave.

Seminole custom is to bury the dead person with the head toward the west and the feet facing east. During earlier times, a small wooden stake was placed in the ground near the head of the burial, and a small fire kindled a few feet away. Family and friends would stay by the fire until midnight for four nights to show their love and respect. They believed that the soul required four days and nights to reach the afterworld.

Some people would fast, going without food or drink for this period. On the fourth morning, the fire in the mourner's home was extinguished, the hearth was cleaned out, and a new fire was rebuilt to cook food for a feast. All pots and utensils were also washed and sprinkled with bayberry leaf tea; then all of the remaining tea was poured out on the ground.

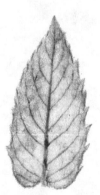

Spearmint
Mentha spicata

Today as in the past, after the mourning period, the family provides a feast, usually at the deceased's home. On the grave, they place a small "spirit plate," containing a tiny portion of the feast foods to feed the departed spirit of the loved one. To banish sadness and protect them from arthritis—which may develop at this time—mourners drink brewed herbal teas of gray or prairie willow *(Salix humilis)*, called *hoyvnijv*, and spearmint *(Mentha spicata)*, called *kofutcka*. They also bathe their hands and faces with the teas.

Traditional favorite foods are like powerful medicines and sweet prayers; they play a significant role in ceremonies for the dead. The inclusion of these special foods at births, deaths, and all other important ceremonial times is reassuring and offers additional blessings. At feasts and festival times, small spirit plates may be prepared and placed upon people's graves with particular prayers of remembrance. Some of these old-time favorite Seminole foods are frybread, venison, frogs' legs, turtle, and other wild game meats, as well as wild seeds, fruits, and vegetables.

In the past, alligator, which is so widely associated with the Florida Seminole today, was rarely hunted or eaten because it was considered sacred and associated with a number of religious traditions and taboos. Twentieth-century tourist and trade pressures have changed this. Now alligator tail meat is cooked and sold at contemporary Seminole fairs and powwows as "gator nuggets," deep-fried and delicious. And alligator now occasionally appears on Seminole spirit plates.

Handling of medicines associated with the dead is especially sensitive, so as not to offend the spirits. According to Josie Billie, when a sick person dies, anything that remains of that person's herbal medicine must be disposed of carefully so it doesn't harm anyone else. Frequently it is poured over stones or a large rock in order to dissipate its energies.

Navajo Dance Hall of the Dead

The Navajo believe there is a detailed cosmic order to life and death. They live in ways they hope will ensure a death from old age. When a person lives a long time and dies of natural causes, it means she died without faults and without inner turmoil or anger. If she has such an esteemed death, her soul is free to return to Dawn Woman and to be born again into another body.

But when a Navajo dies before his or her time—from sudden illness, suicide, violence, or witchcraft—traditionalists feel great concern. This is not so much a fear of death or of the dead as it is apprehension for the living. An untimely death can cause a *chindi*, a destructive ghost, to arise. The *chindi* makes trouble for the departed's family and relatives. In such cases the dead person's home and belongings may have to be burned or destroyed.

To prevent such unsettling events, the Navajo endeavor to live in a state of peace, without transgressions, and to attain ultimate harmony in life and death. They strive for balance in their life on earth according to the principles of beauty, believing this will give them freedom from trouble in their everlasting life. When people are ill or distressed, Navajo holy people use their sacred rites, with and without special herbs and healing

I want to stay home and die here. Let me die in the house and do not do anything to it; it is an old-age hogan. I'm not dying of anything that you should be scared of; you should not be scared of those who die of old age.

—*final words of Frank Mitchell, famous Navajo chanter*

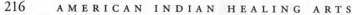

medicines, to bring them back into equilibrium. Their rituals, along with chants and sand paintings, enable people to feel the power of natural and supernatural healing and get in touch with the cosmic forces surrounding Navajo lifeways.

Each tribal group sees the path of death that leads into the realms of the afterlife a bit differently. Some Navajo people believe their souls will travel down into the underworld. Others think they will journey across the Milky Way, which is the Path of Souls, toward the Dance Hall of the Dead, where those who have led a good life will all meet again. This Spirit World is immense and filled with the beauty of eternal life. The spirits who have passed over are in motion or dancing, just as the flickering stars are perceived to dance in heaven.

Anywhere from three to seven days of rites and rituals may follow a person's death. These ceremonies encourage the spirit of the deceased to leave, and enable it to journey safely along its way and be welcomed into the Spirit World.

The way you live your life sets the stage for death and the afterlife. Choosing the appropriate rituals and chants, eating the correct foods, and living properly, with care and concern for others around you, all have an impact. Using the right herbs is also essential; the Navajo have a large and fascinating array of botanicals.

In Navajo regions, a common small shrub that can be used medicinally throughout life and for ceremonial purposes as the Life Way pollen is the rugged broom snakeweed, *Gutierrezia sarothrae*. This vital perennial herb is used in childbirth and to heal wounds and snake, insect, and spider bites. After it is burned, the ashes of this plant are rubbed on the forehead to cure headache, fever, and nervousness. Mixed with other burned herbs, the ashes of broom snakeweed become a blackening agent for the Evil Way, Holy Way, and Hand-trembling Way rites. In fact, it is used in almost all of the more than three hundred different ceremonies associated with the Navajo healing tradition.

Another conspicuous perennial herb of the Navajo is soapweed, *Yucca angustissima*. Fiber from this valuable plant is used to tie Navajo ceremonial equipment and to hold certain paint pigments. Soapweed is also a purifier; its roots provide the suds that people drink and bathe in for cleansing rituals. Soapweed's edible fruits and seeds were also used as counters for the moccasin game (see Chapter 4).

Medicinal and ceremonial uses for desert or Utah juniper (*Juniperus osteosperma*) abound. Perhaps its most remarkable use is as "ghost beads." Navajo mothers string the juniper seeds on yucca thread, making bracelets for their babies to protect them from disturbing dreams. Tourists also seek these natural ghost beads, threaded into dream catchers and strung into necklaces. Juniper has long been a foremost treatment for influenza, headaches, nausea, stomachaches, and postpartum pain; juniper infusions are sometimes used to wash the body of a dead loved one before burial. Tribes all over North America use various species of juniper throughout life and at death.

Hopi House of the Dead

Living a good life in harmony and balance is also considered essential among other tribes in order to attain a comfortable, reassuring death path. The Hopi Sun Trail is a person's main life path; it leads directly into the afterlife. If an individual faithfully follows the Sun Trail and respects and listens to the elders and old people, her soul will pass easily along a smooth highway.

After death, the soul sets out along a Sky Path leading westward. Members of the Warrior Society, Kwanitakeas, wearing a big horn headdress to identify themselves, patrol this passage through the afterlife. They ring bells to draw good souls onward. The more righteous souls travel without incident. Some fly smoothly like clouds to a large celestial village of white houses, where all of their dead loved ones reside in peace and with abundance. These ancestors' souls taste only the essence of any foods they are offered. This keeps them light and free.

But those who have not lived a good life, who have caused grief and pain to others or have committed treachery, will suffer as they make their journey. They may have a dreadful trek, a long, arduous trip that lasts centuries before they can reach the House of the Dead.

When he was discussing Hopi religious practices, Percy Lomaquahu, the late Hopi elder of Hotevilla, Third Mesa, said: "We keep the principles of our traditions in our hearts." The Hopi carefully follow specific burial customs to ensure safe passage for the soul and spirit. They wash the deceased, especially their hair, with natural yucca suds. Then they lovingly dress the body in traditional clothes. A Hopi woman is usually fastened into her white cotton marriage blanket, tied with a big knotted belt. In the Sky World these items will both symbolize and provide clouds and falling rain. The Hopi tie prayer feathers, *ankwakwosis,* around the foreheads of the dead to bless them; these also represent the falling rain. Often people are buried with feathered prayer sticks and other favorite possessions.

Grieving and praying sustain the departing spirits and souls and help the living to deal with the loss. People prepare and serve traditional foods and special herbs; they also place some in the grave.

The way that people view and handle death is a reflection of their lives, their understanding of their origins, and how they honor their traditions. To lead a good life yourself, it is important how you honor those that pass on before you. Once buried, the dead cannot be forgotten.

Pueblo All Souls' Day

In many parts of the Southwest, ceremonies leading up to All Souls' Day celebrate the tribe's dead. During the night of October 31, people light candles in their houses and churches. This is the time when the spirits of the dead return. They visit their families and friends and partake of distinctive food offerings.

Pueblo families bring corn, beans, melons, and meat along with specialty dishes such as *panocha,* a sweet dish made of wheat sprouts, to the churches for their dead relatives and loved ones. They place ripe corn stalks with the ears of corn still attached in their homes and churches. The dead will use these as canes to bless their passage to the *sipapau,* the mystical place where the tribe first came out of the earth. House doors are left open, and each family displays its finest blankets and shawls to please the revenants.

Throughout the Southwest, people extensively use the fragrant evergreen cedars, *Juniperus monosperma, J. communis,* and *J. montana.* Medicinal and practical uses for these trees' berries, leaves, bark, and wood abound. Fragrant cedar oils, salves, and lotions have long been valued skin treatments. And all parts of these plants can be used to ward off illness or bad magic.

After death, cedar water and cedar oil lotions are used to prepare the deceased for burial. Branches, small twig bundles, and cedar-filled pouches may accompany the corpse for cremation or burial. And people carve tiny symbols, called milagros, of cedar wood as special amulets and place them beside a deceased relative or friend to bless their final journey.

Los Días de los Muertos, the Mexican Days of the Dead

Today, one of the most well known ceremonies surrounding death is Los Días de los Muertos, or the Days of the Dead, which evolved from ancient Aztec beliefs and rituals. Mictlantec-uhtli, the Aztec God of Death, rejoiced in death. Death was not frightening or negative; it was part of an eternal cycle of changes, an important step to another stage of existence. Elaborate belief systems supported Aztec culture; when a person died, his soul was said to go to one of thirteen heavens or nine underworlds. Even today we continue to benefit from many of their rich ideas, valuable healing traditions, and delicious foods.

The Days of the Dead distinctively blend many beliefs and practices that predate the Spanish conquest with Spanish Roman Catholic observations of All Saints' Day on November 1 and All Souls' Day on November 2. During these special times, descendants of the ancient Aztec, Zapotec, Mixtec, and other predecessors of today's Mexicans generously share their best offerings with their dead loved ones. They spend many days in hectic and creative preparations for this festive time.

The dead's annual homecoming draws all levels of society together into shared experiences of death and rebirth, although each of Mexico's regions has evolved its own unique customs for this holiday. In celebrating death, the Aztecs enriched life and ensured its continuation. This remains the central thread of meaning for these modern fiestas.

For the creative people who fashion the unique sculptures, candles, candies, and other foods for this major festival, this is one of the most prosperous and happy times of the year. Sugar skulls and marzipan bones, along with "bread of the dead," *pan de los muertos,* a light, sweet specialty shaped and baked only at this time of year, decorate stalls in the town plazas or *zócalos.* Rural markets are filled with gaily decorated tombstones, miniature coffins, skulls, and bones. Vendors display an enormous variety

Milagros (Miracles)

People in the Southwest and parts of Mesoamerica create tiny milagros, or miracles. These are special amulets for good luck, protection, and remembrance. The small carved stone fetishes and tiny clay shapes that accompanied ancient burials may have been their ancestors.

Tribe members fashion milagros of stone, bone, or metal, or carve them out of wood. They are special gifts made in the unique forms and symbols that are significant to each tribe. Many people use them to ask the saints for help and protection. They may offer tiny figures of birds, coyotes, horses, and sheep to ask for fertility or help in healing sick animals. In some churches, people adorn statues of the various saints, the Virgin Mary, or Jesus Christ with these miniatures to petition for prayers or in gratitude for small miracles that have occurred in their lives. Milagros are especially made for each individual and unique purpose, so there is an enormous variety.

of papier-mâché or plastic skeletons. Some are serape-clad dancers or musicians with gold grins and tinfoil eyes. Their hilarious postures and antics make everyone laugh, and laughter is good medicine.

People also lovingly decorate tiny shops and private homes. Women clean and adorn their houses, making special candles and sweet treats and preparing generous amounts of traditional foods for the feasts. Men and children prepare beautiful altars in their homes, bedecked with tiny toys and foods and beverages for their dead loved ones.

At midnight the people leave their homes, carrying glowing candles, flowers, beverages, and precious foods as they walk to the cemetery. Some carry musical instruments and sing favorite songs to accompany the processions. Families arrange flowers and other offerings on the graves of their departed, with whom they spend the long night. The fluttering candle flames are proof that the souls, or *almas,* are with them and partaking of the offerings. Some say that the human souls come back to eat and drink the souls of the foods and flowers.

At daybreak, people eat the remaining foods to celebrate their dead, and to mock death by symbolically consuming it. By portraying death in hilarious ways and eating these ceremonial foods, the people conquer it and feel a sense of rebirth and reverence for life. When they return home after their night of communion and prayer in the cemetery, they spend the day resting, reflecting, and feasting.

Two beans discovered by the Spanish almost five hundred years ago had long been aromatic components of Aztec foods and beverages. These prehistoric foods still influence our contemporary gastronomy, especially at funerals and death feasts. Cacao beans were a noble treasure that the Aztecs called the food of the gods. They introduced Spanish explorers to chocolate, *Theobroma cacao*, which they called *xocolatl*, from *xoco*, meaning "bitter," and *atl*, meaning "water." Many people feel that eating chocolate helps banish sadness and elevates mood, and recent research has shown that chocolate does in fact affect neurotransmitters, chemical message carriers in the brain.

Vanilla beans come from the seed pods of several South American wild orchids, but mainly *Vanilla planifolia*. Vanilla comes from the Spanish *vainilla*, meaning "little sheath," referring to the appearance of the ripe bean pod. It is often used as a flavoring for beverages and desserts. Both of these native tropical foods must be dried, fermented, and aged to develop the distinctive aromatic fragrances so characteristic of festival foods.

Will I leave only this:
Like the flowers that wither?
Will nothing last in my
 name—
Nothing of my fame here
 on Earth?

At least flowers!
At least songs!

*—From the Songs of
Huexotzingo, a fifteenth-
century Aztec poetic lament*

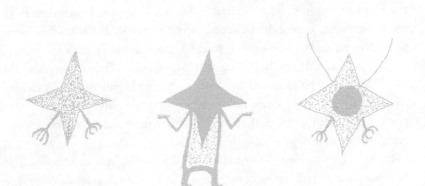

Used in a variety of ways, a number of natural substances attend an American Indian who has died. Sweetgrass, *Hiërochloe odorata* and spp.; sage, *Artemisia* spp. and *Salvia* spp.; tobacco, *Nicotiana* spp.; red cedar, *Juniperus virginiana;* bearberry, *Arctostaphylos uva-ursi;* and *kinnikinnik* mixtures, along with sacred cornmeal and pollen, often accompany prayers. These substances can be used independently or they may be grouped together. Sometimes friends or family create and bless a small pouch with some of these herbs to escort the body of their deceased loved one on the journey into the afterlife.

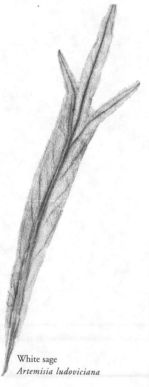

Cancerweed
Salvia lyrata

Smudges and Smudging

Burning herbs is a sacred practice used for prayer and purification that is respected in most American Indian traditions. It is called smudging or smoking, although the intent is not to inhale the smoke or burn up the herbs. Instead you bathe in the smoke and pray with it.

Once ignited, the herbs are not supposed to flame; they should slowly smoke. The aromatic fumes from their volatile oils enhance the smudge. Because smudging involves heat and burning, a fireproof clay pot or large shell, such as that of abalone or sea clam, is a good accouterment to use as a protective vessel.

Sage is a purifier, used to banish all trouble and bad spirits. It cleanses an area and sweeps away negativity. (Select species of wild sage are preferred for smudges; people who substitute culinary sage may find that it can cause headache.) On the other hand, sweetgrass welcomes the good spirits and good energies back into an area or gathering. These two herbs are often burned during healing prayers and ceremonies, helping to connect with spirit helpers. Burned during funerals and death feasts, their smoke carries prayers and sadness upward to the ancestors' spirits.

Sweetgrass is often braided because it signifies the hair of Mother Earth. Many tribes across America use a "sweetgrass" that is not always the same botanical we know as *Hiërochloe odorata.* In some areas a local

White sage
Artemisia ludoviciana

sedge or rush is used. These also have wonderful scents. The importance of sweetgrass at every level of ceremonial life has long made it a valued trade item.

You can use three-foot braids, thick or thin, of fragrant sweetgrass to bless an area or to place on an altar; you can also pack them with regalia and other special objects. Some people carry sweetgrass braids for protection. Many of us place a fresh one in our cars each year. A braid or two often accompany the dead to their graves.

To smudge with sweetgrass, ignite one end of the braid. When the flame dies out, the smoke should continue to rise. Along with prayers, you may first offer the smoke upward to the Creator and then to the four cardinal directions and to the earth.

Finally, you can offer the smoke to yourself. Move the braid so it encircles your head and torso and travels up and down the outer space around you. Cup your hands and draw the aromatic smoke to your heart for love and caring, and to your face and head for clarity of vision and good thoughts. As you brush it down your arms and body, you are sweeping away all anger, tension, and discomfort.

Sage can be loosely crumbled into a smudge pot, but it is usually bundled snugly into "smudge sticks" and tied with bright cotton threads. Sage is frequently bundled with cedar, juniper, or sweetgrass to make beautifully fragrant blends. These are sold in health food stores, New Age shops, at powwows and Indian trading posts, and even at museum shops and religious stores. The soothing scents are considered an incense by many people. They are also highly valued for aromatherapy.

Sweetgrass
Hierochloe odorata

To smudge, ignite your smudge stick or sage wand and gently blow on it to extinguish the flame and enhance the smoking. If you are doing this with other people, position everyone in a circle. Move around clockwise and pass or carry the smudge stick so that you encircle each person. Smudge from head to toe; often people use their cupped hand to draw the smoke into specific body areas. Some people use a feather fan to distribute the aromatic smoke to everyone.

You can also crumble small handfuls of sage and cedar into a smudge pot and burn them together. One person in the group can smudge everyone, one at a time. Or you can pass the smoking pot from one person to the next; everybody smudges himself and takes a moment in silent prayer with the smudge before he passes it. The collective prayers and good energies in gatherings like this are amazing; often a real sense of spiritual healing can overwhelm everyone there.

You can use other herbs for smudging to serve various needs. Mugwort, bergamot and other mints, yarrow, mesquite, bearberry, and tobacco may be used individually or in blends to soothe and relax. These herbs all possess insecticidal and fungicidal properties, too.

MAKE A FRAGRANT SMUDGE STICK

2 fresh stalks mugwort, with leaves and blossoms

2 fresh stalks yarrow, with leaves and blossoms

2 fresh stalks bergamot, with leaves and blossoms

1 large sheet newspaper

2 rubber bands, or long pieces of string

Gather several fresh stalks of your favorite herbs. Some of the most common herbs yield the best fragrances. Mugwort makes a fine smudge on its own. You may also want to try cedars, junipers, sumac, osier, mesquite, tansy, and pinyon. Each of these botanicals has its own savory aroma. Experiment with different combinations to suit your various needs. This recipe makes an aromatic smudge that is wonderful for meditation. It also makes a fine insect repellent and helps to banish mildew.

Lay the sheet of newspaper open. Gather the selected herb stalks together and hold them tightly in one hand. Bend them gently back over onto themselves 6 to 7 inches from one end. Quickly bend the remaining lengths back on themselves again in this same 6- to 7-inch-long wand. Holding this all together well, place it on the newspaper at an angle. Roll it up tightly, like a big cigar, and secure it snugly with the rubber bands or string.

Place the stick in a warm place, out of direct sun, to dry for at least several days and preferably a week. You may unwrap it in a day or two to check it, then wrap it again more snugly. Let it dry out thoroughly for a few more days. If it is very humid, it may take a couple of weeks to dry.

Unwrap the stick, discard the paper, and tie the herb bundle securely with fine cotton cord or thread. When ready to use, ignite one end and get it smoking. You can use this as a ceremonial smudge. To make a mosquito repellent, perch it upright in a clay pot or coffee can filled with an inch or two of sand. If you want to burn the smudge for only several minutes, you can snuff out the smoking end by rubbing it

Yarrow
Achillea millefolium

inside the pot or shell, or pressing it into the sand. Don't use water to extinguish it.

Caution: Do not use this in a closed, confined area. Before use, make sure that no one has allergies or asthma, which could be aggravated by the smoke. This is not advised for pregnant women, babies, or young children, who might develop respiratory difficulties.

Make a Kinnikinnik

Kinnikinnik is an old Algonquian Indian word for special botanical mixtures used for ceremonial offerings and in ritual. The term also signifies the highly esteemed plant bearberry, *Arctostaphylos uva-ursi*. The small, oval, leathery leaves of bearberry are so prized that they are often smudged alone. Bearberry may also be part of a larger mixture that includes tobacco or thirty or more other botanicals. Each herb is prepared and dried separately; then they are mixed together and carried in leather pouches.

Kinnikinnik is not always burned. Sometimes it is carried as an offering substance or worn for its healthy aroma and to ward off harmful influences. *Kinnikinnik* may also be packed in baskets and bags with ceremonial items to keep them nurtured and healthy.

To make a *kinnikinnik*, select your favorites from the list below and balance their scents to suit your own needs. Fragrances sometimes build slowly; the constituents of some botanicals become enhanced as they dry, and others only release their best perfume in combination with others, or when they are smudged.

Angelica, *Angelica atropurpurea,* leaves
Asters, *Aster* spp., leaves and blossoms
Bayberry, *Myrica* spp., leaves
Bergamot, *Monarda* spp., all plant parts
Birch, *Betula* spp., bark
Blueberry, *Vaccinium* spp., leaves
Bristly crowfoot, *Ranunculus pensylvanicus,* leaves and fruits
Canadian hemlock, *Tsuga canadensis,* needles

Coltsfoot, *Tussilago farfara*, leaves
Dittany, *Cunila origanoides*, leaves
Dogwood, *Cornus* spp., bark and leaves
Goldenrod, *Solidago* spp., leaves and blossoms
Horseweed, *Erigeron canadensis*, leaves and flowers
Indian tobacco, *Lobelia inflata*, leaves
Juniper, *Juniperus* spp., leaves, bark, and berries
Licorice, *Glycyrrhiza glabra*, root and bark
Life everlasting, *Gnaphalium polycephalum*, leaves
Meadowsweet, *Spiraea alba* and spp., leaves and bark
Mints, *Mentha* spp. and vars., all plant parts
Mountain mints, *Pycnanthemum* spp., all plant parts
Mullein, *Verbascum thapsus*, leaves and roots
Partridgeberry, *Mitchella repens*, leaves
Pearly everlasting, *Anaphalis margaritacea*, leaves
Pussytoes, *Antennaria neglecta* and spp., leaves and blossoms
Sage, *Artemisia* spp. and *Salvia* spp., leaves and bark
Spicebush, *Lindera benzoin*, leaves, berries, and bark
Sumac, *Rhus* spp., leaves, bark, and berries
Sun chokes, *Helianthus tuberosa*, leaves
Sunflower, *Helianthus annuua*, leaves
Sweet clover, *Melilotus* spp., blossoms and leaves
Sweet coltsfoot, *Petasites palmata*, leaves
Sweet fern, *Comptonia peregrina*, leaves, twigs, and bark
Tamarack, *Larix laricina*, needles and bark
Tansy, *Tanacetum vulgare* and *T. huronese*, all plant parts
White cedar, *Thuja occidentalis*, leaves, bark, and berries
Wild lettuce, *Lactuca virosa*, leaves
Willow, *Salix* spp., bark and leaves
Yarrow, *Achillea* spp., all plant parts
Yerba santa, *Eriodictyon californicum*, leaves

Certain tribes, such the Great Lakes Algonquian and the Iroquois, developed fabulous formulas for their *kinnikinniks,* and their mixtures became valued trade items. Many California tribes also blended their smoking mixtures and smudges in notable ways. Today there are numerous *kinnikinnik* blends all over tribal America. Often they contain a few or many of the botanicals listed. Some also have tobacco in them, but this is not necessary.

> Naked you came from Earth the Mother.
> Naked you return to her.
> May a good wind be your road.
> —*Omaha song*

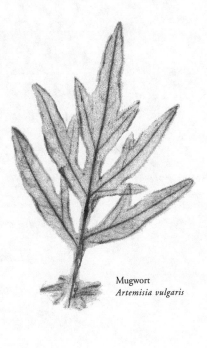

Mugwort
Artemisia vulgaris

Mullein
Verbascum thapsus

An American Indian Medicine Chest

GIFTS FROM MOTHER EARTH

Foxglove
Digitalis purpurea

Foxglove
Digitalis purpurea

Earth teach me stillness

as the grasses are stilled with light.

Earth teach me suffering

as old stones suffer with memory.

Earth teach me humility

as blossoms are humble with beginning.

Earth teach me caring

as the mother who secures her young.

Earth teach me courage

as the tree which stands alone.

Earth teach me limitations

as the ant which crawls on the ground.

Earth teach me freedom

as the eagle which soars in the sky.

Earth teach me resignation

as the leaves which die in the fall.

Earth teach me regeneration

as the seed which rises in the spring.

Earth teach me to forget myself

as melted snow forgets its life.

Earth teach me to remember kindness

as dry fields weep with rain.

—UTE PRAYER

Foxglove
Digitalis purpurea

Across North America native healers closely studied their indigenous environments. Their knowledge of the many medicinal plants they found has been handed down through countless generations of ancestors and elders. American Indians have been adding, subtracting, and otherwise changing elements of this earth-based wisdom far longer than our collective memory can reveal. Much has been lost, but many aspects of native wisdom and herbal healing continue to enrich our modern lives; in every region, healers developed precursors or complements to contemporary conventional medicines.

American Indian herbalism is aimed at maintaining general wellness and at strengthening any areas of weakness in order to restore balance. Treatments are holistic, centering on bringing mind, body, spirit, and nature into harmony.

Native healers use all kinds of natural substances—plants, minerals, animals, and fungi—individually or combined in complex formulas. In these prescriptions, each chosen for a particular person and situation, every element contributes its own beneficial attributes, and the synergy of the combined ingredients further enhances the treatment. Not all medicines are curative; some are spiritual and symbolic. And American Indians have long been practitioners of preventive medicine, using a host of natural materials for their restorative, tonic, and prophylactic properties.

Today, the therapeutic virtues of plants, fungi, and minerals are well acknowledged. One in four modern-day prescription drugs contains an ingredient derived from a flowering plant, and one in five plants has a documented medicinal use. Most plants have a complex assortment of benefits: roots have one use, flowering tops and leaves have another, stems another, and so on. Cautious, well-informed use of plants can enable most of us to maintain good health and balance.

A variety of bumps, bruises, and simple ailments, such as coughs, colds, cuts, burns, and rashes, span the life cycle. Our medicine cabinets are full of the products we buy to treat these everyday complaints. Using readily available yet often overlooked natural ingredients, we can create American Indian–inspired alternatives to use as stomach calmatives, relaxants, and healing salves as well as treatments for headache, cough, fever, and dermatitis. Easy-to-make recipes for nontoxic shampoos, astringents, tooth powders, and skin washes bring native wisdom to personal hygiene and general well-being.

Note: Do not self-diagnose or self-treat serious long-term problems without consulting a qualified doctor or medical herbalist. If you are taking prescription medication, seek professional advice before using herbal remedies. Carefully identify plants and fungi, and never use anything you have not positively identified. Finally, most herbs and herbal preparations should not be taken with caffeine; nor should they be taken during pregnancy and while nursing an infant unless recommended by professional health care providers.

Medicine Bags

Personal medicine bags are powerful, sacred objects that have long been part of American Indians' private accouterments. A person can wear one openly around his neck or suspended from his waist. Some people conceal them.

An individual can make her own medicine bag, or relatives or friends may make it for her. Many American Indians create a medicine bag to help them accomplish a formidable task, or something they feel is a long shot; others keep special medicine bags in their house, car, or truck.

Medicine bags are important throughout life, but especially during illness or other major changes. Because these are times of accentuated self-awareness, sensitivity, and sometimes quandary, making someone a medicine bag is a way to honor his identity and provide reassurance.

People may create entirely new medicine bags or add to existing ones. These cherished possessions are created from soft-tanned animal skins or from red cloth, calico, or muslin. Some are plain, but they may also be ornately beaded, quilled, or painted with clan or dream symbolism, medicine plants, or totems. While he cuts and stitches it together, the bag's maker prays for the health and happiness of the recipient. He carefully chooses the items that will go into it and directs a particular prayer or good thought into each one.

Some medicine bags are blessed and begun with a pinch of tobacco or pollen, sweetgrass, sage, or red cedar. Less is better: It is not the amount but the energy that counts. You might choose to add special seeds, a small stone or crystal specific to a sacred place, or a pinch of earth from your home, wrapped or tied in a tiny piece of red flannel.

Medicine bags are works in progress. You can add to or subtract from the unique personal items they contain throughout your life, depending upon events. Invested with prayers and healing energies, they often retain their power for a lifetime or beyond.

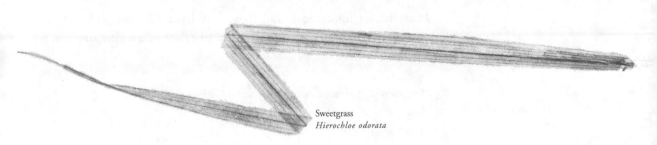

Sweetgrass
Hierochloe odorata

Making Basic Herbal Preparations:
A Lexicon and General Recipes

Native herbs have provided natural remedies for countless life needs since earliest human time. The best treatments have evolved through generations of empirical use and people are still improving upon them today. When you make recipes with healing botanicals, use the finest ingredients available, as well as sterile utensils and containers, and work with a sense of peace, understanding, and respect for everything you handle. The more love and goodwill you put into your creative efforts, the finer the healing benefits will be.

It's always a good policy to learn about each individual herb or fungus, how it responds to your personal needs, and how your body reacts to it before mixing them in formulas. Herbs and mushrooms are complex organisms. Most target specific regions of the body, but when they are combined, their synergistic effects may provoke uniquely different responses in people with varying body types.

Here are some of the basic techniques used to prepare herbal remedies, from the simpler to the more complex.

INFUSIONS

Teas

Many herbal tonics, teas, and tisanes are basic infusions. The simplest preparation of leaves and blossoms for one dose of a revitalizing tea, or a tisane of blossoms, is as follows.

    1 teaspoon (2–3 g) dried or two teaspoons (4–6 g)
      fresh cut or bruised herbs
    1 cup boiling water

Put the herbs in a cup, pour the boiling water over them, and steep or infuse the mixture, covered, for three to five minutes. Strain; if you like, add some raw honey to taste.

For an 8-cup pot:

1 ounce (20–28 g) dried herbs or 1¹/₂–2 ounces (30–42 g) fresh herbs
8 cups boiling water

In a warm pot, pour water that has just boiled over the herbs. Cover and infuse for 10 minutes, then strain, cool, and refrigerate. You can use this infusion as a primary ingredient for other salves or ointments. You can also freeze it in snap-and-seal bags or ice cube trays.

Infused Oils

Infused oils make fine massage oils; they are also frequently added to creams, salves, or ointments. You can extract the herbs' fat-soluble ingredients in either of two ways. Cold-infused oils are heated naturally in the sun. Hot-infused oils are simmered. The standard infusion is:

8 ounces (250 g) dried or 16 ounces (500 g) fresh herbs
24 ounces (750 ml) olive, sunflower, corn, safflower, or
   other good-quality vegetable oil

Simmer the herbs gently in the oil for 2 to 3 hours, or allow the mixture to rest, covered, in the sun (a sunny windowsill will do) for two to four weeks.

Strain and filter off the pure oil. Store in sterile, dark glass bottles.

Infused Vinegars, Wines, and Syrups

To draw out the herbal constituents when you make these items, use the cold-infused (solar) method and the same measurements as listed in the infused oils recipe above. Place the fresh or dried herbs in bottles or crocks covered with your choice of vinegar, wine, or syrup. Depending on your preference, infuse for anywhere from two to six weeks. At that point you can strain off and remove the botanicals or leave them in for their appearance.

Rather than using the solar method, infuse honey, maple syrup, and sugar syrup by gently heating them in a pot with your choice of therapeutic or culinary herbs or spices for 30 minutes. Because they are more prone to ferment, store these infusions in sterile jars or bottles with corks to avoid the possibility of exploding screw-top bottles.

DECOCTIONS

This technique is used to extract the deeper essences from roots, barks, stems, and berries, or from mature coarse herbs, such as angelica, echinacea, curly dock, or yarrow.

1 ounce (20–28 g) dried or 2 ounces (40–56 g)
   freshly chopped botanicals
3 cups (750 ml) of water

Combine and simmer the ingredients, uncovered, for about 20 to 30 minutes, until the liquid is reduced by about one third.

Strain and use, or pour into a covered glass jug and refrigerate for two to three days. The decoction may last for a week or more, but it is best to make herbal preparations in small amounts and use them right up or freeze them for future use. This will ensure that you use them at peak vitality.

To store this for later use, you can cool the decoction and pour it into ice cube trays. Freeze the trays overnight, then turn them out and store the cubes in marked plastic bags.

TINCTURES

Tinctures are stronger preparations of herbs and some fungi. They provide stronger healing action and have a longer shelf life than other preparations—up to two years or more. It is best to use all homemade preparations within a prescribed amount of time, which is usually specific to the herb, and then make a new supply.

When you buy herbal tinctures, they come in 1- and 2-ounce amber-brown bottles with dosage recommendations on the label. Depending upon the herb, the dose is usually 10 to 30 drops, taken three times daily. You should not exceed the maximum number of drops. A smaller dose may work just as well, which is why you are given a range.

When using a tincture, measure it into a cup of water, hot water, or herbal tea and then drink it. Focus your attention on the process and concentrate your mind on wellness, healing, and good energy.

Alcohol-sensitive patients and pregnant women should add the recommended tincture dosage to a cup of hot water or herbal tea and allow it to stand, uncovered, for 5 minutes. This will allow the alcohol to evaporate.

Here is a basic recipe.

$7^1/_2$ ounces (200 g) dried herb or fungi, or 11 ounces (300 g)
   fresh material, chopped
1 quart (1 liter) alcohol, preferably vodka, rum, or brandy

In a tightly covered, sterile jar, soak the herbs or fungi in the alcohol for three days to as much as six weeks. This will depend upon whether you are infusing something like rose petals or other leafy herbs—which take only three days—or bark or other woody material, which will take much longer. Gently shake the jar once or twice each day.

To filter the tincture, pour it through a cloth-lined sieve or sterile filter. Store in dark, sterile jars, tightly capped.

Note: Never use rubbing alcohol (isopropyl) or industrial alcohol (methyl) in tinctures. This would make them poisonous. Most commercial tinctures are made in grain alcohol, usually 60 percent by volume, with distilled water.

COMPRESSES

A simple way to use herbs externally is to soak a cloth in an herbal infusion or decoction and hold it against areas of irritated skin. You can also use both hot and cold compresses to reduce fevers, soothe inflammations, treat sports injuries, and ease eyestrain and headache.

FOMENTATION

This hot external application of healing herbs is generally used to treat colds, flu, pain, and swelling. Soak a towel or cloth in a hot herbal infusion or decoction, wring it out, and place it on top of the affected area. It should be as hot as can be tolerated without burning the skin. Cover it immediately with a large dry towel or wool cloth and leave it in place for 10 to 20 minutes, or until cool. Repeat as needed.

POULTICE

This is a mixture of fresh, dried, or powdered herbs that you can apply directly to your skin to reduce the swelling of sprains or broken bones, ease nerve or muscle pains, or draw out the pus from infected wounds. Macerate or bruise fresh herbs such as plantain, heal-all, St. John's wort, or slippery elm bark to release their healing properties and place them on your skin. If you like, you can quickly simmer fresh herbs for two minutes and use them while they are still warm. Hold the herbs in place with large grape or coltsfoot leaves or a cloth bandage. You can renew a poultice every two to three hours as needed.

PLASTER

Similar to a poultice, a plaster is an herbal bandage used on highly sensitive skin. You make a dressing of selected botanicals, place it between two pieces of clean cloth, and apply it directly to the affected area. You can renew a plaster every half hour as needed or leave it on overnight.

POWDERED HERBS AND CAPSULES

You may prefer to take powdered herbs in capsules, which provide a precise dose while avoiding a bitter taste.

To make your own capsules, buy size 00 gelatin or vegetarian capsules. You can dry and powder your own herbal materials, or purchase them from reputable herbal suppliers. Pour the powdered herbs into a clean saucer and slide the two halves of the empty capsule together while scooping up the herb powder. Join the two halves and store the capsules in airtight containers.

You can also dust powdered herbs on foods, over wounds, or on the skin. Herbs that are so finely processed deteriorate more rapidly, so prepare only small amounts and use them up quickly.

SALVES

A salve sits on the skin surface and provides protective healing benefits. Here is how to make a simple salve.

3 ounces powdered herbs

7 ounces cocoa butter or pure vegetable shortening

1 ounce beeswax, more or less, depending upon the consistency desired

1 ounce raw honey (optional)

2 or 3 drops vitamin E oil (optional)

Mix the herbs, cocoa butter, and beeswax and heat in a small covered pot over low heat for one to two hours, stirring frequently. If you like, you can add the honey and vitamin E oil toward the very end of cooking.

Blend the mixture thoroughly and pour it into small containers or onto clean foil in little cookielike pools. Allow it to cool and become firm and ready to use.

VARIATION: To make a cooling, pleasant lip balm, add a drop or two of fragrant essential oil of mint or cedar during the final process.

CREAMS

Creams are absorbed into the skin. They provide natural cooling and soothing relief, which is enhanced if you chill the cream before applying it. This can be especially pleasant in the heat of summer.

Creams are composed and simmered in a double boiler for about three hours to create a fine emulsion.

$2^1/_2$ ounces (70 g) glycerin

5 ounces (150 g) emulsifying wax

$2^1/_2$ ounces (80 ml) water

1 ounce (20–28 g) dried or $2^1/_2$ ounces (50–70 g) fresh herbs

Measure all ingredients into the top of a double boiler. Heat at a low simmer. At the end of the cooking time, strain out the herbs. Pour the cream into a clean bowl and stir or whip it continuously until it cools and sets.

Spoon the whipped cream into sterilized dark glass jars, label, and refrigerate. Use it within three months.

To counter mold growth or spoilage and extend the shelf life of the cream, you can add one of the following at the very end of the cooking process: 1 ml of an essential oil; 5 ml of fine borax; or several drops of tincture of benzoin.

LOTIONS

Homemade herbal lotions are different from those you buy at the store. The basic homemade variety is lighter and more watery. You can easily make these water-based herbal preparations to treat specific skin ailments by adding more water to infusions or decoctions. Add the lotions to your daily bath or measure them into sterile bottles and refrigerate them to use as topical skin treatments. Herbal lotions are good for facials and to comb through your hair for additional luster and healthy texture and growth.

OINTMENTS

These preparations combine heated oils or fats with selected herbs. Unlike creams or lotions, they do not contain water. Ointments bond with the skin, providing a protective layer against moisture. This makes them useful for diaper or heat rash, chapped lips, and sunburn.

2 ounces (60 g) dried or 5 ounces (150 g) fresh herbs
2 cups (500 g) petroleum jelly or soft paraffin wax
1 ounce (28 g) raw honey

Heat the herbs, petroleum jelly, and honey together in the top of a double boiler. Simmer, stirring well, for about 15 minutes. Acting quickly, while it is still hot, filter the ointment through clean cheesecloth. Pour it into sterile jars before it sets. Cover when cool, label, and date.

A Basic American Indian Medicine Chest

These herbal preparations will cover most of your normal daily needs.

Arnica oil for bruises, muscle pains, and sore feet
Calendula cream for inflammations, sunburn, and skin disorders
Cedar lotion for general skin treatment and facial care
Corn silk for kidney and bladder pains and infections
Echinacea capsules and tincture for colds and infections
Echinacea-goldenseal salve for chapped skin and lips
Puffballs for headache treatments, styptics, and wound dressings
Sage leaves for smudging, purification, and antiseptic use
Slippery elm bark powder for coughs and digestive problems
Sweetgrass braid for smudging, purification, and antiseptic use
Witch hazel lotion for rashes and skin problems
Yarrow powder for pain relief, anesthetic, and antiseptic use
Yucca root for soapy cleansing and hair care

Strengthening the Immune System

Good health depends upon having a healthy immune system, which controls your ability to resist infection and recover from illness and injury. Several species of the prairie or purple coneflower, *Echinacea purpurea* and *E. angustifolia,* are primary strengthening herbs for the immune system.

Echinacea has a long history of healing use among many tribes. Plains Indians ate the whole plant, especially the perennial roots, as a vegetable. The Sioux chewed the roots to treat sore throat, toothache, and stomach problems, and made them into poultices for snakebite and other infections. The Comanche also chewed the roots to treat toothache and sore throats. At ceremonial times, medicine men applied the macerated roots to their hands as a local anesthetic before handling glowing coals or boiling meat. People burned or smudged the dried herbal plant parts and inhaled their smoky essence to relieve headaches and depression, as well as treat congestion and respiratory distress.

Today science bears out what American Indians have long known. The effectiveness of echinacea as an immune system stimulant has been extensively studied and the plant is widely used, especially in Germany and other parts of Europe. It has also gained considerable popularity in the United States, where many people use it in herbal teas, as a powder in capsules, or as tinctures.

You should not take echinacea routinely. Instead, use it periodically or when you are feeling under the weather, extremely tired, or weak. As an immune stimulant, echinacea helps fight allergies, asthma, and other respiratory ailments. A tincture provides a soothing throat treatment to ward off infections. And an echinacea decoction makes a valuable healing gargle.

You are likely to find echinacea in many commercial herbal tea and tincture formulas. It is often worked into various creams, salves, and oils to treat external skin problems such as acne, boils, rashes, and canker and cold sores.

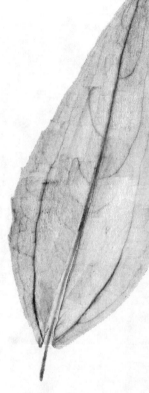

Purple coneflower
Echinacea purpurea

ECHINACEA ROOT TINCTURE

This is a basic therapeutic and preventive treatment when used on its own. It can also be added to other herbal, mushroom, and mineral preparations. High-quality, fresh echinacea root should produce a tingling sensation on the tongue.

7^1/$_2$ ounces (200 g) dried or 11 ounces (300 g) fresh,
  finely chopped echinacea roots
1 quart (1 liter) vodka, with 35 to 40 percent alcohol content or less

Combine ingredients in a large, sterile quart jar and cover securely. Shake vigorously for 1 to 2 minutes. Store in a cool, dark place for two weeks, shaking it daily.

Pour the mixture through fine cheesecloth or a filter, squeezing all liquid from the roots. Discard the spent roots. Pour the fresh tincture into dark-colored, sterile bottles and cap securely. Label and date the bottles.

To use: Take ^{1}/$_2$ teaspoon (2 ml) in water or hot tea, one to three times daily as needed. Do not take it every day or for more than seven days in a row. Instead, use it sparingly as an immune stimulant.

VARIATION: To make a gentle, effective echinacea herbal tincture, another immune stimulant, use this same recipe. Instead of the roots, substitute an equal amount of the aboveground herbal parts of the plant, including the blossoms.

ECHINACEA PRAIRIE SPRAY MIST

This simple recipe provides therapeutic relief from sore throat and upper respiratory distress. Measured into small 1- or 2-ounce spray bottles, it is great for home use and also makes a thoughtful gift.

1 teaspoon echinacea root tincture (above)
1 teaspoon raw honey
2 ounces mineral or spring water

Combine ingredients in a covered spray bottle and shake well to blend. Spray your mouth and throat to relieve irritation and infection. Use sparingly, as needed. Keep refrigerated.

Pau D'Arco

The early Incas and other Andean tribes knew the many virtues of their native evergreen tree, called lapacho by the Spanish and pau d'arco by the Portuguese. The inner bark of two species, *Tabebuia avellanedae* and *T. impetignosa,* possesses immune stimulant, antitumor, and antibiotic actions, as well as antidiabetic properties. Among the many remarkable benefits it provides for people around the world today are treatments for chronic fatigue syndrome, leukemia, and other cancers.

The dried inner bark of pau d'arco can be worked into valuable decoctions, tinctures, ointments, and medicinal teas. The natural antibiotic nature of this herb is vital for treating yeast and fungal conditions, and ongoing research shows that it also lowers blood pressure. Native peoples in South America prized pau d'arco as a cure-all, and continuing research is providing validation for their ideas.

TONIC HERBAL VINEGARS AND WINES

During the lushness of the growing season, herbalists eagerly harvest the best botanicals at peak strength from meadows, hedgerows, woods, and gardens and prepare them for future use. Many are easily and quickly dried, packaged, labeled, and dated. They infuse some herbs, and tincture others in alcohol, wine, vinegar, or glycerin for more concentrated use. Infused wines and vinegars make a nice addition to your American Indian medicine chest.

Caution: Remember never to collect botanicals from roadside margins.

Drinking tonics is an easy and agreeable way to take herbs for improving digestion, increasing vitality, cooling and soothing some inflammations, and adding calcium to your daily diet. Poured into a spray bottle, these products can be used as a moisturizer for hair or skin. When dabbed or poulticed on the skin, some will calm insect bites, dermatitis, or fungal problems.

Herbal Anti-inflammatory Vinegars

You can extract natural salicylates, which provide pain relief and reduce inflammation, from the leaves of wintergreen, *Gaultheria procumbens,* and the twigs and bark of birches *(Betula* spp.), black haw *(Viburnum* spp.), poplar *(Populus* spp.), or willow *(Salix* spp.).

Fill an 8-ounce jar with the fresh harvested or dried botanical or a combination of herbs. Cover with cider, white, or wine vinegar and cap tightly. Infuse, shaking daily, for three to four weeks. Strain through a fine filter into another sterile jar, cap tightly, and label. A therapeutic dose of these vinegars is 1 teaspoon a day, taken as needed.

Herbal Calcium-rich Vinegars

To make a nutrient-rich tonic, follow the previous recipe, using one or more of the herbs below. Allow the mixture to sit and infuse for one to two weeks, shaking it gently every day. Once it's done, take 1 teaspoon to 1 tablespoon daily in a small glass of cool water before or 30 minutes after a meal.

Dandelion, *Taraxacum officinale,* roots
Nettle, *Urtica and Laportea* spp., leaves, stems, and blooms
Plantain, *Plantago* spp., roots and leaves
Raspberry, *Rubus* spp., leaves
Red clover, *Trifolium pratense* and other species, blossoms
Yellow dock, *Rumex crispus,* root

Tonic Tinctures

Some botanicals contain natural steroids, a large group of chemicals with powerful medicinal effects. For example, the steroid digitoxin, a cardiac stimulant and diuretic, is obtained from common foxglove. Those with estrogenic qualities affect female body functions. You can make tinctures of these plants in vinegar or vodka, but they should be used with caution. **Note: Be sure to consult a medical professional or qualified herbalist before using these remedies because of their strong action.** Tincture each of these herbs separately.

Sarsaparilla, *Smilax* spp., is a hormone-balancing herb and a purifier for toxic or sluggish systems.

American ginseng, *Panax quinquefolia,* is a tonic for men and women. It provides a stress-relieving boost when you're feeling depleted and is particularly helpful in cases of exhaustion.

Black cohosh, *Cimicifuga racemosa,* is an antispasmodic, used to relieve menstrual cramps, stimulate labor, and decrease menopausal hot flashes.

Devil's club, *Oplopanax horridum,* is used to balance blood sugar, and it provides tonic action for the pituitary and hypothalamus.

Poke, *Phytolacca americana,* is used in **very small amounts** to clear lymph congestion, relieve swollen nodes, and cleanse the blood.

Wild yam, *Dioscorea villosa,* treats threatened miscarriage, intestinal and menstrual cramps, and pain from passing stones.

To make a tincture, follow the recipe for the basic tincture on pp. 240–41. Chop the fresh roots and pack them into sterile glass jars. Cover with cider vinegar or vodka and infuse for one to two weeks. Take 10 to 25 drops or ¹/₂ teaspoon daily, mixed in cool or warm water or tea.

Headaches

To successfully prevent or treat a headache, it helps to know the mechanisms that can trigger this sometimes debilitating ailment. Headaches can be caused by tension and stress, food allergies, toothache, and many other factors. Pay close attention to how and where your headaches begin. Careful self-analysis may help you pinpoint the cause and then prevent or relieve your headache.

Migraine headaches can be so crippling that it is crucial to prevent their onset as well as treat their symptoms. Feverfew, *Chrysanthemum (Tanacetum) parthenium,* is a perennial summer daisy that was introduced from Europe and is now widespread throughout North America. It has long been used as an effective remedy for headaches, a valued treatment for arthritic and rheumatic pain, and an herb of parturition. Numerous contemporary studies have confirmed its ability to decrease the pain and frequency of migraine attacks. **Note: This herb can cause mouth ulcers or mild dermatitis in some people. Feverfew should not be given to children under twelve years old or taken during pregnancy.**

To prevent migraines, chew one to two small leaves daily, either fresh or dried. Some people prefer to take feverfew capsules or tablets. Unfortunately, these preparations are not standardized, so they have varying amounts of parthenolide, the active constituent. You may need to try varying the daily dose, using the manufacturer's recommendations as your guide, until you settle on what is right for you. People with fair complexions may have a greater tendency to skin irritation with this herb.

The Cherokee and other southern tribes used their native skullcap, *Scutellaria lateriflora,* to relieve pain, stimulate or regulate menstruation, and ease childbirth. They chewed the fresh leaves of this perennial mint and made strong teas from its leaves, stems, and flowers. The sedative action of this herb on the nervous system led to its early appreciation as a nerve tonic. In addition to providing headache relief, it is used to treat anxiety, panic attacks, tension, depression, epilepsy, convulsions, and hysteria.

Drunk as a hot tea, an herbal infusion of skullcap is most effective if you take it first thing in the morning, before each meal, and just before bedtime, as needed. Skullcap has an astringent, slightly bitter taste. It makes a welcome, calming treatment for insomnia, too. It's best to harvest skullcap's aboveground parts from mature three-year-old plants when they are in flower during the summer. Tinctures, capsules, and tablets extend the availability of this herb, which is sometimes formulated with other nervines.

Black willow
Salix nigra

Willow bark, *Salix nigra* and other species, possesses significant fever-reducing and pain relief properties due to its salicin content. Salicin is metabolized within the body much like its synthetic sister, aspirin. American Indians chew on fresh willow twigs to ease pain and headache; willow bark teas and tinctures provide stronger analgesic effects. The bitter essence from willow soothes sinus passages and stimulates the body to counteract internal pain. Fresh willow twigs also make good dentifrices.

A number of other soothing, relaxing botanicals are useful in treating tension and sinus headaches. Choosing the right herb or herbal formula may require professional health care guidance. Among them are several that were introduced into North America from the Mediterranean and other parts of the world. However, they have been here so long that they have made their way into native herbalists' formularies. The essential oils of both lavender, *Lavendula officinalis,* and rosemary, *Rosmarinus officinalis,* provide topical general relief when you massage one or two drops on your temples. Many people find just the fragrance of one or the other of these classic Mediterranean herbs to be very soothing. Also, a warm cup of a mild rosemary herbal infusion (1 teaspoonful dried herb per cup) before or during each meal, as needed, will help relieve migraine and general headache discomfort.

Used in teas and tisanes, the fragrant yellow flowers of American basswood, *Tilia americana,* and European linden, *Tilia cordata,* also provide relief for headache and stress. In addition, they soothe colds and flu, reduce fevers, lower blood pressure, and calm the mind. You can take advantage of the emollient qualities of these flowers by working them into lotions and creams for skin irritation. **Caution: To prevent developing sensitivities, consume these herbs in moderation.**

Herbal infusions or teas made from one or more mints, or a few drops of a mint tincture in water, offer cooling relief from food-related headaches and digestive disorders. American pennyroyal, *Hedeoma pulegioides,* and European pennyroyal, *Mentha pulegium,* are among the strongest therapeutically, but they should be avoided by pregnant and nursing women and all children under five years old. When used in mild teas, our native bee balm, *Monarda didyma;* wild bergamot, *Monarda fistulosa;* cultivated peppermint, *Mentha piperita,* and other mints also provide varying degrees of relief.

Basswood
Tilia americana

BASIC HERBAL STEAM INHALANT

The volatile oils of many mints can be used to make a helpful steam inhalant to relieve headaches associated with sinus congestion or colds. These oils are antiseptic, antifungal, antibacterial, and generally cooling for the skin, but higher concentrations may irritate people with sensitive skin.

5 cups boiling water

1 small handful fresh bee balm leaves (or half as much, if dried)

1 medium Pyrex or heatproof, broad-mouthed pottery bowl

1 large towel, baby quilt, or blanket

Place the bowl and assembled ingredients on a table at which you can easily sit for about 10 to 15 minutes. Sitting comfortably, put the herbs in the bowl and pour the boiling water over them. Position your face and head about 12 to 18 inches above the steaming bowl, or whatever distance is most comfortable for you. Cover your head and the bowl with the towel. Be sure this covering hangs down around you, trapping the steam inside.

Gently breathe in the vapors of the escaping volatile oils. As you adjust and feel initial relief, breathe in more deeply and exhale completely for about 10 to 15 minutes. Concentrate on breathing, relaxation, recovery, and wellness. You can repeat this process two or three times a day, depending upon your needs and comfort level.

You can also alter this basic recipe by substituting other beneficial herbs, such as eucalyptus, to relieve other head and respiratory ailments.

Respiratory Ailments

As shown by the growing popularity of aromatherapy and other herbal fragrance treatments, the aromas and odors from herbs and foods trigger certain memories and physical responses for people as well as animals. With your doctor's permission, you can use the basic inhalant recipe in the previous section to treat mild forms of respiratory problems, along with conventional medical treatments.

The native herbs echinacea and skullcap, discussed on pp. 240 and 245, in simple decoctions or teas taken once or twice a day, provide relief for respiratory congestion. You can also take the recommended tincture or capsule doses of either herb two to three times a day for a one- to two-week period. A tablespoon of the dried, chopped aboveground herbal parts of echinacea or skullcap, or a small handful of the fresh chopped herbs, may be added to the basic steam inhalant recipe for more relief. For persistent respiratory problems, seek professional advice.

Simple tinctures of either cramp bark or highbush cranberry, *Viburnum opulus,* or black haw, *Viburnum prunifolium,* afford some relief for breathing difficulties. You can try ½ teaspoon of either tincture in tea or water, repeated six to eight times throughout the day.

American Indians used the roots and aboveground parts of New Jersey tea or red root, *Ceanothus americanus,* for fevers, colds, and stomach problems. The astringent roots of this plant, in tincture or tea, provide valuable relief for bronchitis, tonsillitis, sore throats, and asthma. You can use these tinctures directly on the tongue or put them in tea or water. For younger patients, you can make a small spray bottle of one part tincture and one part water, add a few drops of maple syrup or honey, and mist it onto the sore throat.

Before they are quite ripe, many puffballs are choice edible foods, but once they ripen, American Indians use them medicinally. Inhaling the dark spores of ripe white puffballs treats headache, respiratory problems, and nosebleeds. The underripe white gemmed puffballs, *Lycoperdon perlatum;* the spiny puffball, *L. echinatum;* and the pear-shaped puffball, *L. pyriforme,* have long been collected, threaded together, and worn by many Indians for protection and breathing relief. Their fragrances as they dry out become remarkably strong, robust, and pleasant. **Caution: Avoid the pigskin poison puffball, *Scleroderma citrinum.***

Be careful: Many fungi absorb quantities of toxic materials from the soil or substrata in which they grow, making otherwise trustworthy specimens toxic. It's essential to be sure of the environments where you gather mushrooms for foods or medicines. Even choice morels and chanterelles tested in the laboratory have proven to be contaminated by serious levels of toxins when harvested from railroad margins, roadsides, and areas where herbicides were sprayed or illegal dumping took place.

Additional herbs that relieve and treat respiratory distress and asthma are the root teas of cup plant, *Silphium perfoliatum;* compass plant, *S. laciniatum;* wild potato vine, *Ipomoea pandurata;* Indian physic, *Gillenia trifoliata;* and spikenard, *Aralia racemosa,* along with species of sarsaparilla. The root teas of cow parsnip, *Heracleum lanatum;* American angelica, *Angelica atropurpurea;* pearly everlasting, *Anaphalis margaritacea;* sweet everlasting (rabbit tobacco), *Gnaphalium obtusifolium;* and

Highbush cranberry, or crampbark
Viburnum opulus

plantain-leaved pussytoes, *Antennaria plantaginifolia,* also provide considerable relief. Inhaling the fragrant smoke of *kinnikinniks* or smudges made of healing botanicals (see Chapter 9) also relieves upper and lower bronchial congestion.

Sore Throats and Colds

Many herbs relieve the distress of colds, flu, and fevers. And although coughing is a natural reflex that helps to clear the respiratory tract, easing extended coughing bouts can help speed recovery. You can make herbal gargles to soothe a sore throat, tonsillitis, coughs, and bronchitis, and try formulating syrups with a mucilage content to coat raw, irritated areas. Herbal lozenges can provide relief through the slow release of their healing properties.

The aromatic, spring-harvested inner bark of wild cherry, *Prunus serotina,* was used extensively by American Indians to treat colds, sore throats, fevers, and bronchitis. Their herbal remedies were the ancestors of modern over-the-counter preparations. **Caution: The bark harvested in fall can be highly toxic, and contains a cyanidelike glycoside.**

WILD CHERRY COUGH SYRUP

Spring-gathered inner bark of native wild cherry is your best choice for this soothing elixir, but you may substitute slippery elm bark or combine both.

2 teaspoons chopped or powdered dried wild cherry bark

2 teaspoons chopped dried marshmallow root

2 cups water

1 cup raw honey

1 cup maple syrup

Wild cherry
Prunus serotina

Combine the first three ingredients in a small pot and bring to a boil over medium-low heat, stirring carefully. Lower the heat and simmer, stirring occasionally, for about 20 minutes or until the decoction has reduced by half.

Strain the liquid through a filter into a clean saucepan—there should be about 1 cup—and return to low heat. Simmer slowly, stirring in the honey and maple syrup, for about 5 minutes, until thick.

Pour the hot syrup into a sterile jar; cover when it is cool. To soothe a bad cough, use it as needed, about 1 teaspoon to 1 tablespoon (depending upon body size) every four hours.

VARIATION: You may substitute mullein leaves, sea dulse, kelp, alaria, bladderwrack, or bee balm, depending upon your personal tastes and the ingredients you have available.

To make soothing lozenges, add 1 cup of the prepared decoction to 1 cup of honey and blend well. Slowly boil to the hard crack stage. Pour the mixture out in small dollops on a cookie sheet covered with aluminum foil and allow it to dry. If you like, wrap each lozenge individually.

RED RASPBERRY LEAF AND SAGE GARGLE

This strong astringent tea or herbal infusion makes a fine gargle to ease soreness in the mouth and throat and relieve annoying tickles. The fruits, leaves, blossoms, and roots of red raspberry, *Rubus idaeus,* are cherished for use in many herbal medicines. The leaves and roots are especially astringent. Sage, *Salvia officinalis,* and our native big sagebrush, *Artemisia tridentata,* are aromatic herbs long used to treat sore throats and colds.

    1 tablespoon dried, crushed raspberry leaves
    1 tablespoon dried, crushed sage leaves
    2 cups boiling water
    1 teaspoon raw honey (optional)

Place the dried herbs in a warm teapot and pour the boiling water over them. Cover and steep for 10 to 20 minutes. Strain the infusion into a sterile jar and cool to lukewarm.

Pour 4 ounces into a glass, and try it, unsweetened, as a gargle and mouthwash. If you prefer, sweeten it with the honey. Repeat the process every two hours until your discomfort has passed. Do not use this gargle for more than a week. If your condition persists, consult a health care professional.

Store the remaining infusion, covered, in the refrigerator. Discard the unused portion after six days.

VARIATIONS: You can substitute other astringent, tannin-rich herbs, such as the leaves or roots of canker root or goldthread, *Coptis groenlandica;* Virginia strawberry, *Fragaria virginiana;* elderberry flowers, *Sambucus canadensis* or *S. nigra;* and selections of the various sea algae or seaweeds. In a pinch, warm, mildly salted water will suffice as a fine gargle. Many tribes use the fragrant leaves, bark, and ripe, red berry-like fruits of winged sumac, *Rhus copallina;* fragrant sumac, *R. aromatica;* smooth sumac, *R. glabra;* and staghorn sumac, *R. typhina,* for colds and sore throat relief. Their lemony fruits are high in vitamin C and other trace minerals. You can use these botanicals to make therapeutic herbal teas, decoctions, lotions, and smoking mixtures to treat upper respiratory distress.

Echinacea teas, tinctures, and spray mists (see p. 241) also provide anti-inflammatory relief for sore throats and colds. And if you are brave and determined, you can chew small cloves of raw wild or cultivated garlic, followed by several sprigs of fresh parsley or cilantro to help purify your mouth and counter the garlic.

Elderberry
Sambucus canadensis

Skin Remedies

The skin is the largest organ of the body and the best barrier against harm. Because the skin mirrors internal health, treatments for its ailments are sometimes taken internally to restore a healthy balance in the body. It's important to pay close attention to this extensive protective covering and to maintain it well. To keep the skin and the rest of your body well hydrated, drink plenty of water—at least eight 8-ounce glasses—daily; in several, stir in a teaspoon or two of lemon juice or herbal vinegar for internal cleansing.

A number of fairly common plants and mushrooms are of value for soothing and clearing skin troubles. Selectively knowing the best ones, as our ancestors did, is relatively easy. You can dust the green-gold spores of club moss, *Lycopodium clavatum,* and other related species on skin irritations for relief of itchy, irritating rashes. The olive-brownish spores from ripe puffballs, *Lycoperdon, Calvatia, Calbovista,* and *Bovista* spp., promote healing when used as a dry talc and dusted on irritated skin. **Note: Avoid the pigskin poison puffball, *Scleroderma citrinum.***

The antibiotic properties of purple loosestrife, *Lythrum salicaria,* make it a good plant for poultices and skin washes to use on skin ulcers, minor wounds, and eczema. A strong infusion of yarrow, *Achillea millefolium,* used chilled, is another fine antiseptic skin wash.

The gel of aloe vera, *Aloe vera,* used right from a raw leaf, is a calming, healing burn treatment. Many of us keep aloe plants for this and other good reasons.

DANDELION-DOCK ROOTS DECOCTION FOR CLEAR SKIN

Two herbs that can promote skin healing and soothe many minor irritations are dandelion root, *Taraxacum officinale,* and yellow dock root, *Rumex crispus.* Make a mild decoction (see p. 234) of 2 teaspoons of each of their dried roots in 10 ounces of water. Drink two cups a day and use the remaining liquid, once it has cooled, as a surface wash or mist on irritated skin. Repeat this for a week until you experience relief. If problems persist, see a medical professional. **Caution: Do not use this during pregnancy.**

You can use this dandelion-dock decoction and other cooling herbal antiseptic washes to soothe most minor burns and keep them from becoming infected. Soak a clean cotton cloth in the cooled decoction, then place it over the burned area for two to three hours to quiet inflamed skin.

CALENDULA BURN WASH

This decoction is another useful remedy for treating burns.

2 tablespoons each fresh calendula petals, witch hazel leaves, and
plantain leaves
16 ounces boiling water

Combine all ingredients and steep, covered, in a large teapot until the mixture cools, about 20 minutes. Strain and use.

Keep a labeled jar of this burn wash in the refrigerator for summer sunburns, heat rashes, insect bites, and other common skin irritations. You can use it as a topical wash and as a dressing. Put a few ounces in a spray mist bottle and keep it in the refrigerator to refresh your face, neck, and arms after strenuous workouts.

By itself, calendula is a fine burn treatment. You can also make this healing decoction into a soothing cream, lotion, or ointment (see pp. 238-39).

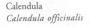

Calendula
Calendula officinalis

HERBAL VINEGAR SKIN WASH

This jewelweed vinegar wash is an excellent antidote for poison ivy. If you dab it on your skin with cotton swabs immediately after contact with the plant, it may prevent your breaking out with the itchy, irritating rash. You can also use this product as a treatment for ringworm and athletes' foot by dabbing or poulticing it directly on the affected skin. And adding 1/4 cup of this vinegar wash to a warm foot bath or bathtub soothes irritated skin.

8 ounces freshly gathered, clean, whole
jewelweed plants, without roots
6 ounces, more or less, apple cider vinegar

Press the plants down into an 8-ounce sterile glass jar, packing them tightly until the jar is full. Pour in the vinegar, covering the plants and filling the jar to the top. Cover the jar securely and shake gently. Label with the name and date. Place the jar in a cool, dark area, and remember to shake it once a day.

You can begin to use this skin wash after a week. If you want it to be stronger, leave it for two weeks. Filter off the vinegar from the herbs and store it in a clean, labeled glass bottle.

Treatments for Cuts and Scrapes

Various cuts, scrapes, and other wounds are a normal part of everyday life. Most get better by themselves, but some require antiseptic care to minimize irritation and prevent infections. A large fresh leaf of English plantain, *Plantago major;* coltsfoot, *Tussilago farfara;* grape, *Vitis* spp.; or witch hazel, *Hamamelis virginiana,* makes a soothing bandage or poultice when held lightly in place over the injured skin.

You can also use a light tea made from the leaves and blossoms of yarrow, *Achillea millefolium,* or the leaves and roots of comfrey, *Symphytum officinale,* for a cooling wash and lotion. These rugged botanicals clean and heal most wounds, burns, rashes, and other skin problems. Decoctions and ointments of arnica, *Arnica cordifolia,* and witch hazel clear bruises, reduce swellings, and help erase old scars.

English plantain
Plantago major

BASIC HERBAL HEALING DECOCTION

This is a basic product from which you can make your own lotions, salves, creams, lip balms, and hair treatments.

Combine freshly cut, organically grown herbs in the general proportions of:

2 parts boneset, leaves, stems, flowers
2 parts echinacea, leaves, stems, flowers
1 part mountain mint, leaves, stems, flowers
1 part prickly ash, roots

Gently crush the botanicals together and place them in a deep enamel or stainless steel pot. Barely cover with fresh water and simmer, uncovered, for 30 minutes. Allow the fragrant, dark decoction to cool. Strain it and measure it. At this point, if you want, you can bottle and store some for a time, refrigerated or frozen.

Return the herbal liquid to a clean pot with an equal amount of good-quality vegetable oil (corn, sunflower, or peanut) and simmer for several hours, stirring occasionally, until all of the water has evaporated and a rich herbal oil results. Once you cool the oil, you can use it as is for topical treatment of dermatitis, eczema, chapped hands, and sore feet.

If you wish, you can add beeswax, honey, and a few drops of vitamin E oil to the herbal oil and simmer it into a fine lip balm. A few drops of tincture of benzoin will help preserve this product.

Note: Homemade products like these, without emulsifiers and lots of preservatives, have a limited shelf life; some will last longer if refrigerated. It is best to make your kitchen cosmetics and natural remedies seasonally and renew them as you can. Another good rule of thumb is to dry and package your best healing botanicals—roots, blossoms, leaves, and seeds—so that you can readily make up necessary preparations out of season. Remember that herbs and botanicals are more concentrated when dried; therefore you may use less of each ingredient.

SAMPSON'S SNAKEROOT HERBAL DIGESTIVE TONIC

The roots of the native perennial wildflower Sampson's snakeroot, *Gentiana villosa,* are a wonderful digestive aid, and can be used in place of European gentian, which is more commonly known and frequently used.

10 drops gentian root tincture, *Gentiana villosa*
5 drops mint tincture, *Mentha piperita* or another species

Add the tinctures to a 6-ounce glass of warm water. Drink this two to three times a day until symptoms ease.

Tinctures of Oregon grape root, *Mahonia* spp.; wild yam root, *Dioscorea villosa;* hops, *Humulus lupulus;* and licorice root, *Glycyrrhiza glabra,* also improve digestion and help relieve irritable bowel syndrome, which is often related to stress or food allergies. Some people will need a modest "cocktail" like the one above. Others may require only a few drops of one tincture placed on the back of the tongue after a heavy meal. Everyone is different, and these guidelines are cautious indicators. For persistent problems or conditions, consult a professional health care provider.

STRAWBERRY-MINT DIGESTIVE TEA

This delicious blend will aid digestion and ease gas. Fresh leaves are best, although dried will do. If you use dried herbs, cut the amounts almost in half.

3 strawberry leaves (3 leaflets of three)
9 large bergamot, peppermint, or spearmint leaves
2 cups boiling water

Gently crush the leaves as you put them in a small, warm teapot. Pour in the boiling water and cover the pot. Let this steep for 10 minutes.

Sip the tea slowly. Try drinking a cupful before each big meal, two to three times a day.

VARIATION: For any of these herbs, you can substitute 3 large dandelion leaves, 1 teaspoon of crushed fennel seeds, or 1 teaspoon of dried gentian root.

Maintaining Healthy Teeth and Gums

There are a multitude of native-based ways to clean and strengthen teeth and gums. The stems and twigs of a broad array of beneficial trees and shrubs are always available as dentifrices. When chewed and rubbed on the teeth and gums, they promote good dental hygiene (see page 46). There are also homemade products you can make, based upon early Indian wisdom.

Caution: Skin Sensitivities

When it comes to skin, one area of growing concern is photosensitivity, which is heightened sensitivity to sunlight. This can be caused by environmental factors, foods, or drugs. In addition, a few plants can cause photodermatitis, or skin burns. Because of their particular chemistry, some of these unique plants are being investigated as treatments for psoriasis, leukemia, and AIDS. The following plants can cause photodermatitis in some people and animals:

Cow parsnip, *Heracleum lanatum*, foliage and roots[1]
Poison hemlock, *Conium maculatum*, foliage and roots
St. John's wort, *Hypericum perforatum*, all parts[2]
St. Andrew's cross, *Hypericum hypericoides*, all parts[2]
Wild parsnip, *Pastinaca sativa*, all parts[3]

Contact with the roots, juices, or other parts of numerous plants can cause dermatitis or other skin irritations and rashes. But with most of them, being forewarned is usually enough to avoid trouble. The plants listed above are more problematic. Both of the Hypericums are frequently used in tinctures, salves, oils, and formulas that have beneficial, calming effects, both internally and externally. They are also important ingredients in many valuable skin care products. And the Hypericums are among the best herbal antidepressants known. Because it's hard to avoid them, people using products containing the Hypericums should be especially careful in the sun and use extra protection for eyes and skin.

Other problems may occur when these wild plants are mowed in and around the wet areas where they tend to grow. Unsuspecting people and farm animals have exhibited skin blotching, burning irritations, and lesions from swimming in streams, ponds, and lakes where these plants may have gotten into the water.

Treatments for Indigestion

How you process and digest your food governs how you feel. If your digestive system is in good working order, you'll feel healthier and have more energy. If you do not fully process and eliminate the wastes from the foods you eat, lingering toxins can cause headaches, skin problems, arthritic inflammations, and irritability.

Herbal teas, infusions, and tinctures can relieve many simple ailments. Seek professional help for persistent problems or recurring abdominal pain.

[1]Psoralen is the active compound in the roots. The acrid sap can cause blisters on contact.
[2]Hypericin, taken internally or externally, can cause skin burns on sensitive people when they are exposed to sunlight.
[2]Xanthotoxin can cause photodermatitis.

NATIVE HERB AND SPICE TOOTH POWDER

Our common native sage, *Artemisia tridentata,* or rugged sagebrush, and the unique native allspice, *Pimenta officinalis,* lend aromatic qualities to this traditional mixture, which is wonderfully cleansing and refreshing. It cleans and brightens your teeth and also makes a fine gargle and mouthwash to clear up bad breath, or halitosis. Make this tooth powder in small amounts and use it right up. You can use it every day or, if you prefer, alternate with your conventional toothpaste.

1 tablespoon baking soda
$^1/_2$ teaspoon sea salt or kosher salt
$^1/_2$ teaspoon allspice, powdered or ground fine
$^1/_2$ teaspoon sage, ground fine

In a small glass or ceramic dish, measure and blend together all the ingredients. When well mixed, store in a shallow nonmetal container with a nonmetal, airtight top. Some people make small individual jars so they can dip a damp toothbrush directly into the mixture.

To use this, sprinkle a pinch of the powder on your wet toothbrush. If you prefer, place a dab of fresh aloe gel on your toothbrush first. Brush as you would normally.

To use as a mouthwash, stir a teaspoon of the mixture into a cup of warm water.

ALOE-SAGE LIP BALM OR GLOSS

The succulent plant aloe, *Aloe vera,* provides a generous quantity of natural healing gel that works fine alone or, as in this recipe, in combination with other substances. You can use this lip balm year-round for protection from chapping.

1 teaspoon cocoa butter, grated
$^1/_2$ teaspoon pure beeswax, grated
$^1/_2$ teaspoon pure almond oil

$^1/_2$ teaspoon dried sage, ground fine

1 teaspoon raw honey

1 teaspoon aloe gel

3 drops vitamin E oil

Measure the cocoa butter, beeswax, and almond oil into a Pyrex cup. Melt them carefully in the microwave, using full power, for 15 seconds. Do this twice, checking and mixing well between heatings. Alternatively, you can heat the mixture over boiling water in the top of a double boiler.

As soon as the beeswax has melted, quickly mix in the remaining ingredients. Blend well. Pour into a tiny container or by generous drops onto foil or waxed paper and allow to cool and solidify. Use as needed.

Herbs and Their Actions

In this chapter we have given you an easy-to-assemble selection of home remedies. But the herbs and recipes above only hint at the wealth of botanical resources available to American Indian healers. Their work and that of other healers is covered in the fields known as **phytotherapy,** the treatment of illness with plants and plant-derived substances, and **pharmacognosy,** the branch of pharmacy that deals with the drugs and medicines made from plants and other natural sources. These remedies are often complements to pharmaceutical drugs, which are included in the field of **pharmacology.**

Because herbs and fungi can act strongly, it's best to know how they work. Today healing herbs are grouped into primary categories of use. Here are some more of the primary resources, by category, that are used by American Indians.

The effects of stress on physical, mental, emotional, and spiritual health are often only too apparent. To help your body withstand the strains of everyday life, you can use **adaptogens,** substances that help people adapt to stressful conditions. Perhaps America's most famous (and costly) adaptogen is American ginseng, *Panax quinquefolius.*

Numerous food, beverage, and health care products center on wild American ginseng roots and berries. Other health preparations combine our native ginseng with herbal complements such as sarsaparilla, goldthread, American ginger, and echinacea. Oriental ginseng species are sometimes formulated with American ginseng as a tonic to target special health and energy needs.

Perennial herbs used as **analgesics,** or pain relief, are the roots and leaves of American white hellebore, *Veratrum viride,* and blue flag, *Iris versicolor,* both of which are extremely poisonous. Others are black birch, *Betula lenta;* slippery elm, *Ulmus rubra;* partridgeberry or squaw vine, *Mitchella repens;* yarrow, *Achillea millefolium;* devil's bit, *Chamaelirium luteum;* and queen-of-the-meadow, *Spiraea ulmaria,* which contains the chemical forerunner of aspirin, salicylic acid. Many other botanicals are used for pain relief, especially the inner bark of most willows and alders growing along the marshy edges of rivers. Analgesics often help regulate the menses, assist uterine contractions during childbirth, and serve as digestive aids in herbal teas.

Antibiotic and **antiseptic** agents kill or inhibit the growth of harmful organisms such as bacteria. Many plants possess these properties. Among them are round-leaved sundew, *Drosera rotundifolia;* bloodroot, *Sanguinaria canadensis;* Seneca snakeroot, *Polygala senega;* hops, *Humulus lupulus;* blue cohosh, *Caulophyllum thalictroides;* the strongly aromatic sweet flag, *Acorus calamus;* and horsemint, *Monarda punctata.* Also useful are root teas made from wild indigo, *Baptisia tinctoria;* sweet goldenrod, *Solidago odora;* rattlesnake weed, *Hieracium venosum;* common juniper, *Juniperus communis;* Virginia snakeroot, *Aristolochia serpentaria;* and Canada lily, *Lilium canadense.*

Bloodroot
Sanguinaria canadensis

Rattlesnake weed, common juniper, Virginia snakeroot, and Canada lily are also valuable snakebite remedies. And not only are our native wood sage, *Teucrium canadense;* bee balm,

Monarda didyma; and American dittany, *Cunila origanoides,* valued antibiotics and antiseptics, but their leaf teas also treat problems of menstruation and digestive difficulties.

Antidiabetic herbs are those that may act therapeutically on diabetes, a disease that is marked by metabolic disorders and is sometimes characterized by excessive urination and intense thirst and hunger. Insufficient insulin production within the body can also trigger various other problems. American Indian medicine people explored the diverse uses of natural plants, singly and in carefully balanced formulas, to help the body regulate itself.

Native botanicals used in this field have been the roots and leaves of American barberry, *Berberis canadensis;* Canada fleabane, *Erigeron canadensis;* daisy fleabane, *E. philadelphicus;* alum root, *Heuchera americana;* joe-pye weed, *Eupatorium purpureum* and *E. maculatum;* red trillium, *Trillium erectum;* and wild ginger, *Asarum canadense.* The Jerusalem artichoke tuber, *Helianthus tuberosus,* one of our most common and delicious plants, contains inulin, a substance that may aid diabetes treatment. The leaves and roots of clintonia, *Clintonia borealis;* bugleweed, *Lycopus virginicus;* and flowering spurge, *Euphorbia corollata,* have proven to be beneficial when made into herbal teas.

Many plants have valuable **astringent** properties. They cleanse the skin and cause it to tighten and contract. One of our foremost astringents is witch hazel, *Hamamelis virginiana.* This rugged shrub grows densely in many parts of the eastern United States. It can reach heights of ten to twenty feet. Botanicals from the understory whose leaves and roots can be used as astringents are bearberry, *Arctostaphylos uva-ursi;* wintergreen, *Gaultheria procumbens;* goldthread, *Coptis groenlandica;* and Canada anemone, *Anemone canadensis.* Other common healing botanicals in this category are striped pipsissewa, *Chimaphila maculata;* shinleaf, *Pyrola elliptica;* tall cinquefoil, *Potentilla arguta;* bugleweed, *Lycopus virginicus;* and American bugleweed, *L. americanus.*

Nervines are agents that strengthen or calm the nerves. They are sometimes called nerve tonics. Examples are jimsonweed, *Datura stramonium,* which is highly poisonous; wild cucumber, *Echinocystis lobata;* wild clematis, *Clematis virginiana;* Indian pipes, *Monotropa uniflora;* black haw, *Viburnum prunifolium;* ground pine (club moss), *Lycopodium clavatum;* basswood, *Tilia americana;* rattlesnake plantain, *Goodyera pubescens;* and

Alum root
Heuchera americana

Healing Plants with Poisonous or Toxic Qualities

Along with the beneficial synergy of some botanicals, there may be harmful side effects. Many valuable medicinal plants have toxic or poisonous properties. An increasing number of plants are known to cause dermatitis or other allergic reactions in some people. Others can trigger photosensitivities, which cause skin blisters and skin pigmentation changes. And some herbs are known to contain potential carcinogens. Of course, many prescription medicines also have side effects.

If you use herbs in moderation and with a full understanding of all of their facets, it's unlikely that you will experience problems. But it is important to be aware that some herbs have many personalities. Just because something is natural doesn't mean it's good for you or that it isn't strong medicine. In general, for most things, less is better.

This is a selection of key medicinal plants that have a broad range of applications. Those marked with an asterisk are toxic in some situations.

Common Name	Botanical Name	Also Known As
Blue Cohosh*	Caulophyllum thalictroides	Squawroot
Poke*	Phyolacca americana	Pigeonberry
Hops*	Humulus lupulus	
Pipsissewa*	Chmaphila maculata	Wintergreen
Ground Pine*	Lyopodium clavatum	Club moss
Sassafras*	Sassafras albidum	Aguewood
Indian Balm*	Trillium erectum	Birthroot
Jack-in-the-Pulpit*	Arsaema triphyllum	Indian turnip
Indian Tobacco*	Lobelia cardinalis	Cardinal flower
Indian Tobacco*	L. siphilitica	Blue Lobelia
Witch Hazel	Hamamelis verginiana	Snapwood
Maidenhair Fern	Adiantum pedatum	
Pitcher Plant	Sarracenia purpurea	Turtle socks
Spahgnum	MossSphagnum magellanicum	Peat moss
Milkweed*	Asclepias syriaca	Indian broccoli
Dogbane*	Apocynum cannabinum	Indian hemp

moccasin flower, *Cypripedium acaule,* which is the pink lady's slipper. The ripe seeds, mature leaves, and perennial roots and blossoms of these unique botanicals are prescribed in varying ways, depending upon the medicine person, the season of use, and the age, body weight, and condition of each patient. At times their effects might seem paradoxical, but many of our most powerful medicines produce sharply contrasting effects in different individuals. For example, an herb may have a sedating effect on one person but cause anxiety in another.

Angel's trumpets, or jimsonweed
Datura stramonium

GLOSSARY OF TRIBES

More than five hundred American Indian tribes and additional groups of native peoples are indigenous to and currently live in North America. Most tribes have their own traditional names, which characteristically mean "people" or "people of a particular place." The tribal names by which these groups have become known were often given to them by other tribes or by European observers; when that is the case, we've noted it in parentheses.

This word map is a brief tour of the tribes mentioned in this book. We have also included a few historical and prehistoric groups in order to explain their relationships to living peoples of the Americas. There is no intent to exclude anyone.

Abenaki, "People of the Dawn," are Algonquian Indians of the Northeast who live in Vermont, New Hampshire, and southern Quebec. They were part of the great Wabanaki Confederacy (about 1750–1850), which also included the Penobscot, Passamaquoddy, Micmac, Maliseet, and Pennacook peoples.

Absaroka, "Bird People" (Siouan), are now known as the **Crow** Indians of the high northern Plains. They were noted allies who at one time were related allies of the Hidatsa. Their heartland today is the "Greasy Grass" region of southeastern Montana along the Little Big Horn River. The capital of the Crow Nation is Crow Agency.

Acoma are Pueblo people and one of the oldest groups in the Southwest. They are noted potters, artists, craftspeople, and farmers. Acoma Pueblo's Sky City is one of the most ancient inhabited settlements in New Mexico and the United States.

Adena were an ancient Mound Building culture (about 1000 B.C. to A.D. 200), who lived in what is now the Ohio River valley. There they built the Great Serpent Mound, which is over 1,330 feet long, and numerous other earth mounds.

Alabama, "Plant Gatherers," are an early tribe in the Southeast who were members of the powerful Creek Confederacy during the colonial period. Both the state and a prominent river are named for them. Today their central tribal unit shares a reservation with the Coushatta Indians in Polk County, Texas.

Aleut, "Islanders," are native peoples of the Aleutian Archipelago, a chain of about a hundred islands stretching almost 1,200 miles between Alaska and Siberia. The Aleuts are famous fishermen, artists, and basket weavers who live today in villages on mainland Alaska.

Algonquian (also Algonkian or Algonquin) is the name of a native language group. It is also the name for a large group of tribes and bands in the Eastern Woodlands who speak similar dialects. Some of the eastern Algonquian tribes were among the earliest to meet European explorers. Today they are known as the Narragansett, Nipmuc, Wampanoag, Mohegan, Pequot, Paugussett, Schaghticoke, Abenaki, Penobscot, Passamaquoddy, and Maliseet, as well as many others.

Anasazi, "Ancient Ones," were prehistoric Cliff Dwellers and farmers in the Desert Southwest who built huge planned towns at Pueblo Bonito and along Chaco Canyon from about 900 B.C. to A.D. 1100. Centered in the Four Corners region, they were distant ancestors of the Hopi.

Anishinabe, "First People," are Algonquian-speaking Indians of the Great Lakes area, also known as **Chippewa** (**Ojibway** in Canada). They are skilled hunters, fishermen, and herbalists as well as noted producers of wild rice. Their reservations are in Michigan, Minnesota, Wisconsin, North Dakota, Montana, Manitoba, and Ontario.

Apache, "Enemy" (from a Zuni name given because of the fear they inspired), included numerous tribes and bands in the Southwest who roamed broadly, traded widely, and adapted various lifestyles. They now live in Oklahoma, New Mexico, and Arizona. They are known as the Chiricahua, Cibecue, Mescalero, Lipan, Mimbreno, Jicarilla, San Carlos, Tonto, and White Mountain Apaches, as well as the Kiowa-Apache in Oklahoma.

Arapaho, "Traders" (from a Pawnee name), are western Algonquians who lived across the Great Plains. They were noted horsemen, warriors, medicine people, artists, and traders. Today they live in Oklahoma and on the Wind River Reservation in Wyoming.

Arctic peoples are Aleut, Inupiat, and Inuit (Eskimo) peoples as well as numerous other groups, villages, and bands who are distinct from other American Indians. These groups share many cultural traits that enable them to live in some of the world's harshest, most beautiful environments. Their homelands extend more than five thousand miles from the Aleutian Islands to Labrador and Greenland.

Arikara, "Horns," refers to the early hairstyle of the men of this tribe. These traditional buffalo hunters were once aligned with the Hidatsa and the Mandan. Today these Three Affiliated Tribes share reservation lands around Fort Berthold, North Dakota.

A:shiwi, "Flesh," are **Zuni** Pueblo peoples in western New Mexico. Modern descendants of the ancient Mogollon Culture, they are noted for their distinctive kachina rites, dances, silver work, fetishes, and art. Their dry farming and knowledge of the land is widely respected and is the basis of many of their healing rituals.

Assiniboine, "Those Who Cook with Stones," is a reference to the early cooking methods of these Plains Indians, who are a branch of the Sioux. Today they share settlements in Montana and Canada with the Sioux, Gros Ventres, Cree, and Ojibway. They are centered on Fort Belknap Reservation in northern Montana.

Athapaskan is another of the major language families and the name given to the many tribal groups who spoke it, from the sub-Arctic to the desert Southwest. Some of these tribes are the Apache and Navajo in the Southwest, and the Koyukon and Dogrib in the north.

Aztec are native Nahuatl-speaking Indians of central Mexico, whose dynamic empire flourished from 1200 until the Spanish conquest, about 1500. Their language and bloodline survive in many contemporary Mexicans.

Bannock are Indians who were originally part of the Paiute tribe in the Great Basin region beyond the western Plains. Sometimes called Sho-Bans, they are kin to the Shoshone Indians, with whom they share lands on the Fort Hall Reservation in Idaho.

Bella Coola are a distinctive Northwest Coast tribe who live in British Columbia. They are noted for their ceremonial objects and potlatches (large-scale giveaways with special feasts). They are centered in Bella Coola, British Columbia, today.

Blackfeet, also **Blackfoot,** were a powerful Plains confederacy of noted buffalo hunters and warriors, including the Blood, Piegan, and Siksika. Today they are centered in Canada and around Browning, Montana.

California Indians include the Yokut, Yurok, Hoopa, Pomo, Maidu, Miwok, Mission Indians, and others who settled densely in these lush areas. The bountiful environments in this part of the continent supported a greater diversity of native tribes than in any other region in North America.

Catawba, "People of the River," are Indians who settled in the river valleys of the Southeast. Today they are centered in reservation lands in South Carolina. Many also live in Oklahoma among the Choctaw Indians.

Cayuga, "People of the Marsh," are one of the five original tribes in the Iroquois League. They continue to live in their settlements (reservations) in central New York and southern Canada.

Cayuse were noted horse breeders whose name is synonymous with *pony*. These were Indians of northern Oregon and southeastern Washington in the Columbia Plateau, also known as the Great Basin region. Today, many live on the Umatilla Reservation in Pendleton, Oregon.

Cherokee, "People of the Different Speech," were skilled hunters, farmers, and medicine people, probably named by their neighbors the Creek Indians. Most were forced to walk the Trail of Tears in 1838–39 because of the United States government's removal policy. The Cherokee were the largest of the southeastern tribes and remain one of the biggest tribes today. Tribal headquarters are in Tahlequah, Oklahoma, in the West, and Cherokee, North Carolina, in the East.

Cheyenne, "People of a Different Speech" or "Red Talkers," were an early farming people from the Great Lakes regions who migrated to the Great Plains. Modern-day northern Cheyenne live on a reservation in Lame Deer, Montana; the southern Cheyenne share federal trust lands with the southern Arapaho in Concho, Oklahoma.

Chickasaw were southeastern Mississippian people with close ties to the Creek and Choctaw Indians. The Chickasaw were an early farming tribe noted for their hospitality. During the early 1800s most Chickasaw people relocated west of the Mississippi River into Indian territory, where they became known as one of the Five Civilized Tribes. Today they are centered in south-central Oklahoma, and their nation's seat is in Chickasaw.

Chinook are numerous tribes and bands of Indians who share a common language and live along the Columbia River in Oregon and Washington. The name also applies to a species of Pacific salmon as well as to the strong, moist winds that blow from the western Pacific inland across the high plateau regions. These famous fishermen, traders, and artists live with the Chehalis Indians on reservation land near Oakville, Washington.

Chippewa (Ojibwa or **Ojibway** in Canada) call themselves **Anishinabe,** "First People." This is the largest Algonquian tribal group in the Great Lakes region. Noted farmers, fishermen, artists, and healers, they are famous for their Grand Medicine Society, also called Midewiwin (or Mide). Many live on reservations in Wisconsin, Minnesota, Michigan, Montana, North Dakota, Ontario, and Manitoba.

Chitimacha are a southeastern tribe of skilled fishermen and farmers who have long lived in the Mississippi delta regions of lower Louisiana. They were noted for their blowguns and intricately plaited split-river-cane baskets and mats. They are descendants of the ancient Mound Builders and closely related to the Creek and Choctaw.

Choctaw are descendants of the ancient Mound Builders and closely related to the Creek and Chitimacha. Skilled farmers, plant gatherers, hunters, and artists, their homelands are in the Southeast. They were relocated to the West in 1830, suffering great losses along the way. Today the eastern Choctaw have a reservation near Pearl River, Mississippi, and the western Choctaw Nation seat is in Durant, Oklahoma.

Chumash are Pacific Coast fishermen, plant gatherers, and artists who are noted for their long cedar-plank boats. They originated in south central California near present-day Santa Barbara, but settlement pressures and diseases drove them to the brink of extinction.

Cochiti are one of the nineteen Pueblo groups along the Rio Grande valley south of Santa Fe, New Mexico. They are noted farmers, potters, jewelers, and drum makers, famed for their contemporary works, especially their cottonwood drums and clay storyteller dolls.

Coeur d'Alene, whose name means "Pointed Heart" in French, are a Salish tribe once noted for their salmon fishing and plant gathering along the Coeur d'Alene and Spokane Rivers. Their tribal headquarters today is in Plummer, Idaho.

Comanche were noted horsemen and buffalo hunters, once called "Lords of the Southern Plains" because of their power and grace. The tribe is now centered in Lawton, Oklahoma, where they share lands with their allies the Kiowas and Apaches.

Coushatta or **Koasati,** village farmers, artists, and basket weavers, were members of the Creek Confederacy who once lived in Alabama. Many were removed to Indian Territory (Oklahoma) in the 1830s, where a great number still live today. Many other Coushatta live in Louisiana, Texas, and Alabama.

Cree are widespread bands living across Canada, where they were once vital to the fur trade. These Algonquian hunters, traders, artists, and scouts of the sub-Arctic regions are more particularly known by their place names, like the Plains Cree, Swampy Cree, Western Wood Cree, Eastern Wood Cree, and James Bay Cree. The latter have garnered much support for their campaign against a Canadian hydroelectric project destined to destroy their homelands.

Creek are descendants of the ancient Temple Mound Builders of the Southeast, so named because their villages were located along rivers and creeks. Along with many similar tribes, such as the Alabama, Muskogee, Coushatta, and a number of small bands, they formed the Creek Confederacy. Many migrated or were removed from their homelands during the early 1800s. The Creek Nation seat is at Okmulgee in eastern Oklahoma, although many remain in their original homelands.

Crow, also **Absaroka** or **Apsaroke,** "Bird People," were early relatives of the Hidatsa of the upper Missouri River regions. The Crow were noted buffalo hunters, scouts, and plant gatherers of the Great Plains. In August, during its famous annual fair and rodeo, the Crow Reservation in Montana briefly becomes the "Tipi Capital of the World."

Dakota, "Allies," are also called **Lakota** or **Nakota.** The Santee Sioux and their four bands (Sisseton, Mdewkanton, Wahpeton, Wahpekute) are the Dakota Indians for whom two of the northern Plains states are named. These eastern Sioux blend many woodland and prairie Indian traditions in their culture. Their reservation is in eastern South Dakota.

Delaware, or **Lenni Lenape,** "True People," originally lived in the regions that became the states of New York, Delaware, New Jersey, and Pennsylvania. They were considered by many other eastern tribes to be the "Grandfather People" because of their peaceful leadership. Named for Lord de la Warr, the first governor of Virginia, these tribal groups suffered early settlement pressures and most moved to Canada and Oklahoma.

Desert People and **Cliff Dwellers** were prehistoric Indians of the desert Southwest. They are also called the Mogollon, Hohokam, and the Anasazi, among other names. From about 1000 B.C. to A.D. 1500, these complex ancient cultures farmed and hunted across the arid regions and built multistory mud, wood, and masonry homes in the high plateau and cliff areas. Ancestors of contemporary Pueblo and some other southwestern Indians, they were noted for their artistic accomplishments and social organization.

Diné, "People," are commonly called **Navajo** or **Navaho.** This is the biggest tribal nation in the United States, with more than 250,000 members. They migrated from the North to the Southwest about a thousand years ago. Noted horsemen, herders, farmers, jewelers, and weavers, the Diné are also respected herbalists and healers. They are centered in Window Rock, Arizona, and on Navajo reservations covering almost 16 million acres in the Four Corners region of Nevada, Utah, Arizona, and New Mexico.

Erie, "Nation of the Cat" or "Wild Cats," were a northern Iroquois group living in southern Canada until the mid-1600s, when their tribal numbers were decimated by conflicts over the rich fur trade.

Eskimo, "Eaters of Raw Meat" in the Algonquian language, call themselves **Inuit, Inupiat,** or "Real People." These native peoples are closely related to the Aleuts and other groups who live in the Arctic and sub-Arctic regions. Their elaborate masks, artistry, and social and ceremonial customs continue to influence our own concepts of art and healing. Numerous Eskimo villages are organized into six native corporations in Alaska, and the Inuit in Canada have the extensive Nunavut region in the Northwest Territories.

Flathead. Although they were Salish, the Flathead Indians did not follow the unusual custom of head-shaping practiced by some of the Salish Indians of the Northwest; hence their name. (The Salish flattened the back of the head to produce a distinctive dome shape.) They were fishermen and horsemen whose homelands were the territory that became Montana and northern Idaho. The Flathead Reservation today is shared with the **Kootenai** tribe, south of Flathead Lake, near Dixon, Montana.

Fox, also **Mesquakie,** "Red Earth People," were semi-nomadic prairie Algonquians of the western Great Lakes regions. They were also known as "People of the Calumet" because of the sacred pipes (calumets) they used in ceremonies. The Fox were close allies of the

Sac (Sauk) Indians, and today they share reservations and trust lands in Oklahoma, Kansas, and Iowa.

Great Basin Indians were the Bannock, Paiute, Ute, Washo, and Shoshone tribes, who shared an immense desert basin, including Death Valley and a broad area that touched ten western states and enveloped most of what is now Nevada, Idaho, Utah, Wyoming, and Colorado. Sometimes referred to as the Digger Indians because of their foraging practices, these tribes shared a common lifestyle and language group.

Great Lakes Indians were a group of Algonquian tribes, including the Chippewa (Ojibway), Fox, Sac (Sauk), Kickapoo, Ottawa, Menominee, and Potawatomi, who lived around the broad, fertile Great Lakes regions. They shared a common language family and way of life.

Gros Ventre, whose name means "Big Belly" in French, are a northern Plains tribe who call themselves **Atsina.** They were once members of the Blackfeet Confederacy and were skilled buffalo hunters and artists. Today they share the Fort Belknap Reservation in northern Montana with the Assiniboine.

Haida, "People," were a Northwest Coast tribe who lived on Queen Charlotte Island, off the coast of British Columbia. Noted woodworkers, boat builders, totem pole carvers, and fishermen, the Haida built huge spruce and cedar-plank houses in which they hosted potlatches (ritual gift-giving events). Contemporary Haida live in several coastal villages in Canada and Alaska; many are famous for their distinctive artwork.

Haudenosaunee, "People of the Longhouse," are the **Iroquois** of upper New York state and Canada. These are the Onondaga, Oneida, Cayuga, Seneca, Mohawk, and Tuscarora, referred to as the Six Nations of the Iroquois. They are noted for their clan system, farming, longhouse traditions, artworks and crafts, and their early democratic system of government.

Havasupai, "People of the Blue-Green Water," are descendants of ancient farmers along the Colorado River who grew corn, melons, squash, beans, sunflowers, and tobacco in irrigated fields in the desert Southwest. Their reservation near Supai, Arizona, along the rim of the Grand Canyon, embraces one of the most awesome landscapes in North America.

Hawaiians are descendants of prehistoric Polynesians and other Pacific Islanders who settled the eight tropical Hawaiian Islands. Early Hawaiians were village farmers, fishermen, and artists ruled by royal kings and queens. Two hundred years of exploitation and settlement pressures have thinned the native populations, but they remain strong in their traditions.

Hidatsa, also known as the **Minitari,** were village farmers and traders who built earth lodges on bluffs overlooking the Missouri River. They are one of the Three Affiliated Tribes, sharing reservation lands with the Mandan and Arikara in North Dakota near Fort Berthold.

Hohokam, "Vanished Ones," were prehistoric desert farmers in the ancient Southwest. They lived in the Gila and Salt River valleys from 100 B.C. to about A.D. 1500. Their distinctive pottery, etched shells, weavings, and earthen mounds remain as vivid reminders of a sophisticated early culture and may also reflect an association with early Mesoamerican cultures.

Hoopa (Hupa) are village Indians in the northern California highlands, closely related to the Karoks and Yuroks, with whom they share many traditions. Fishing, hunting, gathering, fine basketry, and cedar-plank houses are distinctive accomplishments of this tribe. They continue to live in the Hoopa Valley in northern California, retaining many of their unique cultural customs.

Hopewell Culture were ancient Mound Builders centered in the prehistoric Ohio, Illinois, and Mississippi River valleys more than two thousand years ago (from 300 B.C. to about A.D. 700). These skilled Stone Age craftspeople established widespread trading networks and left us haunting reminders of their artistic presence. They may have been ancestors of the Eastern Woodland Indians (today's Algonquian and Iroquoian Indians).

Hopi, "Peaceful Ones," are the westernmost Pueblo peoples, who farm near their ancient village settlements on the mesas and in the valleys of northeastern Arizona. They are probably descendants of the Anasazi. Their remarkable kachina rites and *kiva* ceremonies are part of one of the oldest healing cultures in North America.

Hualapai (Walapai), "Pine Tree People," are named after the rugged pinyon pine, which produced one of their staple foods. These Colorado River region hunters and gatherers were also noted herbalists and medicine people whose powers often came from dreams. Their tribal center today is Peach Springs, Arizona, near the Grand Canyon.

Huron, "Rough," also called **Wyandot,** "Islanders" or "Peninsula Dwellers," were various clans of northern Iroquois hunters and fur traders in the Great Lakes regions. They were also noted farmers who built their longhouses along river plateaus. They were nearly exterminated during the Fur Trading Wars in the 1600s. Their descendants live today in both Canada and the United States.

Illinois, "People," were various bands of prairie Algonquians who hunted and traded across the plains. Conflicts, diseases, and westward expansion thinned their numbers. Today their descendants are settled in the northeast corner of Oklahoma.

Inuit, "Real People," sometimes called Eskimos, are Arctic and sub-Arctic native peoples who live in villages and bands across northern Canada. They are closely related to the Aleut, Inupiat, and others in these circumpolar regions. Canada has set aside considerable lands, called Nunavut, in the Northwest Territories for them.

Inupiat (Inupiaq), "Real People," are Arctic and sub-Arctic native peoples of Alaska, often called Eskimos. Closely related to the Inuit, they are skilled hunters, fishermen, and craftspeople whose villages were organized into six native corporations by the Alaska Native Claims Act of 1971.

Iowa, "Sleepy Ones" (the name is from the Sioux), were early farmers, horsemen, and buffalo hunters across the Missouri and Mississippi River valleys who suffered great losses from conflicts, diseases, and westward expansion. Their descendants are settled on trust lands in Kansas, Nebraska, and Oklahoma.

Iroquois, "Real Adders" or "Poisonous Snakes" (French/Algonquian), call themselves **Haudenosaunee,** "People of the Longhouse." The Iroquois League of Six Nations included the Onondaga, Oneida, Cayuga, Seneca, Mohawk, and Tuscarora. The Iroquois were noted farmers, warriors, statesmen, and leaders in the tribal Northeast. Their reservations and reserves stretch across upper New York state and southern Canada.

Karok are closely related to the Hoopa and Yurok Indians of northern California. Noted for their hunting,

fishing, acorn gathering (an important staple food), and finely woven baskets, they were famous for their annual World Renewal Ceremonies and other medicine rites. They live in the Hoopa Valley in northern California.

Kickapoo, "Moving About," are Great Lakes Algonquians of the Wisconsin River regions who are closely related to the Fox and Sac Indians. True to their name, they moved about throughout their history. Today their various groups are settled in Mexico, Kansas, and Oklahoma.

Kiowa, "Main People," were seasonal hunters and warriors who ranged across the Great Plains. They were and are noted leaders, artists, and medicine people. They were allies of the Apache and Comanche, with whom they farm and share trust lands and oil leases in Carnegie, Oklahoma, today.

Klamath, "People," were hunters and gatherers of the Oregon Plateau regions. Noted resistance fighters and warriors, the Klamath suffered many losses as a result of federal government policy changes, especially the termination policies of the 1950s.

Kwakiutl were Northwest Coast people living on northern Vancouver Island. These skilled hunters, fishermen, and craftsmen were noted for their potlatches (feasts and giveaways) and mystical religious societies with elaborate masks, rites, and stories. They were also mask and totem pole carvers whose works expressed complex tribal traditions. Ten Kwakiutl bands remain in British Columbia today. The salmon industry is central to their economies.

Lakota, "Allies," were mainly the Teton Sioux bands of the Brule (Sichangu), Oglala, Hunkpapa, Blackfeet, Two Kettles, Miniconjou, and Sans Arcs. In the past, they were noted horsemen and warriors of the western Plains. Today their reservations are in the Dakotas and surrounding regions.

Makah, "Cape Dwellers," are rugged Northwest Coast people living on the Olympic Peninsula of Washington state. They are noted fishermen, whalers, hunters and gatherers, as well as fine weavers and carvers. Their reservation is in Neah Bay, Washington.

Malecite (Maliseet), "Broken Talkers" (the name comes from the Micmac), are Eastern Woodland Algonquians who were allies of the Micmac and early members of the Wabenaki Confederacy. They were known as hunters, trappers, traders, and artists. Today their bands maintain reserve lands in Maine and Canada.

Mandan were early Plains Indians who settled along the Missouri River, where they were successful farmers and gatherers as well as dynamic buffalo hunters. Along with their neighbors, the Arikara and Hidatsa Indians, they are called the Three Affiliated Tribes. They share lands and a similar way of life at Fort Berthold, North Dakota.

Maya were a sophisticated early culture that developed more than two thousand years ago in Mesoamerica. The Maya built vast temple and ceremonial sites, irrigated fertile farmlands, and developed calendars, astronomy, and detailed hieroglyphs to record their ideas. Their descendants live in Mexico, Guatemala, and Belize and are noted for their healing traditions.

Menominee, "Wild Rice People," were Great Lakes Algonquians, noted for their hunting, fishing, trading, and artistry. The *kinnikinniks* (smoking/smudging mixtures) that they used in their calumets (special pipes) were highly esteemed. Centuries of settlement pressures and federal termination policies have pushed the Menominee into decline; they continue to work for proper restitution.

Metis, "Mixed Blood" (the word is French), is a historical term usually meaning someone of Cree-French ancestry. This stems from the 1700s, when Canadian backwoods trappers traded with the Cree and other tribes to supply the European demand for North American fur pelts.

Miami, "People of the Peninsula," were prairie Algonquians of the southern Great Lakes regions who were noted warriors, traders, and artists. They were known for their calumets (peace pipes) and war clubs. Several bands of Miami Indians live in northeastern Oklahoma and are known as the Wea and Piankashaw.

Micmac, "Allies," were maritime Algonquians, allies of the **Maliseet** and members of the Wabenaki Confederacy in the Northeast. Woodland hunters, gatherers, herbalists, and fishermen, they are noted for their fine craftsmanship. They live mainly on reserves in Nova Scotia, New Brunswick, and Prince Edward Island.

Mikasuki (Miccosukee) are close relatives and allies of the Seminole Indians in Florida. These fishermen, hunters, herbalists, and artists maintain their traditional ways on their own reservation along the Tamiami Trail (Alligator Alley).

Mississippi were ancient Temple Mound Builders who flourished throughout the broad Mississippi River valley from about A.D. 700 to 1150. Their great site at Cahokia, Illinois, covered about four thousand acres, with more than eighty-five different mounds; it may have housed almost forty thousand people. Ancestors of today's Creek Indians and other southeastern tribes, these prehistoric peoples were probably influenced by the ancient Olmecs, Toltecs, Maya, and Aztecs, whose cultures flourished in Mesoamerica.

Missouri (Missourias), "People with Dugout Canoes," were probably once Woodland Indian farmers who migrated to the Great Plains and became horsemen and buffalo hunters. Intertribal warfare dispersed them and reduced their numbers during the 1800s and 1900s. Today the Missouri are affiliated with the Otoe, with whom they share settlements in Oklahoma.

Mogollon Culture were prehistoric Southwestern farming people who cultivated the high mountain valleys between 300 B.C. and about A.D. 1300. These early gardeners raised corn, squash, beans, cotton, sunflowers, peppers, and tobacco. They also built pit houses and *kivas* (underground ceremonial chambers) and were noted for their weavings and stylized black-on-white pottery.

Mohawk, or Ganiengehaka (in their own language), were "People of the Flint Country" and "Keepers of the Eastern Door" for the Iroquois League. Easternmost of the Six Nations, the Mohawk were longhouse village farmers, warriors, hunters, traders, and basket weavers. They are known today as "walkers of high steel," teachers, artists, and storytellers. The Mohawk are centered on their reservations and reserves in upstate New York and Canada.

Mohegan, "Wolf People," were Eastern Woodland Algonquians who were noted for their hunting, trading, medicine, farming, and whaling. Today they continue their traditions in eastern Connecticut. They have also developed economic enterprises based on their gambling casinos.

Mojave (Mohave), "Beside the Water," were desert Southwest people who lived along the Colorado River along with their neighbors the Yumans, Havasupais,

Hualapais, and Yavapais. They farmed and hunted the fertile bottomlands near the Mojave Desert, and were also noted warriors, weavers, artists, and potters. They are centered today on three reservations in Arizona, Nevada, and California, which they share with other related tribes.

Montagnais, whose name is French for "Mountaineers," were Canadian Algonquian hunters and fishermen of the north who traveled seasonally across the vast sub-Arctic regions and traded with their neighbors the Cree and Naskapi. Today they live on reserves in northern Quebec.

Montauk, "People at the High Land," were East Coast Algonquians on Long Island who established a confederacy of neighboring Algonquian tribes in the 1700s. They were noted whalers, fishermen, farmers, and gatherers. Their descendants still live in southeastern Long Island.

Mound Builders were prehistoric Indians of three distinct cultural groups who lived in central and eastern America from about 1000 B.C. until about A.D. 1500. Today they are known as the Adena, Hopewell, and Mississippi cultures. Although they were skilled hunters, farmers, artists, and potters, they are especially well known as builders of fabulous earthen mounds and villages.

Narragansett, "People of the Point," were eastern Algonquian hunters, gatherers, fishermen, whalers, warriors, medicine people, and traders who lived in stockaded villages in what is now Rhode Island. Settlement pressures and warfare thinned their numbers, but the Narragansett are still centered in Charlestown, Rhode Island, where their tribal headquarters, church, and longhouse are located.

Natchez were Temple Mound Builders who maintained well-organized villages along the lower Mississippi River. Their economy was based on hunting and gathering. Early settlement pressures dispersed this powerful tribe; their descendants settled among and intermarried with other southern tribes.

Navajo (Navaho), who call themselves **Diné,** "People," are the largest tribal group in Native America. Noted warriors, herdsmen, gardeners, weavers, artists, and medicine people in the Southwest, they are famous for their intricate sand paintings and the ceremonial objects that accompany their healing chantways. They

are centered in the Four Corners region around their capital in Window Rock, Arizona.

Nez Perce, "Pierced Noses," who call themselves **Nimipu,** "People," were hunters, gatherers, fishermen, and horsemen of the northern plateau regions around the Snake and Salmon Rivers. Settlement pressures and federal persecution drove them off much of their homelands. Their tribal centers today are the Nez Perce Reservation near Lapwai, Idaho, and the Colville Reservation near Nespelem, Washington.

Northeast or Eastern Woodland Indians are a broad cultural group of Indians who shared similar ways of life. It includes the various Iroquois and Algonquian tribes throughout the northeast, from the Atlantic Ocean west to the Mississippi River, and from southern Canada south to North Carolina. Although many were displaced, descendants of most of these tribes continue to live in their homelands.

Northwest Coast Indians are a diverse group of tribes who share a lush and narrow (150 miles across) strip of Pacific Coastal terrain stretching almost two thousand miles from northern California to southern Alaska. These are the dynamic totem pole and potlatch peoples known as the Chinook, Makah, Nootka, Kwakiutl, Tsimshian, Haida, Tlingit, and others, who hunted for salmon, halibut, seals, and whales. They are famed for their fantastic masks, ceremonial rituals, and artwork.

Ojibway (Ojibwa), also known as **Chippewa,** are Great Lakes Algonquians who call themselves **Anishinabe,** "First People." These noted hunters, trappers, farmers, medicine people, and healers were famous for their Grand Medicine Society, the Midewiwin, which continues to exert traditional healing influences in countless ways. The Ojibway and Chippewa are centered on their reserves in Canada and on reservations in the Great Lakes area.

Omaha, "Those Going Against the Current," were a Missouri River tribe of village farmers on the Great Plains who lived in earth lodges most of the year. They are gathered today on lands in Nebraska near the Winnebago Indians, where their traditions continue to flourish.

Oneida, "People of the Standing Stone," are one of the Iroquois tribes. They were successful village farmers, hunters, and artists as well as traditional longhouse people. Today they hold lands in New York, Wisconsin, and Canada.

Onondaga, "People of the Hills," are also "Keepers of the Council Fire" and "Keepers of the Wampum" for the Iroquois League in upstate New York and Canada. The Onondaga are the "Faith Keepers" and the most central of the six tribes of the Iroquois. They are based near Nedrow, New York.

O'Odham, "Desert People," are also known as the **Papago,** "Bean People," and the **Pima,** "River Dwellers." Descendants of the ancient Hohokam, the "Vanished Ones" of the desert, they live in the desert Southwest, sharing the Salt River and Gila River Reservations with the Maricopa, and the Ak Chin Reservation with the Papago.

Osage call themselves **Ni-U-Ko'n-Ska,** "Children of the Middle Waters." These seminomadic prairie Indians were once buffalo hunters and village farmers. They are centered near Pawhuska, Oklahoma, today, where oil reserves and other economic resources benefit their lives.

Oto were seminomadic, like many tribes of the prairie and Plains regions. They were closely aligned with the Winnebago, Iowa, and Missouri Indians. Settlement pressures during the 1800s caused hardships and land losses for them. Today the Oto and Missouri have combined into the Otoe-Missouria tribe and share trust lands near Pawnee, Oklahoma.

Ottawa, "Traders," were Great Lakes Algonquians and allies of the Hurons, who were part of the great fur trading networks in the 1600s and 1700s. Today their descendants live in Kansas, Michigan, and Oklahoma, but they do not have reservations or trust lands.

Paiute, "Water Ute" or "People of the Rushes," were numerous bands who ranged widely across the rugged Great Basin region fishing for salmon, hunting, and gathering. Their reservations today are in Arizona, California, Nevada, Oregon, and Utah.

Papago, "Bean People," called themselves **Tohono O'Odham,** "Desert People." They lived in the Sonoran Desert near the Gulf of California. These seminomadic farmers and gatherers coaxed life from harsh environments. Today they still inhabit their homelands as well as three reservations in Arizona.

Passamaquoddy, "People of the Pollack," were northeastern Algonquian fishermen, farmers, hunters, and gatherers, who were once members of the Wabenaki Confederacy. One of their dependable staples was pollack. They have two reservations near Calais, Maine.

Pawnee, "Horns" or "Hunters," were noted farmers and village traders of the Plains and prairies who were relatives of the Arikara, Caddo, and Witchita. Driven from their historic lands in Nebraska and Kansas, they are centered today in Pawnee, Oklahoma. They are noted for their hospitality, farming, artwork, and dancing.

Penobscot, "People of the Rocky Place," were northeastern Algonquian hunters, gatherers, fishermen, and medicine people of the Wabenaki Confederacy. Their reservation, centered on Indian Island, near Old Town, Maine, also includes numerous other islands in the Penobscot River. They are noted for their sports, traditional crafts, carvings, and artworks.

Pequot, "Destroyers" or "Fox People," were northeastern Algonquian hunters, gatherers, fishermen, warriors, and traders. This powerful tribe dominated early trading until their numbers were decimated by colonial warfare. They are based in Connecticut, with the Mashantucket tribal headquarters in Ledyard and Mashantucket, and the Paucatuck Pequot Reservation in North Stonington. Successful tribal enterprises, especially gambling, not only have enriched their financial well-being but have also contributed to the economy of the state and southern New England.

Pima, "River Dwellers," were successful hunters, gatherers, and village farmers in the desert Southwest. Considered to be descendants of the ancient Hohokam, the Pima irrigated their broad fields and grew corn, squash, melons, beans, cotton, sunflowers, and tobacco. Today they share the Salt River and Gila River Reservations with the Maricopa Indians.

Plains Indians were mounted horsemen, buffalo hunters, and tipi dwellers who ranged across the Great Plains, an area reaching from central Canada south to Texas, and from the Mississippi River west to the Rockies. More than twenty unique tribes, each with its own traditions, history, and ways of life, hunted across this continent's broad midsection. Today they are known as the Assiniboine, Arapaho, Gros Ventre,

Crow, Plains Chippewa, Plains Cree, Blackfeet, Cheyenne, Sioux, Kiowa, Comanche, Tonkawa, and others.

Pomo were village traders, hunter-gatherers, and noted medicine people in California. They made some of the finest baskets in Indian America, an artistic tradition that continues today. The Pomo live on several reservations, the largest of which is in Mendocino County.

Ponca were peaceful Prairie Indians who migrated west from southern Minnesota to Nebraska to farm and hunt buffalo. Settlement pressures, diseases, and conflicts caused many changes for these leaders, statesmen, and artists. The Ponca live on allotted lands in Oklahoma and Nebraska today.

Potawatomi, "People of the Fire," were Great Lakes Algonquians who were noted hunters, gatherers, medicine people, and artists. Their history of hardships includes the migration from Indiana in 1838, which was called the Trail of Death because so many people died. Today various Potawatomi bands have reservations and lands in Wisconsin, Michigan, Ontario, Kansas, and Oklahoma.

Powhatan, "At the Falls," were about thirty bands of eastern Algonquians living in over two hundred villages in the region that became Virginia. They banded together into the Powhatan Confederacy during the 1500s and 1600s. Powhatan is also the name given to their powerful chief, who was the father of Pocahontas. Today some of their descendants live on the Pamunkey and Mattaponi Reservations in Virginia; others, now called the Rappahannock, Potomac, Nansemond, and Chickahominy, live throughout the East.

Prairie Indians were many different tribes who lived and hunted across the grasslands of the Missouri and Mississippi River regions. Some of these tribes lived in permanent villages with extensive farms, where they made pottery, carvings, and weavings. They also hunted buffalo, antelope, and other wild game and fish. Some of the eastern bands of the Sioux, as well as the Arikara, Hidatsa, Mandan, Iowa, Oto, Missouri, Kaw, Omaha, Osage, Ponca, Pawnee, Quapaw, and Wichita, are their descendants.

Prehistoric Indians were the many ancient peoples who lived throughout North America before the coming of Columbus and "recorded history," probably for more than twenty thousand years. Many of the names by which they are known today are based upon the types of stone, bone, ivory, and pottery that have been found in their sophisticated ancient sites. These were the earliest ancestors of today's native peoples.

Pueblo Indians, "Villages," were the diverse village dwellers of the desert Southwest, who are today known as the Hopi, Zuni, and the nineteen New Mexico Pueblo tribes of the Rio Grande River regions. They are thought to be the descendants of the ancient Anasazi and Mogollon peoples. The unique architecture of their Arizona and New Mexico pueblos includes dwellings made of adobe and stone in multistory, terraced villages, often built on high plateaus or mesa tops.

Quapaw, "Downstream People," were peaceful people of the lower Mississippi River valley who lived in bark-covered houses inside palisaded villages. Settlement pressures and federal relocation policies forced them to move to trust lands in the northeast corner of Oklahoma, where mineral desposits found on their land help support contemporary tribal members.

Sac (Sauk), "Yellow Earth People," were village Algonquians of the western Great Lakes and close allies of the Fox. Their seasonal ways of life were based on hunting and farming until settlement pressures and conflicts disrupted their traditional existence. Today they share small reservations and trust lands in Iowa, Kansas, and Oklahoma with the Fox.

Seminole, "Unconquered" or "Runaways," were southeastern Creeks who were driven out of their homelands in Georgia and Alabama. They settled and intermarried with other southern tribes in Florida in order to continue their hunting, farming, and village traditions. Federal settlement pressures and wars reduced their numbers and forced many to walk the Trail of Tears in 1838–39, bringing them to Indian Territory, which later became the state of Oklahoma. But many fought to remain; they now have five reservations and trust lands in Florida as well as lands in Texas and in Seminole, Oklahoma.

Seneca, "People of the Great Hill" and "Keepers of the Western Door" for the Iroquois League, were noted farmers, hunters, statesmen, artists, and medicine people. They now have three reservations in western New York near the city of Buffalo and additional parcels of leased lands.

Shawnee, "Southerners," were groups of eastern Algonquians who ranged over considerable territory in the western Cumberland Mountains. These farmers, hunters, fishermen, and statesmen were also warriors, as settlement pressures threatened to displace them. Today they share trust lands in Oklahoma.

Shinnecock were noted fishermen, whalers, and farmers who were sought after for their wampum (shell beads) during the fur trading era. These Algonquian people are centered on their reservation in Southampton, New York (on the south fork of Long Island), where they continue to develop tribal enterprises.

Shoshone were diverse groups who lived, hunted, and foraged in the high, arid Great Basin region west of the Rocky Mountains. They share reservations and trust lands today in Idaho, Utah, Nevada, and California.

Sioux, "Adders," call themselves Dakota, Lakota, or Nakota, which means "Allies." Four major branches of this dynamic horse culture, each with distinct bands, migrated from the Woodlands onto the Great Plains centuries ago. Despite the impact of settlement pressures and warfare, the Sioux have remained enduring leaders. They have eight reservations in South Dakota, two in North Dakota, four in Minnesota, and more in other states, as well as reserve lands in Canada.

Southeast Indians included the Creek, Cherokee, Choctaw, Coushatta (Koasati), Chickasaw, Catawba, Chitimacha, Alabama, Seminole, Yuchi, Natchez, and other tribes who shared similar ways of life in the diverse environments of the Southeast. In the 1700s and 1800s many were forced to relocate to Indian Territory west of the Mississippi but a number of their descendants remain in or near their original homelands.

Southwest Indians are the many tribes who populated the arid environments in the Southwest. Among them are the Hopi, Zuni, Acoma, Jemez, Cochiti, Taos, Isleta, Laguna, Picuris, Pojoaque, Sandia, Santa Ana, Santa Clara, San Felipe, San Ildefonso, San Juan, Santo Domingo, Tesuque, Zia, and Nambe Pueblos, as well as the Navajo, Papago, Pima, Yuma, Yaqui, Yavapai, Havasupai, Hualapai, Mojave, and Apache.

Tlingit were numerous bands of fishermen, traders, weavers, and warriors on the Northwest Coast; they were neighbors of the Haida and Tsimshian. In southern Alaska, where the salmon were central to their economy, Tlingit woodcarvers were noted for their totem poles.

Tsimshian, "People of the Skeena River," were Northwest Coast fishermen, carvers, and artists who gathered much of their livelihood from the Pacific Ocean. Today there are seven Tsimshian bands in western Canada as well as many who live on their reservation on Annette Island, near the coast of Alaska.

Tuscarora, "People of the Hemp," were the sixth tribe to join the Iroquois League when they migrated north from the Carolinas in the early 1700s, seeking to escape settlement pressures and other conflicts. Today they have a reservation in northwestern New York, and they share reserve lands in Canada and North Carolina.

Umatilla, of the high western plateau regions, were related to the Cayuses, Modocs, Wallawallas, Yakimas, and Nez Perces living in what is now northern Oregon and southern Washington. The Umatilla Reservation, established in 1853 near Pendleton, Oregon, is shared with Cayuse and Wallawalla. These tribes sponsor dance and art pageants, a popular annual rodeo, and have built a fine new cultural center.

Ute, "People of the Sun" or "Land of the Sun," were the tribal neighbors of the Paiute and Shoshone in the Great Basin region. These nomadic hunters and gatherers were sometimes called Digger Indians because they knew the art of gathering many wild foods and medicines from the earth. Today they are centered on three reservations in Colorado and Utah (which takes its name from the tribe).

Wabenaki, "People Living at the Sunrise," was an Algonquian Indian confederacy during the historic period (about 1750–1850). It brought together the Abenaki, Penobscot, Passamaquoddy, Micmac, Maliseet, and Pennacook peoples.

Walapai, "Pine Tree People" (see **Hualapai**).

Wampanoag, "People of the Dawn," were coastal Algonquian fishermen, farmers, and warriors in the Northeast, where they formed strong alliances during the settlement periods. Displacement, conflicts, and diseases thinned their numbers and eroded their lands. Today, the Gay Head Wampanoags are centered on Martha's Vineyard, and the Mashpee Wampanoags are based in Mashpee, Massachusetts, on Cape Cod.

Winnebago, "People of the Dark Water," were Great Lakes Algonquian fishermen and village farmers as well as noted medicine people. They have reservations in Wisconsin and Minnesota and share reservation lands with the Omaha in Nebraska.

Wyandot, "Islanders" or "Peninsula Dwellers" (see **Huron**).

Yakima, "Runaway," were Plateau Indians who lived along the Yakima River, a tributary of the Columbia River. These fishermen, hunters, gatherers, and weavers were also noted warriors who endured countless conflicts. Their reservation, which they share with the Paiutes and other native peoples, is based in Toppenish, Washington.

Yaqui, "Chief River," were farmers, fishermen, medicine people, and foragers in an area of the desert Southwest that straddled the United States-Mexico border. They suffered from countless raids, settlement conflicts, and missionary pressures. Today their descendants live in six communities in southern Arizona as well as in Mexico.

Yavapai, "People of the Sun," were numerous bands of nomadic people in the desert Southwest who foraged for seasonal wild foods and medicines. They resisted missionary and settlement pressures but were drawn into conflicts during the 1800s. They share reservation lands today with the Apache and Mojave in western Arizona.

Yuma, "People of the River," were southwestern village farmers, fishermen, and hunters who lived along the Colorado River. They banded together to prevent the Spanish and European settlements that eventually split their resistance. They share reservation lands today with the Maricopa and Cocopah in California and Arizona.

Yupik were Arctic people related to the Aleut, Inuit, and Inupiat. Their ancestors migrated across the Bering Strait from Siberia more than ten thousand years ago. Sometimes called Eskimos, there are distinctive settlements of Yupik in Alaska, Siberia, and along the Pacific Arctic regions.

Yurok, "Downstream People," were northern California people who fished and hunted along the Klamath River with their neighbors the **Karoks,** "Upstream People." Today these tribes have several small reservations (rancherias) in Humbolt County, California.

Zuni, "Flesh," also **A:Shiwi,** are traditional Pueblo farmers, hunters, and artists of the upper Zuni River in western New Mexico, where they originally had seven villages. They are descendants of the ancient Mogollon Culture. Noted stonecutters, carvers, silversmiths, and jewelers, they are especially famous for their festival dances at Zuni Pueblo, where they host an annual fair.

LEXICON OF HERBS, FUNGI, AND MINERALS

Native peoples use countless herbs, botanical parts, and fungi throughout the life cycle. On the next few pages are some of their key substances, along with a listing of their diverse uses. Some of these materials are still being investigated for their pharmacological properties and other possible benefits.

Key to the Charts

A = Art and symbolism

B = Beverage

C = Cordage and fiber

D = Dentifrice

E = Dyes and inks

F = Food

G = Fumigants

H = Seasonings

I = Insecticides

J = Preservatives

K = *Kinnikinniks,* smoking/smudging mixtures

L = Love medicines and charms

M = Medicines

N = Cosmetics

O = Fuel

P = Poisons

Q = Contraceptives and abortifacients

R = Birthing

S = Sacred and ceremonial

T = Tools

HERBS

Common Name	Latin Name	Uses
1. American angelica	*Angelica atropurpurea*	A, F, H, L, M
2. American ginger	*Asarum canadense*	A, B, F, H, J, L, M, S
3. American ginseng	*Panax quinquefolia*	A, B, F, L, M, S
4. Arrow-wood	*Euonymus americanus*	C, D, M, O, T
5. Bearberry	*Arctosphylos uva-ursi*	B, G, K, L, M, S
6. Bee balm	*Monarda didyma*	B, D, F, G, H, I, J, L, M, N
7. Black birch	*Betula lenta*	B, D, H, I, M, O, T
8. Black cohosh	*Cimicifuga racemosa*	I, L, M, P, R
9. Black haw	*Viburnum prunifolium*	D, F, M, T
10. Blue cohosh	*Caulophyllum thalictrioides*	B, L, M, R
11. Bloodroot	*Sanguinaria canadensis*	A, D, E, I, L, M, N
12. Boneset	*Eupatorium perfoliatum*	B, D, L, M
13. Broom snakeroot	*Gutierrezia sarothrae*	I, L, M
14. Cardinal flower	*Lobelia cardinalis*	L, M, P
15. Chaparral	*Larrea tridentata*	G, K, M, O
16. Colicroot	*Aletris farinosa*	M, R
17. Coneflower	*Echinacea angustifolia*	A, B, D, F, K, L, M, N
18. Cotton	*Gossypium hirsutum*	C, M, Q
19. Cranesbill	*Geranium maculatum*	I, L, M
20. Culver's root	*Veronicastrum virginicum*	L, M, Q
21. Dogwood	*Cornus florida*	D, F, K, L, M, O, S, T
22. Elderberry	*Sambucus canadensis*	B, E, F, I, M, N, P
23. Evening primrose	*Oenothera biennis*	F, K, L, M, R
24. Figwort	*Scrophularia marilandica*	G, M, I, P
25. Fireweed	*Epilobium angustifolium*	A, C, D, G, K, M
26. Fringe tree	*Chionanthus virginicus*	A, C, D, M, T

COMMON NAME	LATIN NAME	USES
27. Golden ragwort	*Senecio aureus*	E, G, M
28. Goldenrod	*Solidago odora*	B, D, E, F, G, I, K, M
29. Goldenseal	*Hydrastis canadensis*	D, E, L, M, N
30. Goldthread	*Coptis groenlandicus*	E, I, M, R
31. Hemp dogbane	*Apocynum cannabinum*	C, I, M, T
32. Hops	*Humulus lupulus*	J, K, M
33. Horsetail	*Equisetum arvense*	B, M
34. Horseweed	*Erigeron canadensis*	E, G, M
35. Iceland moss	*Cetraria islandica*	F, H, M, N
36. Indian breadroot	*Psoralea esculents*	F, M
37. Indian cup	*Silphium perfoliatum*	C, E, G, I, M, R
38. Indian pink	*Spigelia marilandica*	A, M, N
39. Indian tobacco	*Lobelia inflata*	G, K, M
40. Juniper	*Juniperus communis*	B, C, F, G, H, I, J, K, L, M
41. Kelp	*Laminaria digitata*	B, D, F, H, M
42. Mayapple	*Podophyllum peltatum*	F, L, M, P
43. Meadowsweet	*Filipendula ulmaria*	B, D, G, K, L, M, R
44. Milkweed	*Asclepias syriaca*	C, F, M
45. Mistletoe	*Phoradendron flavescens*	L, M, P, R
46. Moccasin flower	*Cypripedium calceolus*	A, L, M
47. Mountain tobacco	*Arnica fulgens*	G, I, K, M, P, S
48. Passionflower	*Passiflora incarnata*	B, F, L, M
49. Pipsissewa	*Chimaphila umbellata*	B, M
50. Prickly ash	*Zanthoxylum americanum*	B, M
51. Sagebrush	*Artemisia tridentata*	B, D, G, I, J, K, L, M, S
52. Slippery elm	*Ulmus rubra*	C, D, M, O, T
53. Spicebush	*Lindera benzoin*	B, D, F, H, I, K, M
54. Spikenard	*Aralia racemosa*	B, M, R

COMMON NAME	LATIN NAME	USES
55. Sweet flag	*Acorus calamus*	H, I, K, M, S
56. White oak	*Quercus alba*	C, E, M, O, T
57. White pine	*Pinus strobus*	B, C, D, M, O, S, T
58. White willow	*Salix alba*	B, C, D, M, O, T
59. Wild indigo	*Baptisia tinctoria*	E, G, I, M, P
60. Wild licorice	*Glycyrrhiza lepidota*	H, M, R
61. Wild senna	*Cassia marilandica*	M, P, Q
62. Wild strawberry	*Fragaria vesca*	B, F, L, M, R, S
63. Wild yam	*Dioscorea villosa*	F, M, P, Q
64. Wintergreen	*Gaultheria procumbens*	B, H, I, M
65. Witch hazel	*Hamamelis virginiana*	D, I, M, N, R
66. Wormseed	*Chenopodium ambrosioides*	F, H, I, M
67. Yarrow	*Achillea millefolium*	B, D, G, I, K, M, Q
68. Yellow jessamine	*Gelsemium sempervirens*	A, I, M
69. Yellowroot	*Xanthorhiza simplicissima*	E, M, Q

FUNGI

Common Name	Latin Name	Tribal Name	Uses
1. Indian paint fungus	*Echinodontium tinctorium*		A, E, G, M, N
2. Tinder polypore	*Fomes fomentarius*	Punk	G, P
3. Larch polypore	*Fomitopsis officinalis*		F, G, I, M
4. Red-belted polypore	*Fomitopsis pinicola*		A, E, M
5. Earthstar	*Geastrum pectinatum* and spp.		G, L, M
6. Giant puffball	*Calvatia booniana* and spp.		A, F, G, L, M, S
7. Gem-studded puffball	*Lycoperdon perlatum*	Snake bread	A, F, G, L, M, S
8. Tough puffball	*Mycenastrum corium*	Frog's navel	E, G, M
9. Buried-stalk puffball	*Tulostoma simulans*	Devil's snuffbox	A, M, S
10. Desert stalked puffball	*Battarrea phalloides*		A, M, S
11. Meadow mushroom	*Agaricus campestris*	Ghost ears	F, H
12. Turkey tails	*Coriolus versicolor*	Tree ears	A, F, M
13. Morels	*Morchella esculenta*	Star sores	F
14. Maize mushroom	*Ustilago maydis*	Cuitlacoche	B, F, H, M, P, R
15. Emetic russula	*Russula emetica*		M, P, Q
16. Oak comb	*Daedalea quercina*		N, O, S, T
17. Beefsteak polypore	*Fistulina hepatica*	Bleeding turtle	E, F, N
18. Artist's shelf	*Ganoderma applanatum*		A, G, I, J, K, M
19. Birch conk	*Piptoporus betulina*		A, F, G
20. Swamp beacon	*Mitrula paludosa*		A, G, L, S
21. Orange earth tongue	*Microglossum rufum*		A, G, L, S
22. Moose antlers	*Wynnea americana*		A, G, L, S
23. Potent psilocybe	*Psilocybe baeocystis*		A, M, P, S

COMMON NAME	LATIN NAME	TRIBAL NAME	USES
24. Blue-foot psilocybe	*Psilocybe caerulipes*		A, M, P, S
25. Common psilocybe	*Psilocybe cubensis*	Flesh of the gods	A, M, P, S
26. Hen of the woods, maitake	*Grifola frondosa*		B, F, M, S
27. Chicken of the woods	*Laetiporus sulphureus*		F, M
28. Wood ears	*Auricularia auricula*		F, M
29. King bolete	*Boletus edulis*		A, F, M
30. Ash tree bolete	*Boletinellus merulioides*		E, F, M

MINERALS

These ten minerals are used by tribal groups across the continent. Some are especially important when carved or worked into amulets and fetishes. Others are used to bind herbal and fungal preparations for the skin and hair or to ease their transit through the body.

1. *Argillite* is a compact stone of sedimentary rock composed mainly of clay materials. It is easily carved and polished into healing amulets and ceremonial accouterments.
2. *Basalt* is a dark, dense igneous rock of a lava flow or intrusion composed of labradorite and pyroxene; it often has a columnar structure. This hard, shiny rock was carved or pecked and etched with mnemonics—symbols of healing and calendar importance.
3. *Clay* is a natural earthy material of hydrated silicates of aluminum that is plastic when wet. It is used for making pottery and bricks and is frequently found in cosmetics and medicines.
4. *Mineral water* contains dissolved salts or gases, like carbonated water, and is used in numerous native healing preparations and formulas.
5. *Mineral oil* is composed of hydrocarbons obtained by distilling petroleum. It is extensively used as a laxative in medicines such as liquid petrolatum, and in external skin treatments.
6. *Petrolatum* or *petroleum jelly* is a yellowish or whitish translucent, gelatinous semisolid obtained from petroleum. It is used in making medicines, and especially as a protective dressing, emollient, and ointment base. It also has extensive cosmetic and industrial uses.
7. *Peridot* is a transparent gemstone that is usually a green variety of olivine, much used in the Southwest by native healers in divining the source of an illness. In some instances it is pulverized and used in sand paintings and in internal and external medicines.
8. *Quartz* is one of the most common minerals. It has many variations in color and luster, such as agate, bloodstone, chalcedony, and jasper. It occurs in crystals such as amethyst and citrine. Sought after by many native healers, quartz continues to have countless valuable uses.
9. *Steatite* or *soapstone* is a large, soft stone variety of talc, with a soapy or greasy feel. It is easily carved, sanded, and polished into bowls, pipes, and healing accouterments.
10. *Turquoise* is an opaque mineral of hydrous copper aluminum phosphate, often containing a small amount of iron. It is usually sky blue to greenish blue in color. This is a special stone for most native peoples. It is often worn for safety and good health, as well as ground and employed in sand paintings and healing formulas.

A DIRECTORY OF RESOURCES AND SUPPLIERS

Your own local health food stores, herb farms, and garden centers are important sources for buying and ordering plants and mushrooms and for investigating the locations of other area resources. These days, supermarkets are also carrying many more herbs and mushrooms. Ask your produce manager about locating additional resources. They are often willing to order items for you if they can.

These stores and companies are good sources of herbal and/or mushroom and mineral products. We've also included some food suppliers.

Ellen's Own Herbals
P.O. Box 176
Kelly, WY 83011
1-307-739-9717

Essiac International
164 Richmond Road
Ottawa, Ontario
Canada K1Z 6W2
1-613-729-9111

Franklin Mushroom Farms
Route 32
North Franklin, CT 06254
1-860-642-3000

Herb Research Foundation
1007 Pearl Street, Suite 200
Boulder, CO 80302
1-800-748-2617

HerbalGram: Journal of the American Botanical Council and the Herb Research Foundation
P.O. Box 201660
Austin, TX 78720
1-512-331-8868

Indian River Herbs
R.R. 4, Box 268A
Millsboro, DE 19966-9804
1-302-945-HERB

Jason Wild Yam Products
8468 Warner Drive
Culver City, CA 90232
1-800-JASON-05

Kneipp Corporation of America
Valmont Industrial Park
675 Jaycee Drive
West Hazelton, PA 18201
1-800-937-4372
Fax 717-455-2442

Maitake Products, Inc.
P.O. Box 1354
Paramus, NJ 07653
1-800-747-7418

Manitok Wild Rice
Box 97 (Chippewa Indians)
Callaway, MN 56521
1-800-726-1863

Materia Medica, LLC
112 Hermosa SE
Albuquerque, NM 87108
1-800-553-4165
Fax 505-232-3162

Native Seeds/Search
2509 North Campbell Avenue
Tucson, AZ 85719
1-520-327-9123

Nature's Plus
P.O. Box 91719
Long Beach, CA 90809
1-800-937-0500

Northland Native American Products
(a Native American–owned company)
P.O. Box 265
Lake Elmo, MN 55402
1-800-229-4007
1-612-436-4499

Polarica/The Game Exchange
P.O. Box 880204
San Francisco, CA 94124
1-800-GAME-USA

The Quinoa Corporation
P.O. Box 1039
Torrance, CA 90505
1-310-530-8666

Quintessence Botanicals
P.O. Box 26400
Federal Way, WA 98093
1-800-776-8366

Vitality Works, Inc.
134 Quincy NE
Albuquerque, NM 87108
1-800-403-4372

World Variety Produce, Inc.
P.O. Box 21127
Los Angeles, CA 90021
1-800-468-7111

You can also try the following places for more information:

- Individual native tribal centers on their reservations throughout North America. Many tribes have their own cultural and heritage centers/museums and independent native crafts shops.
- American Indian centers/councils in all of our major cities.
- American Indian museums and research centers, especially:

  Indian Pueblo Cultural Center (owned and operated by the nineteen Pueblo tribes of New Mexico)
  2401 12th Street NW
  Albuquerque, NM 87102
  1-800-766-4405
  1-505-843-7270

Institute for American Indian Studies
38 Curtis Road, P.O. Box 1260
Washington, CT 06793
1-860-868-0518

National Museum of the American Indian/Smithsonian Institution
George Gustav Heye Center
One Bowling Green
New York, NY 10004
1-212-668-6624

National Museum of the American Indian Center in Washington, D.C.
1-800-242-NMAI [6624]

The network of thirty American Indian colleges is another vital avenue for detailed information.
Contact:

American Indian College Fund
21 West 68th Street, Suite 1F
New York, NY 10023
1-212-787-6312

SELECTED BIBLIOGRAPHY

Albers, Patricia, and Medicine, Bea, eds. *The Hidden Half: Studies of Plains Indian Women.* Washington, DC: University Press of America, 1981.

Arvigo, Rosita, with Nadine Epstein and Marilyn Yaquinto. *Sastun: My Apprenticeship with a Maya Healer.* San Francisco: HarperSanFrancisco, 1994.

Arvigo, Rosita, and Balick, Michael. *Rainforest Remedies: One Hundred Healing Herbs of Belize.* Twin Lakes, WI: Lotus Press, 1993.

Balick, Michael J., and Cox, Paul Alan. *Plants, People, and Culture: The Science of Ethnobotany.* New York: Scientific American Library, 1996.

Beck, Peggy V., Walters, Anna Lee, and Francisco, Nia. *The Sacred Ways of Knowledge, Sources of Life.* Tsaile and Flagstaff, AZ: Navajo Community College Press and Northland Publishing, 1990.

Blumenthal, M., ed., S. Klein, trans. *Gernam Commission E Therapeutic Monographs on Medicinal Herbs for Human Use.* Austin, TX: American Botanical Council, 1996.

Bourke, John G. *Apache Medicine-Men.* New York: Dover Publications, 1993.

Chevallier, Andres. *The Encyclopedia of Medicinal Plants.* New York: DK Publishing, 1996.

Conley, Robert J. *The Witch of Goingsnake and Other Stories.* 1981. Reprint ed., Norman, OK: University of Oklahoma Press, 1991.

Credit, Larry P., Hartunian, Sharon G., and Nowak, Margaret J. *Your Guide to Complementary Medicine.* Garden City Park, NY: Avey Publishing Group, 1998.

Croft, Jennifer. *Careers in Midwifery.* New York: Rosen Publishing Group, 1995.

Crosby, A. W. *The Columbian Exchange: Biological and Cultural Consequences of 1492.* Westport, CT: Greenwood Press, 1972.

Davis, Mary B., ed. *Native America in the Twentieth Century: An Encyclopedia.* New York: Garland Publishing, 1994.

Dobelis, Inge N., ed. *Magic and Medicine of Plants.* Pleasantville, NY: Reader's Digest Association, 1990.

Erichsen-Brown, Charlotte. *Medicinal and Other Uses of North American Plants.* New York: Dover Publications, 1979.

Fawcett, Melissa Jayne. "Shantok: A Tale of Two Sites" in Cultural Resources Management (CRM) 18(7)1995: *"Working Together to Preserve the Past."* Washington, D.C.: National Parks Service, U.S. Department of the Interior.

Fitzhugh, William W., and Crowell, Aron. *Crossroads of Continents: Cultures of Siberia and Alaska.* Washington, DC: Smithsonian Institution Press, 1988.

Foster, Steven. *Herbs For Your Health: A Handy Guide for Knowing and Using 50 Common Herbs.* Loveland, CO: Interweave Press, 1996.

Gladstar, Rosemary. *Herbal Healing for Woman.* New York: Simon & Schuster, 1993.

Gold, Peter. *Navajo and Tibetan Sacred Wisdom: The Circle of the Spirit.* Rochester, VT: Inner Traditions, 1994.

Greaves, T. *Intellectual Property Rights for Indigenous People: A Source Book.* Oklahoma City, OK: Society for Applied Anthropology, 1994.

Green, Rayna, ed. *That's What She Said: Contemporary Poetry and Fiction by Native American Women.* Bloomington, IN: Indiana University Press, 1984.

Griffin, Judy. *Mother Nature's Herbal.* St. Paul, MN: Llewellen Publications, 1997.

Hartwell, J. L. *Plants Used Against Cancer.* Lawrence, MA: Quarterman Publications, 1982.

Heiser, C. B., Jr. *Of Plants and People.* Norman, OK: University of Oklahoma Press, 1985.

———. *Seed to Civilization: The Story of Food.* Cambridge, MA: Harvard University Press, 1990.

Hobbs, Christopher. *Medicinal Mushrooms: An Explosion of Tradition, Healing and Culture.* Santa Cruz, CA: Botanica Press, 1995.

Howard, James H., in collaboration with Willie Lena. *Oklahoma Seminoles: Medicines, Magic and Religion.* Civilization of the American Indian Series, vol. 166. Norman, OK: University of Oklahoma Press, 1984, 1990.

Hudson, Charles. *The Southeastern Indians.* 1979. Reprinted. Knoxville, TN: University of Tennessee Press, 1989.

Josephy, Alvin M., Jr. *500 Nations.* New York: Alfred A. Knopf, 1994.

Kavasch, E. Barrie. *American Indian EarthSense: Herbaria of Ethnobotany and Ethnomycology.* Washington, CT: The Institute for American Indian Studies, 1996.

———, ed. *EarthMaker's Lodge: Native American Folklore, Activities, and Foods.* Peterborough, NH: Cobblestone Publishing, Inc., 1994.

———. *Enduring Harvests: Native American Foods and Festivals for Every Season.* Old Saybrook, CT: Globe Pequot Press, 1995.

———. *Native Harvests: American Indian Wild Foods and Recipes, Revised and Expanded Ed.* Washington, CT: The Institute for American Indian Studies, 1998.

———. *Native Harvests: Recipes and Botanicals of the American Indians.* New York: Random House, Vintage Books, 1979.

Kindscher, Kelly. *Medicinal Wild Plants of the Prairie: An Ethnobotanical Guide.* Lawrence: University Press of Kansas, 1992.

Klein, Barry T. *Reference Encyclopedia of the American Indian.* 6th ed. West Nyack, NY: Todd Publications, 1996.

Kreig, M. B. *Green Medicine.* Chicago: Rand McNally, 1964.

Lenz, Mary Jane. *The Stuff of Dreams: Native American Dolls.* New York: Museum of the American Indian, 1986.

Lewis, W. H., and Elvin-Lewis, M.P.F. *Medical Botany: Plants Affecting Man's Health.* New York: John Wiley & Sons, 1977.

Leung, A. Y., and Foster, S. *Encyclopedia of Common Natural Ingredients Used in Food, Drugs, and Cosmetics,* 2nd ed. New York: John Wiley & Sons, 1996.

Lincoff, Gary H. *The Audubon Society Field Guide to North American Mushrooms.* New York: Alfred A. Knopf, 1981.

Lyon, William S. *Encyclopedia of Native American Healing.* New York: W. W. Norton & Company, 1996.

Mails, Thomas E. *The Mystic Warriors of the Plains: The Culture, Arts, Crafts and Religion of the Plains Indians.* Garden City, NY: Doubleday, 1972.

Miller, Jay, ed. *Mourning Dove: A Salishan Autobiography.* American Indian Lives Series. Lincoln: University of Nebraska Press, 1990.

Moerman, D. E. *Medical Plants of Native American Healing,* Vol. I & II. Technical Reports, Number 19. Ann Arbor: Museum of Anthropology, University of Michigan.

Monte, Tom, and the editors of *Natural Health* magazine. *The Complete Guide to Natural Healing.* New York: Berkley Publishing Group, 1997.

Mooney, James. *Myths of the Cherokee and Sacred Formulas of the Cherokee.* Smithsonian Institution, Bureau of American Ethnology, 19th and 7th Annual Reports (reproduction). Cherokee, NC: Cherokee Heritage Books, 1982.

Nabakov, Peter. *Indian Running.* Santa Barbara, CA: Capra Press, 1981.

Nabhan, G. P. *Enduring Seeds.* San Francisco: North Point Press, 1989.

Nelson, Richard K. *Make Prayers to the Raven: A Koyukon View of the Northern Forest.* Chicago: University of Chicago Press, 1983.

Newcomb, Franc Johnson. *Hosteen Klah: Navajo Medicine Man and Sand Painter.* Norman, OK: University of Oklahoma Press, 1964.

Niering, William A. *The Audubon Society Field Guide to North American Wildflowers: Eastern Region.* New York: Alfred A. Knopf, 1979.

O'Connor, Bonnie Blair. *Healing Traditions: Alternative Medicine and the Health Professions.* Philadelphia: University of Pennsylvania Press, 1995.

Ody, Penelope. *Home Herbal.* New York: Dorling Kindersley, 1995.

Oxendine, Joseph B. *American Indian Sports Heritage.* Champaign, IL: Human Kinetics Books, 1988.

Parker, Arthur C. *Parker on the Iroquois.* Syracuse: Syracuse University Press, 1968.

Plotkin, Mark J. *Tales of a Shaman's Apprentice: An Ethnobotanist Searches for New Medicines in the Amazon Rain Forest.* New York: Viking, 1993.

Roberts, Elizabeth and Elias Amidon, eds. *Earth Prayers from Around the World.* New York: HarperCollins, 1991.

Schlesier, Karl H. *The Wolves of Heaven: Cheyenne Shamanism, Ceremonies and Prehistoric Origins.* 1985. Reprint ed., Norman, OK: University of Oklahoma Press, 1993.

Schmid, Ronald F., N.D. *Native Nutrition: Eating According to Ancestral Wisdom.* Rochester, VT: Healing Arts Press, 1994.

Simmons, William. *Spirit of the New England Tribes: Indian History and Folklore, 1620–1984.* Hanover, NH: University Press of New England, 1986.

Soule, Deb. *The Roots of Healing: A Woman's Book of Herbs.* New York: Carol Publishing Group, 1995.

ssipsis. *Molly Molasses & Me: A Collection of Living Adventures.* Turtle Island, ME: Little Letterpress Robin Hood Books, 1988, 1990.

Stevenson, Matilda Coxe. *The Zuni Indians and Their Uses of Plants.* New York: Dover Publications, 1993.

Strickland, Rennard. *Fire and the Spirits: Cherokee Law from Clan to Court.* Norman, OK: University of Oklahoma Press, 1975.

TallMountain, Mary. *The Light on the Tent Wall: A Bridging.* Native American Series, no. 8. Los Angeles: UCLA American Indian Studies Center, 1990.

Tantaquidgeon, Gladys. *Folk Medicine of the Delaware and Related Algonkian Indians.* 1972. Reprint ed., Harrisburg, PA: Pennsylvania Historical and Museum Commission, 1977.

Tyler, V., and Foster, S. *Herbs and Phyto-medicines in Handbook of Nonprescriptive Drugs,* 11th ed. Washington, DC: The American Pharmaceutical Association, 1996.

Underhill, Ruth. *The Autobiography of a Papago Woman.* Memoirs of the American Anthropological Association, no. 46. 1936. Reprint ed., Menasha, WI: Krause Reprint Co., 1974.

Waldman, Carl. *Encyclopedia of Native American Tribes.* New York: Facts on File Publications, 1988.

Wheelwright, Mary C., recorder. *The Myth and Prayers of the Great Star Chant and the Myth of the Coyote Chant.* Edited with commentaries by David P. McAllester. Tsaile, AZ: Navajo Community College Press, 1988.

Woodham, Anne, and Peters, David. *Encyclopedia of Healing Therapies.* New York: DK Publishing, 1997.

Selected Field Guides

Good field guides exist for all major regions and many states. Check your library for more resources in these subjects.

Bessette, Alan E., O. Miller, A. R. Bessette, H. Miller. *Mushrooms of North America in Color: A Field Companion to Seldom-Illustrated Fungi.* Syracuse: Syracuse University Press, 1995.

Dunmire, William W., and Tierney, Gail D. *Wild Plants of the Pueblo Providence: Exploring Ancient and Enduring Uses.* Santa Fe: Museum of New Mexico Press, 1995.

Foster, Steven, and Duke, James A. *A Field Guide to Medicinal Plants: Eastern and Central North America.* Peterson Field Guides Series. Boston: Houghton Mifflin Company, 1990.

Kavasch, Barrie. *Guide to Northeastern Wild Edibles.* Vancouver, BC, Canada: Hancock House Publishers, 1981.

———. *Guide to Eastern Mushrooms.* Surrey, BC, Canada: Hancock House Publishers, 1982.

———. *Introducing Eastern Wildflowers.* Surrey, BC, Canada: Hancock House Publishers, 1981.

Kindscher, Kelly. *Edible Wild Plants of the Prairie: An Ethnobotanical Guide.* Lawrence: University of Kansas, 1987.

———. *Medicinal Wild Plants of the Prairie: An Ethnobotanical Guide.* Lawrence: University of Kansas, 1992.

Lincoff, Gary H. *The Audubon Society Field Guide to North American Mushrooms.* New York: Alfred A Knopf, 1981.

Moore, Michael. *Medical Plants of the Mountain West.* Santa Fe: University of New Mexico Press, 1979.

———. *Medicinal Plants of the Desert and Canyon West.* Santa Fe: University of New Mexico Press, 1989.

Niering, William A. *The Audubon Society Field Guide to North American Wildflowers: Eastern Region.* New York: Alfred A. Knopf, 1979.

SOURCES AND PERMISSIONS

Note: Some traditional prayers and stories in this book are impossible to trace to a single source and have become more precious in their embrace by many people. Most stories are retold in shortened form. However, an extensive effort has been made to locate rights holders and secure permissions. We regret any omissions and gratefully acknowledge the following individuals and/or publishing companies.

Page xx: ssipsis. Excerpt from "The Earth Way" taken from *Molly Molasses & Me: A Collection of Living Adventures* by ssipsis. Copyright © 1988 by ssipsis. Brooks, ME: Little Letterpress, Robin Hood Books, 1988.

Page 7: Omaha prayer for infants. Excerpt from *The Omaha Tribe* by Alice C. Fletcher and Francis LaFlesche, 1911. Washington, D.C.: ARBAE, 27th, Smithsonian Institution, 1905–1906.

Page 13: Zuni prayer. From *Zuni Origin Myths* by Ruth L. Bunzel, 1932. Washington, D.C.: ARBAE, 47th, pp. 611–837, Smithsonian Institution, 1929–1930.

Page 97: "When I listen to the beat of the drum" by Wunneanatsu Lamb. Copyright © 1996 by Wunneanatsu Lamb. Reprinted by permission of the author.

Page 117: Night Way fragment. From *Navajo and Tibetan Sacred Wisdom: The Circle of the Spirit* by Peter Gold. Copyright © 1994 by Peter Gold. Rochester, VT: Inner Traditions International, 1994.

Page 140: Minnie Aodla Freeman. From *Life Among the Quallunaat*. Edmonton, Canada: Hurtig Publishing, 1978.

Page 165: Mountain chant fragment. From *The Sacred Ways of Knowledge: Sources of Life*. Copyright © 1990. Tsaile, AZ: Navajo Community College Press, Navajo Community College, 1990.

Index

Page numbers of leaf rubbings and illustrations appear in italics.

L

lacrosse, 79-80
Lactuca (lettuce), 128, *128, 144*
Lakota Sun Dance, 110
Lamb, Erin, 27
lamb's-quarters (*Chenopodium album*), *145, 178*
Lame Deer, 120, 192
leaf rubbings, xvi
Legends of the Longhouse (Cornplanter), 87
Lena, Willie, 196, 197
Leonurus cardiaca (motherwort), *132, 133*
lettuce (*Lactuca*), 128, *128, 144*
lexicon of herbs, minerals, and fungi, 277-84
life cycle, xiv-xv
lily, Canada (*Lilium canadense*), *148*
linden, European (*Tilia cordata*), 246
Lindera benzoin (spicebush; fever bush), 67, 68, *68*
ling chih (reishi; *Ganoderma lucidum*), 126
lip balm or gloss, aloe-sage, 258-59
Little People, 87-88, 185, 186-87
Little Water Society, 191
lobelia (*Lobelia*), 170-71
    blue (*L. spicata*), 106, *106*
    Indian tobacco (*L. inflata*), 106, *106*
Lomaquahu, Percy, 217
Lomatium species (wild prairie parsley), 54
Longhouse Curing Ceremony, 167-71
Long-Life Ceremony, 6-7
lotions, 238
love medicines, 106-7

M

maize mushroom (corn smut fungus; *Ustilago maydis*), 144
Malva neglecta (dwarf mallow), 143-44
Malva rotundifolia (cheese plant), 143-44
maple, *96*
    sugar (*Acer saccharum*), *19*

syrup, 19
marigold:
    calendula cornstarch body talc, 103
    calendula deodorant cream, 102
    and mint massage oil, 205
marriage, 95, 96, 106
    Southwestern rites, 107-9
mask societies of the Iroquois, 168, 169
massage oils:
    arnica, 203
    goldenrod hot-infused, 150-51
    marigold blossom and mint, 205
Maxidiwiac (Buffalo Bird woman), 188
Mayan cramp relief tea, 71
meadow rue (*Thalictrium polygamum*), 171
Medford, Claude, Jr., 178
medicine bags, 231
medicine chest, *see* remedies and recipes
Medicine Path, middle age and, 164
medicine wheels, 113-14
memory, herbs to assist, 201
menopause, 176-77
menstruation, 64, 176
    Havasupai origin of, 56
    menarche, 55-57, 61-62
    remedies for, 67-68, 70, 71
    taboos regarding, 60-63
Mentha pulegium (European pennyroyal), 246
Mentha spicata (spearmint), *103*, 214, *214*
Mentha suaveolens (apple mint), *102*
Mexican Days of the Dead, 219-21
middle age, 154-81
    Delaware Big-House Curing Ceremony, 171-74
    Hopi Basket Dance, 159-63
    Hopi Prayer Offering Ceremony at winter solstice, 158-59
    Iroquois Longhouse Curing Ceremony, 167-71
    Medicine Path, 164
    Navajo Mountain Way, 164-67
    Plains Indians journey to the Black Hills for renewal, 157
    remedies, 175-81

Y

yam, *see* wild yam
yarrow (*Achillea millefolium*), 123, *129*, 224, *224*,
    252, 254
    smudge stick, 224-25
Yucca angustissima (soapweed), 216
yucca root, 100
    and cornmeal facial mask, 72
Yurok:
    Brush Dance, 147
    World Renewal Ceremonies, 194-95

Z

Zuni:
    childhood teachings, 42-43
    kachina rites and initiations, 88-91
    lightning symbol, *28*
    marriage rites, 107-9
    Sun Child Ceremony, 12, 13

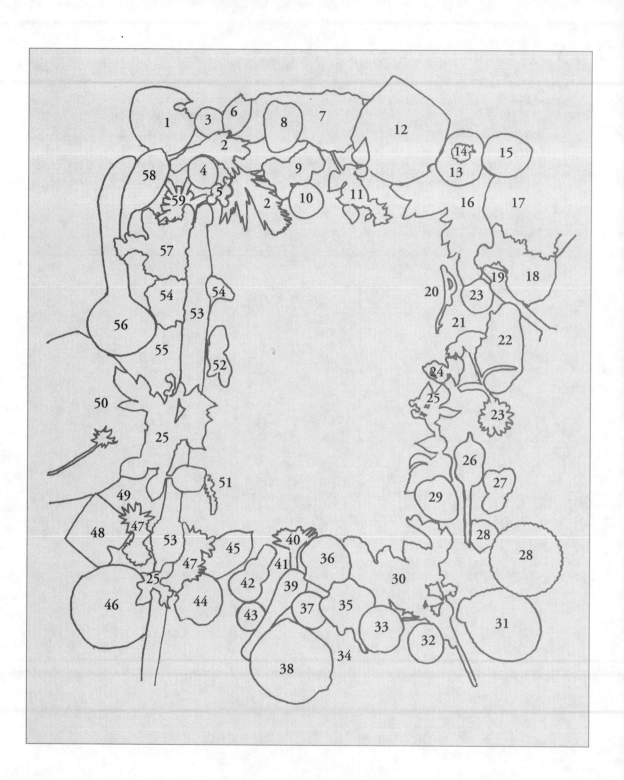

COVER LEGEND

(Clockwise from extreme top left corner)

1. Caddo Indian style incised gourd bowl
2. White cedar and white pine
3. Oregon grape root
4. Goldenseal root
5. Slippery elm lozenges
6. Dried slippery elm bark
7. Dried usnea lichen
8. Dried bearberry leaves
9. Dried polypore fungi
10. Dried wild yam root
11. Wineberry
12. Choctaw cane basket, "Texas Star" pattern, by Claude Medford, Jr.
13. Alibamu-Biloxi-Pascagoula longleaf pine basket by Ethel Robinson
14. Dried coreopsis blossom
15. Dried sassafras bark
16. Fresh sassafras leaves
17. Fresh Oswego tea (red beebalm)
18. Dried calendula blossoms
19. Snipe effigy (spoon handle) carved by Steve Chrisjohn
20. American ginseng root
21. Dried wood ears mushrooms
22. Dried yerba santa leaves
23. Echinacea (prairie coneflower)
24. Black-cap raspberries
25. Red raspberries
26. Gourd effigy rattle, Mound Builders style, by Jeff Kalin
27. Strawberry leaves
28. Akwesasne (Mohawk) strawberry baskets by Mary Leaf
29. Allspice berries
30. Witch hazel leaves and seed pods
31. Sage smudge stick
32. Spicebush berries
33. Cherokee honeysuckle vine bottle-basket by Lucy Teesateskie
34. Dried juniper berries
35. Dried red chili peppers
36. Dried saw palmetto berries
37. Tincture of goldenseal root
38. Turkey tail fungi
39. Popcorn kernels
40. White sage
41. Black walnuts
42. Gourd effigy bottle with corncob stopper by Jeff Kalin
43. Dried corn silk
44. Yellow cornmeal
45. Fresh spicebush leaves
46. Dried hawthorne berries
47. Rudbeckia (black-eyed Susan)
48. Navajo Yei Beichi Medicine Man sand-painting by Ernest Hunt
49. Crow feather
50. Choctaw cane corn-sifting basket by Claude Medford, Jr.
51. Fresh poke leaves and bloom spire
52. Dried morel mushrooms
53. Zuni "Spirit Walker" walking stick by Marcus Banketewa and Lorden Hechilay
54. Fresh yarrow blossoms
55. White birchbark
56. Long-handled gourd dipper
57. Orange butterfly weed
58. Rawhide and deer antler rattle by E. Barrie Kavasch
59. Akwesasne sweetgrass/black ash star by Irene Richmond